For the Common Good

For the Common Good

Philosophical Foundations of Research Ethics

ALEX JOHN LONDON

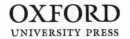

OXFORD
UNIVERSITY PRESS

OXFORD
UNIVERSITY PRESS

Oxford University Press is a department of the University of Oxford. It furthers
the University's objective of excellence in research, scholarship, and education
by publishing worldwide. Oxford is a registered trade mark of Oxford University
Press in the UK and certain other countries.

Published in the United States of America by Oxford University Press
198 Madison Avenue, New York, NY 10016, United States of America.

CIP data is on file at the Library of Congress
ISBN 978–0–19–753483–0

DOI: 10.1093/oso/9780197534830.001.0001

3 5 7 9 8 6 4 2

Printed by Integrated Books International, United States of America

To my children, Joshua, Sophia, and Alexandra.

Contents

II. RESEARCH AMONG EQUALS

III. THE HUMAN DEVELOPMENT APPROACH TO JUSTICE IN INTERNATIONAL RESEARCH

Preface

As I was finishing the manuscript for this book in 2020 the SARS-CoV-2 pandemic was just beginning. As I write this preface, over 115 million people worldwide and nearly 30 million Americans have been infected with COVID-19. Although the United States accounts for less than 5% of the world's population, Americans make up one-fifth of the 2.5 million deaths from COVID-19. As a philosopher who has worked on a range of ethical issues regarding research and public health emergency response, I was concerned that the United States was unprepared for a major disease outbreak. As the pandemic has unfolded it has been a cascade of fears come true.

One of the central messages of this book is that when there is conflict or uncertainty about how best to protect or promote individual or public health, there is a moral imperative to expeditiously carry out research that will provide the evidence and information necessary to ensure that therapeutic intent translates into clinical and public health benefit. Ignoring this responsibility in the face of conflicting judgment and scientific uncertainty and acting quickly from beneficent intent can lead to self-defeating practices. This includes expending scarce time, effort, and resources on, and configuring health systems to deliver, interventions that are ineffective or positively harmful. When large-scale efforts and confident public pronouncements from partisan political figures are subsequently shown to have been based on thin or faulty evidence and to have fallen short of their intended purpose, public trust erodes at the very time when trust and cooperation are both in the short supply and essential to effective pandemic response.

In contrast, the Randomised Evaluation of Covid-19 Therapy (RECOVERY) trial in the United Kingdom represents a paradigmatic example of the way that well-designed research can be used to structure pandemic response and to generate the evidence needed to quickly eliminate unsafe or ineffective strategies and concentrate efforts on those with substantive clinical value. Moreover, that study illustrates how the knowledge generated from scientifically sound and ethically responsible research constitutes a public good. Healthcare institutions around the globe have altered their practices in light of the evidence produced in that study, enabling them to be more effective at advancing patient interests and more efficient in their use of scarce resources.

In a very real sense, the current pandemic illustrates the way that scientifically sound and ethically responsible research constitutes a key tool for responding to uncertainty and generating the causal knowledge that a wide range of actors require in order to discharge key social responsibilities. One of the core claims of this book is that research of this kind is not a morally optional undertaking. The claim that community members have to a social order that protects and advances their ability to pursue a reasonable life plan grounds an imperative to carry out the research needed to effectuate these goals in practice.

In the United States, our reluctance to embrace this idea is rooted in a complex mixture of historical precedent and philosophical argument. We are haunted by the prospect that any imperative to carry out research to advance the common good will inevitably also justify abrogating the rights and welfare of study participants. This specter takes many forms and appears in many different arguments in research ethics. One goal of this book is to show that scientifically sound research and respect for the rights and welfare of individuals are not mutually exclusive. More strongly, the same concern for the common good that grounds an imperative to conduct scientifically sound research in the face of uncertainty and conflicting judgment grounds an equally strong imperative to ensure that this undertaking is organized on terms that respect its various stakeholders' claim to be treated as free and equal persons.

Defending this conception of the common good and the imperatives that it grounds involves understanding research as a social undertaking. This social undertaking is a division of labor between a much wider array of stakeholders than are typically discussed in research ethics. This division of labor often involves important social institutions and produces information that these institutions need in order to discharge their proper social function. As a result, both the ends that research seeks to advance and the means that stakeholders use to advance those ends are ineluctably connected to fundamental considerations of justice.

Although the core claims of this book are centrally relevant to practical problems we are facing in the current pandemic, it is primarily focused on the philosophical foundations of research ethics. The content of the book is drawn from papers I have published over more than two decades. My goal has been to reorganize those ideas into a single narrative that provides a unified and coherent approach to a set of fundamentally philosophical problems that lie at the foundation of an inherently practical undertaking.

My hope is that the book as a whole will be of interest to a wide audience even if significant portions of that audience may not be interested in the whole book. There are places in various chapters where the philosophical arguments are dense, and I have tried to elaborate complex material with care. Readers from research ethics may be surprised to see so much attention paid to abstract questions of justice and comparatively little attention paid to practical problems surrounding informed consent. But my hope is that the rationale for this change in emphasis will be clear, that philosophically minded readers will appreciate these connections and that more practically minded readers will be content to follow their broad outlines.

Similarly, research ethics in the United States is a practical undertaking that arose in a particular historical context profoundly shaped by revelations of scandal and abuse. In chapter 2 I have tried to situate the core problems addressed in the book within a larger historical and conceptual context, recognizing that I am not a historian and that my presentation of that material is necessarily selective. My hope is that this material will be informative for readers who need this background and not too tedious for specialists. Balancing the challenge of writing across disciplines, engaging fundamentally philosophical arguments, and demonstrating their relevance to a very practical undertaking has been a lesson in humility.

Finally, I want to emphasize that my goal in the present work is to articulate a new vision for the philosophical foundations of research ethics. To motivate the need for this project, I identify and elaborate fault lines running through the current foundations of research ethics. These fault lines appear in arguments in both domestic and international research. My positive goal is then to articulate an alternative vision that moves issues of justice from the periphery of the field to the very center. This alternative has the advantage of providing a unified and consistent foundation that makes salient the relationship between research and the larger purposes of a just social order. In this framework the harms and the wrongs of neglect and injustice can be articulated with the same salience as the various threats to participant interests that currently dominate the field.

My goal is to persuade readers that the approach I defend in this book represents a fertile foundation for the field—a better self-understanding and a better foundation for further inquiry. In that sense, the book is not a recipe for dealing with every thorny problem in research ethics. In fact, one goal of the book is to expand both the scope of problems that are seen as falling within the purview of the field and the range of actors whose conduct should be the subject of ethical assessment. Rather than a detailed blueprint, this is an invitation to embark on the process of dealing with old problems and a wide range of new problems from a new starting place in which the social nature of research and its legitimate role in a just social order are central.

Acknowledgments

This project benefitted from the generous support of the Andrew W. Mellon Foundation in the form of a New Directions Fellowship and a supplemental award to support writing this book. My thinking on various topics addressed here has benefitted from numerous conversations and the generous intellectual friendship of my colleagues Jay Kadane, Jonathan Kimmelman, Teddy Seidenfeld, Danielle Wenner, and Kevin Zollman. None of this work would have been possible without the enduring help and support of my partner, Tracy London.

I'm grateful for comments on an early draft of this manuscript from the students in my fall 2019 graduate seminar on philosophical foundations of research ethics, including Natalia Acevedo Guerrero, Tessa Murthy, Tinsley Webster, Suraj Joshi, Alyssa Montgomery, Sarah Dawood, Zina Ward, and Mahi Hardalupas. I am grateful for the copious feedback on an early draft of chapter 5 from the audience at the Harvard Law School Workshop on Health Law Policy, Bioethics, and Biotechnology and for the comments from I. Glenn Cohen and Marc Lipsitch in particular. I am grateful for the excellent feedback on an early version of chapter 4 from the participants in two workshops, including Charles Weijer, Mackenzie Graham, Angela Ballantyne, Danielle Wenner, Jonathan Herington, Ariella Binik, Rieke van der Graaf, Bridget Pratt, Kirstin Borgerson, Douglas MacKay, Benjamin Levinstein, Emily Largent, Michael Da Silva, Derrick Gray, Michael Greer, Brian Hutler, John Lawless, Gopal Sreenivasan, and Sean Valles.

With the exception of chapters 1 and 3, the material in this book includes heavily edited versions of prior work. In the process of turning this work into a coherent manuscript, portions of these papers have been redistributed across different chapters.

Work originally published as London, A. J. (2003). Threats to the common good: Biochemical weapons and human subjects research. *Hastings Center Report*, *33*(5), 17–25 appears in chapter 4.

Material originally published as London, A. J. (2005). Justice and the human development approach to international research. *Hastings Center Report*, *35*(1), 24–37 appears in several chapters including 4, 8, and 9.

Chapters 5 and 6 contain material that was originally published as London, A. J. (2007a). Clinical equipoise: Foundational requirement or fundamental error? In B. Steinbock (Ed.), *The Oxford handbook of bioethics* (pp. 571–596). Oxford: Oxford University Press; London, A. J. (2007b). Two dogmas of research ethics and the integrative approach to human-subjects research. *The Journal of Medicine and Philosophy*, 32(2), 99–116; London, A. J. (2006). Reasonable risks in clinical research: A critique and a proposal for the integrative approach. *Statistics in Medicine*, 25(17), 2869–2885; London, A. J. (2009). Clinical research in a public health crisis: The integrative approach to managing uncertainty and mitigating conflict. *Seton Hall Law Review*, 39, 1173; and London, A. J. (2018). Learning health systems, clinical equipoise and the ethics of response adaptive randomisation. *Journal of Medical Ethics*, 44(6), 409–415.

Chapter 7 is a revised version of the paper originally published as London, A. J. (2012). A Non-paternalistic model of research ethics and oversight: Assessing the benefits of prospective review. *The Journal of Law, Medicine & Ethics*, 40(4), 930–944.

Chapter 8 contains material originally published as London, A. J., and Zollman, K. J. (2010). Research at the auction block: Problems for the fair benefits approach to international research. *Hastings Center Report*, 40(4), 34–45. I am grateful to Kevin Zollman for permission to use this material here.

Chapter 9 also contains some material that originally appeared in London, A. J. (2011). Offshoring science: The promise and perils of the globalization of clinical trials. *IRB: Ethics & Human Research*, 33(1), 18–20; London, A. J. (2008). Responsiveness to host community health needs. In E. J. Emanuel, C. C. Grady, R. A. Crouch, R. K. Lie, F. G. Miller, and D. D. Wendler (Eds.), *The Oxford textbook of clinical research ethics* (pp. 737–744). New York: Oxford University Press; and London, A. J. (2000). The ambiguity and the exigency: Clarifying "standard of care" arguments in international research. *The Journal of Medicine and Philosophy*, 25(4), 379–397.

Socrates: If we could watch a city coming to be in theory, wouldn't we also see its justice coming to be, and its injustice as well? . . . I think a city comes to be because none of us is self-sufficient, but we all need many things. Do you think that a city is founded on any other principle?

Adeimantus: No.

Socrates: And because people need many things, and because one person calls on a second out of one need and on a third out of a different need, many people gather in a single place to live together as partners and helpers. And such a settlement is called a city. Isn't that so?

Adeimantus: It is.

Socrates: And if they share things with one another, giving and taking, they do so because each believes that this is better for himself?

Adeimantus: That's right.

Socrates: Come, then, let's create a city in theory from its beginnings. And it's our needs, it seems, that will create it.

—Plato, *Republic* (Book II, 369b–c)

Political justice means justice as between free and (actually or proportionately) equal persons, living a common life, for the purpose of satisfying their needs.

—Aristotle, *Nicomachean Ethics* (V.vi.4)

PART I
DOES RESEARCH ETHICS REST ON A MISTAKE?

1

Introduction

1.1 Neglected Foundations

The philosophical foundations of research ethics are underdeveloped and riven with fault lines that create uncertainty, ambiguity, and disagreement. The goal of this book is to rethink these foundations and to articulate an alternative in which research is recognized as a collaborative social activity between free and equal persons for the purpose of producing an important social good. Research is a collaborative activity, in part, because it requires the cooperation of a wide range of stakeholders, often extended over time, and often mediated and facilitated by basic social institutions. These institutions impact the rights and welfare of community members and employ a range of scarce social resources. The information that research produces is a social and a public good because it constitutes the evidence base on which a range of stakeholders rely to make decisions that impact the rights and welfare of individuals and that influence the capacity of basic social institutions to safeguard the health, welfare, and rights of persons. It is my contention that research with human participants is thus connected to social purposes of sufficient moral weight that they ground a moral imperative with two aims. The first is to promote a research enterprise that produces information that bridges important gaps between what I refer to as the basic interests of community members and the capacity of the basic social institutions in their community to safeguard and advance those interests. The second is to ensure that, as a voluntary scheme of social cooperation, the research enterprise is organized on terms that respect the status of its many stakeholders, especially study participants, as free and equal.

Defending every aspect of this vision is a larger project than I can complete here. As a result, my main constructive goal is to show that the conception of research ethics articulated here is coherent, that it dissolves or addresses deep tensions at the foundation of orthodox research ethics, and that it places many existing norms and practices on a firmer foundation while fruitfully expanding the purview of the field. It accomplishes these goals, in part,

For the Common Good. Alex John London, Oxford University Press. © Oxford University Press 2022.
DOI: 10.1093/oso/9780197534830.003.0001

by understanding the research enterprise as a voluntary scheme of social co-operation that both calls into action the basic social structures of a community and generates the information on which elements within these social structures rely to advance the basic interests of the community members whose life prospects they shape and influence. As a result, this framework foregrounds issues of justice and fairness that have been neglected within orthodox research ethics.

To establish the need for this constructive project, the main critical goal of this book is to highlight flaws in the conceptual foundations of contemporary research ethics and to illustrate how they threaten to undermine some of the hard-won progress the field has achieved in only a few decades. These flaws are powerfully illustrated in chapter 3 by a series of arguments that are forged out of the foundational values and principles of research ethics, but which effectively undermine a wide range of common requirements that those foundational values are seen as grounding. These arguments reveal a conceptual instability that calls into question the coherence of current requirements and practices. Examining these tensions also reveals arbitrary and often unhelpful limits on the scope of issues that are seen as falling within the purview of the field and on the set of conceptual resources that are used to address them.

In §1.2 I briefly outline eight problematic commitments that shape the conceptual ecosystem of orthodox research ethics and that are discussed at greater length in chapter 2. By the "conceptual ecosystem" I mean the interconnected set of often tacit assumptions that structure the field in the sense that they determine the scope and limits of its purview, the stakeholders whose conduct warrants assessment and oversight, and the terms in which core problems are framed and out of which possible solutions can be crafted. It is against this background set of assumptions that certain ways of formulating problems appear salient or intuitive, certain values appear relevant, and certain strategies for resolving problems appear promising and appealing or irrelevant and inauspicious. Whether they are explicitly stated or tacitly assumed, these eight commitments often reinforce one another and make certain views seem natural and intuitive. Their influence in orthodox research ethics is a recurring theme throughout the book, and it is my contention that we should reject all of them.

Starting in §1.3, the rest of the chapter provides a detailed summary of the core components of the positive program I defend in subsequent chapters. My hope is that this introduction will highlight some of the key respects in which the positive program that I defend here departs from orthodox research ethics and that it will provide a useful roadmap to the main contributions in subsequent chapters of the book.

1.2 Eight Problematic Commitments

1.2.1 An Inherent Dilemma

In this section I outline eight problematic commitments that shape the conceptual ecosystem of orthodox research ethics. One goal of this section is to make these commitments explicit so that it is easier to identify when they emerge in subsequent chapters and to track their influence on a range of issues. Another goal is to bring the outlines of my positive program into sharper relief by explicitly stating some of the often tacitly held positions that it rejects.

First, research ethics has been shaped both practically and conceptually by the widespread perception that there is a fundamental moral dilemma inherent in research involving human participants. This dilemma is expressed in various terms in different contexts. During formative debates that shaped the foundations of the field—discussed in chapters 2 and 4—it was framed as a conflict between the good of the individual versus the common good. In the discussion of high-profile cases of abuse or in guidance documents—discussed in chapters 2 and 5—it is cast as a conflict between respect for the sanctity of the individual versus concern for humanity and the science that will improve the lives of large numbers of future people. In conversations about the reasonableness of research risks—discussed in chapters 5 and 6—it is framed as a conflict between the clinician's duty of personal care and the utilitarianism of the research enterprise.

The idea that research with humans involves a deep moral dilemma helped to shape the origins of the field because it structured the way that both proponents and critics of research oversight framed what was at stake. Early critics of research oversight often treated medical research as an activity with a larger social purpose and argued that this larger social purpose created an imperative to promote research in order to advance the common good. However, because they saw the relationship between the common good and the good of individuals as one of direct conflict—in which efforts to advance one good necessarily required compromising the other—the early critics of research oversight often asserted that the research imperative grounded, if not a duty to override the rights and welfare of individuals, then at least a moral permission to do so. As Walsh McDermott notoriously claimed, "When the needs of society come into headlong conflict with the rights of an individual, someone has to play God" (1967, 39).

In chapter 2 I show that proponents of research oversight and regulation tended to accept this way of framing the problem at least to the extent that they shared the assumption that if appeals to the common good grounded a moral imperative to carry out research with humans, then this imperative would license the abrogation of individual rights and interests. Whereas researchers like McDermott regarded playing God as a part of their rightful social responsibility, proponents of research oversight sought to erect formidable deontological bulwarks around the rights and interests of study participants to protect them from overreach.

The most influential of the early proponents of research oversight, Hans Jonas (1969), went the furthest. He too accepted the claim that if there is a social imperative to conduct research with humans grounded in its ability to advance the common good then it would have sufficient moral force to override the rights and interests of study participants. But Jonas made the bold claim that the antecedent of the conditional is false. In other words, Jonas rejected the claim that research advances the common good and argued that there is thus no social imperative to conduct research with humans. Making this move severed the connection between research with humans and morally weighty purposes that might ground a moral imperative of sufficient weight to override the rights and interests of individuals.

1.2.2 From Social Imperative to Private Transaction

The second commitment that shapes the conceptual ecosystem of orthodox research ethics is that it tends to treat the research enterprise as a morally optional activity of private parties. In chapter 2 I argue that, to some degree, this attitude reflects the success of Jonas's argumentative strategy— if research is not tied to the common good and a moral imperative in the public sphere, then it must be an undertaking in the private sphere that advances more parochial ends. But this attitude likely also reflects the highly pragmatic nature of research ethics and the fact that in the United States it emerged as a distinctive field of inquiry in response to revelations of scandal and abuse at places like Tuskegee, Willowbrook, or the Jewish Chronic Disease Hospital.

Chapter 2 provides a brief introduction to some of the institutions, policies, and regulations created in the wake of these revelations of abuse and suggests that they have contributed to what I refer to as the parochialism of the field. This includes a relatively narrow conception of who the key stakeholders in research are, of the purview of research ethics, and of the terms in which problems in this space are formulated and in which their resolutions are to be crafted.

1.2.3 Two Main Stakeholders

A third aspect of the conceptual ecosystem of orthodox research ethics reinforces the parochialism of the field by framing the moral epicenter of research as falling within what I call the *IRB triangle*, namely, the discrete interactions of researchers and participants that are reflected in study protocols; informed consent forms; and that are evaluated by an Institutional Review Board (IRB), sometimes referred to as a Research Ethics Board (REB) or a Research Ethics Committee (REC). If research has a deep moral connection to a network of social purposes that constitute the common good, then the boundaries of the field cannot be so narrowly constrained. If nothing else, there would have to be some consideration of whether the initiatives and programs that are funded are aligned with and likely to advance these larger social purposes, and such considerations would be likely to implicate the activities of a much wider range of stakeholders. Severing research from these larger social purposes and treating the IRB as the primary focus for moral evaluation limits the focus of the field to issues that arise from the review of individual study protocols and that revolve around the discrete interactions of researchers and study participants.

Treating the IRB triangle as the moral epicenter of research ethics has a number of consequences. In chapters 4 and 7 I show how it treats the activities of a range of stakeholders as falling outside the purview of the field. This includes stakeholders who exert influence on research prior to the formulation of individual protocols or after individual studies are complete. In chapters 4, 7 and 8 I focus specifically on how it encourages the view that the primary moral concerns in the field arise within one-time or single-shot interactions between private parties and that the primary, if not the exclusive, focus of research ethics is on the terms that IRBs use to regulate these interactions. This focus is inadequate, in part, because there are a range of ethical issues that fall squarely within the nexus of concerns that are recognized in orthodox research ethics that simply cannot be addressed through the evaluation of individual protocols (§4.9). More fundamentally, as I show in chapters 2, 4, 7, and 8, this frame obscures the extent to which research is a cooperative social endeavor, extended over time, involving numerous parties, and that the regulation of this activity is an exercise in what economics calls mechanism design—the design of institutions and rules that regulate the conduct of multiple stakeholders and that fundamentally shape the strategic environment in which they interact. This strategic environment includes the goals they are likely to pursue, the constraints on their pursuit, and the incentives that are used to shape stakeholder conduct.

1.2.4 Research as Functional Role

Fourth, the parochialism of orthodox research ethics has been nourished by a tendency to conceptualize research in functional terms. In other words, research ethics tends not to treat research as a social activity involving the distribution of labor across multiple stakeholders over long periods of time. Instead, it treats research as a function—a set of goals and purposes—that an individual adopts or pursues, often in contrast to the goals and purposes that are treated as definitive of clinical medicine.

This functional understanding of research helped to facilitate research oversight by demarcating when a particular individual is acting as a caregiver versus when they are acting as a researcher. In chapter 2 I show how early scandals that shaped the development of the field involved researchers using prerogatives that they enjoyed by virtue of their role as caregiver to advance the ends of research. So, it was useful to demarcate the role of caregiver as making decisions around the goal of advancing the medical best interests of the individual patient while demarcating the role of researcher as making decisions around the goal of generating generalizable scientific knowledge. Conceptualizing research in these terms also allows it to be represented as an activity that fits neatly within the bounds of the IRB triangle. Although this has a certain practical utility, it reinforces a view of the field in which larger social connections, including issues of justice, are difficult to make salient.

In chapter 5 I show how this way of framing matters reinforces the perception that there is an ineluctable dilemma at the heart of research. When research and medical care are understood functionally, they are treated as two sets of goals, purposes, and constraints that are adopted by a single decision maker. Because these goals and constraints are conceptually or logically distinct, they appear to make incompatible demands on the individual professional. If the same decision maker cannot simultaneously maximize what are represented as competing and incompatible demands, then there appears to be a deep dilemma at the heart of research ethics. This idea has played a significant role in structuring discussions of risk in research including the formation of the concept of equipoise and discussions of its strengths and weaknesses.

1.2.5 Two Dogmas of Research Ethics

This functional treatment of research and medicine is closely connected to a fifth feature of the conceptual ecosystem of orthodox research ethics, namely, the widespread acceptance of what I refer to in chapter 5 as two unquestioned dogmas of research ethics. The first is that the fundamental norms in this domain are grounded in, and derive from, the role-related obligations of medical professionals. In particular, to be a clinician is to occupy a social role that is defined by a singular commitment to advancing the medical best interests of the individual patient. The second is that research is an inherently utilitarian activity. To be a researcher is thus to occupy a social role defined by a singular commitment to advancing the ends of science.

Conceptualizing research this way allows it to fit neatly into the confines of the IRB triangle without having to appeal to larger social relationships or obligations, facilitating the practical goals of research oversight. But understanding research and medical practices as goals and ends that are adopted by individuals, abstracted away from any larger division of social labor, makes it appear almost true by definition that research generates a thorny social dilemma by requiring compromises to individual welfare that are inconsistent with the individual clinician's fiduciary duty of care.

1.2.6 Paternalistic Foundations

The sixth feature of research ethics I want to call into question is the widespread perception that its central purpose and normative justification are fundamentally paternalistic. Against the background assumption of an inherent conflict between the interests of study participants and the goals of science, research ethics is naturally portrayed as having one moral purpose—to protect potential and actual study participants from harm or abuse at the hands of researchers. Outside oversight is required because research activities are seen as inherently in conflict with the best interests of study participants and because the complexities of research make it difficult, if not impossible, for study participants to effectively safeguard their own interests.

In chapter 7 I show how understanding the purpose and justification for research ethics in fundamentally paternalistic terms plays a critical role in shaping which issues fall within the scope and purview of research ethics. If the reason for the existence of this field is to protect the rights and interests of study participants, then issues that cannot be cast in terms of safeguarding the interests of study participants are invisible, or must be shoehorned into such terms in order to be seen as relevant. Once again, which questions research addresses, which methods are used to answer those questions, where research takes place, and how the information generated from this process is later used must either be cast as issues related to study participant welfare or be treated as falling outside of the purview of the field.

1.2.7 Justice without Social Institutions

The seventh feature of orthodox research ethics, illustrated in chapter 2, is a conceptual ecosystem in which considerations of justice have almost no substantive role to play. This is ironic in two ways. First, influential documents in research ethics, such as the *Belmont Report* (discussed in detail in chapter 2), list justice as one of the core values or principles of research ethics, alongside respect for persons and beneficence. There it is also recognized that injustice can arise from the way research is embedded in larger social systems. For example, the *Belmont Report* states that "whenever research supported by public funds leads to the development of therapeutic devices and procedures, justice demands both that these not provide advantages only to those who can afford them and that such research should not unduly involve persons from groups unlikely to be among the beneficiaries of subsequent applications of the research." Second, as the philosopher John Rawls (1971, 3) famously said, justice is the "first virtue of social institutions" and research is a social activity that involves a complex division of social labor, carried out over time, often with the participation of important social institutions, and often with the goal of improving the capabilities of actors or agents within those social institutions.

But when research is understood in purely functional terms, and the moral epicenter of the field is located in discrete interactions between researchers and participants, considerations regarding the terms on which important social institutions operate fall entirely outside the purview of the discipline. For example, there is no discussion in the *Belmont Report* about how the use of public funds should shape the priorities for, or nature of, the research that is carried out with those funds. There is a tacit assumption either that research always produces socially valuable knowledge, or that forces external to research ethics—such as the profit motive of firms, the desire for credit on the part of researchers, or some larger humanitarian impulse on the part of each of these parties—are sufficient to ensure that public funds are directed to socially valuable purposes. Notice, however, that if those funds are instead used to support research that is lucrative for firms but lacks social value then the requirement quoted previously from the *Belmont Report* would entail, perversely, that the use of public funds requires that this low-value intervention ought to be made available to those who are unable to pay for it, presumably through some form of social subsidy. This is perverse to the extent that it would require scarce resources to be directed at the purchase and delivery of an intervention that generates revenue for a private actor without producing sufficient social value to warrant its provision.

Although tensions of this sort are often not salient in the context of domestic research, they emerge with powerful force when we turn to research that is sponsored and conducted by entities from high-income countries (HICs) but carried out in communities from low- or middle-income countries (LMICs). As we see in chapters 3 and 8, guidelines governing international research stipulate a range of requirements that implicate the activities of a broad set of stakeholders and that are grounded in the value of justice. One of these requirements holds that research that is carried out in LMICs must be responsive to the health needs and priorities of host communities. Another holds that prior to the initiation of such research, a wide range of stakeholders must agree to the terms on which the fruits of successful research will be made reasonably available to members of the host community. Without a conception of justice as a value that governs the operation of social institutions and their effects on the rights, liberties, and interests of community members, research ethics has struggled to provide consistent justifications for and interpretations of these requirements.

International research represents a context in which it is clear that powerful parties can influence the conduct of research to advance their own interests to the detriment of other stakeholders, including the communities that host such research and the individuals who participate in it. But when research is understood in functional terms, divorced from a larger division of social labor involving diverse parties with their own often quite powerful parochial interests, the field struggles to articulate the moral purpose of research and, with this, the reasons that it is a moral wrong to co-opt the research enterprise to advance the parochial interests of powerful parties. Without established criteria for connecting the research enterprise to some larger social purpose—to some notion of the common good—it is difficult to hold these diverse parties accountable for advancing, or subverting, such larger social purposes.

1.2.8 Reducing Justice to Mutually Beneficial Agreements

Finally, stripped of a diverse set of actors whose activities are morally beholden to some larger set of social purposes, I show in chapters 2 and 8 how research ethics has operationalized justice in terms that reduce it to the satisfaction of the other values that come to function as the twin pillars of research ethics—respect for persons and beneficence. The pragmatic desire to avoid controversial philosophical questions about the nature of justice encourages the tacit acceptance of what I refer to as the minimalist approach to justice. On this view, justice is a function of beneficence and respect for autonomy in the sense that discrete transactions between researcher and participants are regarded as just if they are mutually beneficial and freely undertaken. Although this allows issues of justice to be formulated in a way that fits neatly within the confines of IRB deliberations, reducing justice to a function of the other pillars of research ethics severs important connections between the research enterprise and the institutions of a decent social order.

The allure of this kind of view has been felt most keenly in the context of international research where an approach to the evaluation of cross-national clinical trials with many of these features has been articulated under the banner of the "fair benefits" approach (Participants 2002, 2004). The way that this view follows naturally from core commitments of orthodox research ethics is discussed in chapter 8. Proponents have advocated for this approach on the basis of its ability to satisfy a set of intuitive requirements such as ensuring that benefits to participants and host communities increase as the burdens of research increase, that benefits to sponsors should increase as the benefits to others increase, and that the benefits various parties receive should track their relative contributions to research. Even if these are regarded as ethically appropriate constraints on international research, I argue that there are no grounds to think that the fair benefits approach will jointly satisfy these requirements and that there are compelling reasons to believe that the fair benefits approach will operate in practice in ways that flout each of these requirements.

International research has been at the epicenter of protracted and sometimes divisive debates in research ethics for more than three decades. One reason for this is that the parochialism of orthodox research ethics relied heavily on tacit assumptions about the way that domestic research would connect to a set of domestic institutions and practices whose governance and regulation are treated as falling outside of the scope of the field. When biomedical research began moving in volume from HICs of the Global North to LMICs of the Global South, many of these tacit assumptions could no longer be maintained. As a result, research ethics struggled to find ways to align its overriding focus on ethical issues that arise within the IRB triangle with highly salient concerns about the way that research in settings of deprivation and injustice can be morally problematic. These struggles are discussed in chapters 2 and 8.

The allure of the fair benefits approach, as well as the problems that it faces, stem from tensions latent in the problematic commitments of orthodox research ethics that I have summarized here. The depth of these tensions is illustrated dramatically in chapter 3 in provocative work by Alan Wertheimer. In particular, Wertheimer has argued that even if certain transactions in research are unfair, unjust, or exploitative they should not be prohibited. Instead, "there should be a very strong presumption in favor of principles that would allow people to improve their situations if they give appropriately robust consent, if doing so has no negative effects on others, and this even if the transaction is unfair, unjust, or exploitative" (Wertheimer 2008, 84).

Although the position that Wertheimer articulates is unlikely to garner significant support in the mainstream research ethics community, its philosophical relevance should not be underestimated. Wertheimer's view draws on core assumptions of orthodox research ethics, but from these assumptions it derives conclusions that undermine the field's paternalism and a range of requirements that are typically seen as grounded in this normative foundation. In particular, Wertheimer's view adopts the near exclusive focus on the relationship between researchers and participants that typifies orthodox research ethics. It treats the relationship between these parties as largely private, unmoored from larger social purposes and the imperatives they might ground. Instead, it emphasizes the fundamental importance of the twin pillars of research ethics—namely, the voluntary and informed consent of participants and beneficent concern for welfare understood as requiring a mutually beneficial distribution of a potentially wide range of benefits and burdens.

In effect, Wertheimer uses the core commitments of orthodox research ethics to undermine the deontological bulwarks that are a hallmark of the field. Without a social imperative to conduct research, researchers have broad discretion about whether and with whom to partner in conducting clinical trials. In such a context, strong norms against exploitation, or other forms of unfair, unjust, or disrespectful treatment effectively erect a barrier to conducting studies among desperately needy people by raising the "cost" of conducting such studies. If researchers decide to take their studies elsewhere (depriving potential participants of the associated benefits), this safeguards a vulnerable population from exploitation and unfairness but leaves them prey to the ravages of lethal neglect. But if desperate individuals prefer, and so would choose, exploitative or unfair but beneficial interactions to potentially lethal neglect, then Wertheimer's position—that we ought not to prohibit exploitation even if it is morally wrong—follows from the two values that remain as the pillars of traditional research ethics, namely, beneficence and respect for autonomy. If there is something morally suspect with this conclusion then it reflects a deeper problem with the way the core commitments of orthodox research ethics have evolved in the conceptual ecosystem I describe here.

Wertheimer's revisionist arguments highlight a deep tension in research ethics between the way it balances three moral pitfalls. The first pitfall involves sanctioning neglect. For Wertheimer, erecting deontological barriers around the interests of people who are in desperate situations may protect them from wrongdoing, but it leaves them vulnerable to poverty and disease. The second pitfall involves sanctioning wrongdoing. Orthodox research ethics errs on the side of neglect because of the worry that connecting research to larger social purposes will involve sanctioning wrongdoing in the name of social progress. In contrast, Wertheimer defends permitting some wrongdoing in order to allow desperate people to advance their interests in the face of potentially lethal neglect. The third pitfall is that it is unfair to saddle a narrow range of stakeholders with overly demanding moral requirements. This concern is evoked with special intensity by the prospect that if research ethics requires researchers and sponsors to rectify larger injustices in the world, then it will simply lead them to avoid research in LMICs, consigning more people there to the ravages of neglect.

The eight views just discussed represent sometimes explicit but often tacit presuppositions of orthodox research ethics. They provide the intellectual background that sets the terms in which problems are articulated, the parameters on what an acceptable resolution will look like, and the nature of the considerations that are germane to analysis and reasoning. It is my contention that each of these positions is problematic and the positive program I outline in this book rejects them all.

1.3 The Common Good and a Just Social Order

1.3.1 The Basic Interest Conception of the Common Good

The positive program that I defend here understands research as a scheme of social cooperation that is one small element within a much larger division of labor. In chapter 4 I argue that the role of this larger division of social labor in a just social order is to advance the common good, understood not as the preservation or perfection of the community as an aggregate entity, but as a set of interests that are shared by all persons. In particular, although individuals in a diverse society are likely to embrace different and potentially conflicting conceptions of the good and to find fulfillment in the pursuit of widely different activities, every person can recognize themselves as sharing a more basic or generic interest in being able to form, pursue, and revise a life plan of their own.

To say that a just social order advances the common good, on this conception, is to say that its basic institutions—its social, political, legal, economic, and health-related institutions—are organized on terms that secure and advance the basic interests of that community's members. This conception of the common good thus dovetails with a conception of justice as primarily concerned with the regulation of social institutions, and in chapter 4 I show that this conception of the common good can be formulated within a range of social and political theories that begin from different starting points and cash out its implications within different intellectual and political traditions.

1.3.2 Free and Equal Persons

The basic interests of persons play a dual role in shaping the terms on which the basic structures of a decent social order can operate. In particular, they help to define the social goal that these institutions are required to advance and the constraints under which they are required to advance those goals. This is because they define the respect in which individuals in a diverse society have a claim on one another to be treated as morally free and equal.

Roughly speaking, to say that persons are morally equal is to say that they each have a deep and abiding interest in being able to formulate, pursue, and revise a life plan of their own and that, relative to this interest, there are no grounds for promoting the interests of one person over another. Similarly, the claim to be treated as morally free is understood as a social claim to the physical, social, environmental and other conditions that are necessary to have the real ability to exercise these interests in practice without the arbitrary or unwarranted interference from others.

As a result, justice and fairness require that the basic norms and institutions in a community strive to advance the basic interests of every community member with equal efficacy and efficiency. They also require that efforts to advance these ends must be consistent with respect for the freedom and equality of the community members who take on the responsibility of advancing these goals or whose interests are implicated in their efforts.

1.3.3 Reconnecting to Social Institutions

A wide range of social institutions affect the ability of individuals to function as free and equal persons. In part, this is because the capacity of individuals to formulate, pursue, and revise an individual life plan can be thwarted by a range of threats. These threats include poverty and various forms of indifference or antipathy as well as sickness, injury, and disease. But the ability of social institutions to fill this role depends on the quality of the information that they possess about the sources and nature of such threats and the likely effects of alternative strategies, policies, or interventions for addressing them.

On the view I defend here, the research enterprise is also understood on fundamentally social terms. It is a division of social labor between a diverse range of stakeholders that requires the exercise of social authority and the utilization of social resources in order to fulfill a distinctively social purpose. I argue that the moral purpose of this social enterprise is to generate the knowledge and the means necessary to enable the basic social institutions of a community to effectively, efficiently, and equitably secure and advance the basic interests of their respective members. In the context of health, this means that the social function of the research enterprise is to generate the knowledge and the means necessary to enable the institutions of public health and clinical medicine to secure and advance the basic interests of community members from health-related threats.

1.3.4 Producing a Unique Public Good

Although research may be a conduit for a wide range of benefits, and different actors may be drawn to some of these benefits more than others, the pursuit of these various benefits must not compromise the ability of this scheme of social cooperation to produce a unique social and public good. This good is the knowledge that is required to bridge shortfalls or gaps in the ability of the basic social institutions of a community to safeguard and advance the basic interests of its members.

This knowledge is a *unique* good in the sense that it often cannot be generated by other means. It is a *public* good in the sense that it is nonrival and non-excludable. It is nonrival in that its use by one party does not hamper the ability of others to use it. It is non-excludable in that it is difficult to prevent others from using this information once it has been discovered and disseminated.

It is also a *social* good in the sense that a wide range of stakeholders rely on it to discharge important social responsibilities. Policy makers in government, health systems, and the public or private mechanisms that communities use to pool risk and share resources (such as insurance agencies) rely on this information to make decisions that implicate how scarce resources are allocated. These decisions impact the effectiveness, the efficiency, and the equity with which basic social systems address the needs of the stakeholders who rely on them.

Additionally, health systems, public health experts, clinicians, and other providers rely on this information to understand health needs, to determine the relative merits of alternative strategies for addressing these needs, and to make decisions that impact the ability of individuals to exercise the capacities they need to form, pursue, and revise a life plan in practice. Patients and community members rely on this information to understand their health status, to understand the nature of various threats to that status, and to make momentous decisions that impact their ability to exercise their basic interest. The character and quality of this information is also a critical input into future research. It constitutes the knowledge base used to formulate hypotheses about the pathophysiology of disease and to identify targets and strategies for diagnoses or intervention.

1.4 The Egalitarian Research Imperative

In chapter 4 I argue that the relationship between the information that research produces and the ability of basic social institutions to safeguard and advance the basic interests of community members grounds what I call the *egalitarian research imperative*:

The Egalitarian Research Imperative: There is a strong social imperative to enable communities to create, sustain, and engage in research understood as a scheme of social cooperation that respects the status of stakeholders as free and equal and that functions to generate information and interventions needed to enable their basic social systems to equitably, effectively, and efficiently safeguard and advance the basic interests of their constituent members.

This imperative is egalitarian in two respects. First, it is grounded in the goal of ensuring that the basic social structures of a community have the knowledge and the means necessary to secure and advance the basic interests of community members. These interests define the respect in which community members have a claim to equal moral regard. Second, the division of labor through which these goals are advanced must themselves respect the status of individuals as free and equal.

To secure the cooperation of such diverse stakeholders over time, this enterprise must be justifiable to its various stakeholders as an avenue through which they can advance the common good without being subject to forms of treatment that deny or compromise their status as free and equal. Understanding research as a voluntary scheme of social cooperation among free and equal persons entails that strong norms of respect are not external constraints on this activity. They are integral, enabling components. Together, the arguments in chapter 4 show that a moral imperative to carry out important research with humans can be grounded in a conception of the common good that does not license the abrogation or the denigration of the status of study participants or other stakeholders in this enterprise.

1.5 The Integrative Approach to Risk Assessment

1.5.1 Dissolving the Dilemma

The argument in chapter 4 undermines the claim that embracing an imperative to conduct socially valuable research necessarily requires compromising the rights and welfare of individual participants. Nevertheless, such an abstract, philosophical claim may appear untenable in practice since research participation is widely viewed as antithetical to the interests of individual participants. In fact, the idea that research is an inherently utilitarian undertaking, requiring that the welfare of study participants be weighed against and traded off for benefits to future patients, is so intuitive that it constitutes an unquestioned dogma of research ethics.

Chapter 5 illustrates how some of the common commitments of orthodox research ethics outlined in §1.2 structure the perception that study participation poses a moral dilemma for study participants and for clinicians. This chapter introduces the concept of equipoise and shows why the most common and intuitive way of formulating this concept is also doomed to failure. In particular, its earliest proponents regarded it as a way to use the norms and duties that are treated as definitive of the doctor-patient relationship to constrain the inherent utilitarianism of the research enterprise. But within the conceptual ecosystem of orthodox research ethics, this position is unworkable.

Chapter 5 carefully examines a progression of arguments that purport to show that research with humans requires a compromise or sacrifice of participant welfare. This includes the claim that research participation has the form of a coordination problem known as the prisoner's dilemma. In each case I argue that these arguments rest on questionable presumptions and often reflect an overly paternalistic conception of the norms of clinical medicine and an overly narrow conception of individual welfare. Ultimately, I argue that these arguments fail. At the social level, this means that research can be organized in a way that does not give rise to a prisoner's dilemma.

Instead, I argue that if organized on the terms I defend here, research participation has the structure of a strategic interaction known as a stag hunt—a coordination problem in which it is rational for individuals to participate as long as they are convinced that doing so will produce information that is sufficiently valuable and that enough others will be willing to participate that studies will function as planned. One of the overarching themes of the rest of the book is that we should reject the idea that research ethics and oversight is a fundamentally paternalistic undertaking and instead see their purpose as creating an institutional and social order in which participants are justified in seeing research as an avenue through which they can help to produce an important public good.

1.5.2 The Principle of Equal Concern

In chapter 6, I defend what I call the *integrative approach* to risk management. This approach is integrative in the sense that it seeks to reconcile respect for the basic interests of study participants with the social goals of producing scientifically sound and socially valuable evidence. The integrative approach is grounded in the following principle of equal moral concern:

Principle of Equal Concern: As a necessary condition for ethical permissibility, research with humans must be designed and carried out so as not to undermine the standing of any research participant as the moral and political equal of their compatriots, by either knowingly compromising participant basic interests or by showing less care and concern for their basic interests than the interests of those the research is intended to serve.

When this condition is satisfied, free and equal persons have credible social assurance that research participation offers an avenue for contributing to the common good without making participants subject to neglect, abuse, or domination at the hands of the other stakeholders on whom the research activity depends.

The integrative approach articulates three criteria that give the principle of equal concern greater operational clarity and a set of practical tests for determining whether or not these criteria are met in practice. The first operational criterion ensures that risks associated with research participation are not gratuitous or arbitrary. The second ensures that no study participant receives a level of care for their basic interests that is substandard or medically inappropriate. The practical test for this operational criterion is similar to what Benjamin Freedman (1987) called "clinical equipoise" and it requires that study participants can only be allocated to an intervention if at least a reasonable minority of well-informed expert clinicians would recommend that intervention for that patient.

The third operational criterion for ensuring equal concern ensures that risks to the basic interests of participants that are not offset by the prospect of direct benefit to participants themselves are consistent with the level of risk that is regarded as acceptable in other social activities that are oriented toward advancing meritorious social purposes. The incremental increase in risk associated with study participation should be consistent with socially enforced limits on risk that are incurred in other social activities with a similar structure. In this case, similarity of structure is explicated in terms of activities in which individuals are exposed to risks in the performance of tasks or activities that advance a meritorious social goal.

1.5.3 Integrating Equal Concern and Social Value

In the framework I propose, the egalitarian research imperative and the principle of equal concern work hand in hand to ensure the proper functioning of the research enterprise. The egalitarian research imperative seeks to align research activities with the common good, understood as providing the information necessary to bridge gaps between the health needs of community members and the capacity of the institutions in that community to meet those needs. The principle of equal concern ensures that individuals can contribute to advancing the common good with credible, social assurance that their status as free and equal persons will not be denigrated in that process.

In chapter 6, I connect the integrative approach to risk management with the notion of a learning health system (Institute of Medicine 2007). In particular, the ideal of a learning health system reflects two ambitions. The first is making better use of medical information to continuously improve medical practice. The second is altering clinical practice in ways that will better generate medical information that facilitates this learning process. One way to advance these ambitions is to employ adaptive study designs that adjust the treatments that patients receive on the basis of measured outcomes and that provide a platform for delivering care to patients over a longer term.

These adaptive design features are often thought to be particularly difficult to reconcile with the requirements of clinical equipoise. Since the integrative approach incorporates elements of clinical equipoise, it is thus important to demonstrate that these trial design features are not inconsistent with the approach to risk management defended here. I therefore show that when we explicitly recognize that research is a social undertaking and we design studies to model the behavior of fully informed experts in a diverse community, it is possible to reconcile the egalitarian research imperative, the principle of equal concern, and several additional moral requirements.

1.6 Non-Paternalistic Research Ethics

Within the narrow confines of orthodox research ethics, the idea that the field is grounded in, and charged with advancing, fundamentally paternalistic objectives seems almost analytic. The very rubric of "human subjects protections" evinces a paternalistic goal. Although a system of research ethics and oversight can be grounded in such a moral foundation, it need not be.

In chapter 7, I argue that the broader conception of research ethics that I defend here opens up the possibility for reconceiving research ethics on non-paternalistic foundations. In particular, the view that I defend recognizes that research is a fundamentally social undertaking, often requiring the coordination and cooperation of diverse parties over extended periods of time. Each of the parties to this undertaking often has a range of interests that motivate their participation in the research enterprise. These motives can include profit, fame, career advancement, prestige, and access to medical care including access to investigational agents. Because these parties often do not possess the same information, skills, or abilities, and because they are dependent on one another to achieve their shared and their distinctive ends, their interactions are susceptible to cooptation by powerful parties and to co-ordination problems such as the tragedy of the commons and what is known as the "lemons" problem.

I argue that a better understanding of research ethics is to see its proper social functioning as providing credible public assurance that the division of labor between these parties is organized on terms that satisfy the egalitarian research imperative and the principle of equal concern. In other words, the goal of an effective system of research ethics, policy, and oversight should be to align the parochial interests of these diverse parties with the production of the distinctive social good that provides the normative ground for the social support of the research undertaking and to ensure that this undertaking is carried out in terms that respect the status of study participants, as well as other stakeholders, as free and equal persons.

I argue that even within the paternalism of orthodox research ethics, prospective review before bodies of diverse representation helps to solve the co-ordination problems to which an unregulated system would be prone. But the mismatch between the paternalistic justification for IRB review and the social benefits that it actually provides creates tensions that threaten to un-dermine stakeholder trust. Adopting the framework that I propose here would better align the justification for prospective review with the social benefits that it produces. It would also illuminate the need for new institu-tional structures that incentivize a wider range of stakeholders to advance the twin goals of the egalitarian research imperative.

The argument in chapter 7 constitutes a defense of prospective research review as a mechanism for providing warrant for the social trust on which the research activity crucially depends. However, because the current system of research oversight is so narrowly focused on the IRB triangle, it lacks the ability to hold other stakeholders accountable for the way that they influence the research enterprise. These shortcomings are illustrated in the difficulties research ethics has had in addressing issues of justice and fairness in interna-tional research.

1.7 Justice and the Human Development Approach to International Research

The egalitarian research imperative guides and constrains the way labor is divided between the system that produces practical knowledge and the basic social institutions of a community that put that knowledge into practice. It guides the way labor can be divided by requiring that research activities be directed at advancing the common good of community members. This idea is operationalized, in part, as identifying and then attempting to bridge gaps between the health needs of community members and the ability of the health systems in a community to address those needs. The egalitarian research imperative constrains the activities of stakeholders in the research enterprise by prohibiting activities that might undermine or detract from this social mission, including activities that involve abrogating the status of any stakeholder as free and the moral equal of every other. Activities that might undermine the warrant for public trust in the research enterprise are morally problematic and it is, therefore, a legitimate function of oversight structures to discourage or prohibit such activities.

In chapter 9, I argue for what I call the *human development approach to international research*. In this view, the egalitarian research imperative is understood within the context of a larger conception of human development. Every community has an obligation to undertake a larger program of human development, understood as the project of ensuring that the basic social structures of that community are organized and function on terms that secure and advance the basic interests of community members. Research has a unique role to play in this process by generating the knowledge and the means necessary to bridge shortfalls in the ability of those structures to fulfill this mission.

Although every government has a duty to undertake this process domestically, affluent communities have a duty to support and assist this process in less-affluent communities. This duty includes creating incentives and structures aimed at aligning the parochial interests of stakeholders with the goal of promoting research that targets knowledge gaps that represent development priorities for those communities.

The human development approach extends the egalitarian research imperative into the international context and it connects the requirements of responsiveness and reasonable availability with the conditions of a just research enterprise. In this respect, it provides a coherent foundation for norms that are grounded in justice, in a field that largely lacks a conception of justice that has sufficient content to ground and interpret those requirements.

Additionally, the human development approach provides a coherent and consistent account of the standard of care that should govern domestic research in HICs, domestic research in LMICs, and cross-national research.

Borrowing from the integrative approach to risk assessment and management, it holds that study participants should be provided with what is called the *local de jure* standard of care. This states that participants in research are entitled to a level of care for their basic interests that does not fall below what experts judge to be the most effective strategy for preserving or advancing those interests under conditions that are attainable and sustainable in their community.

1.8 Conclusion

Ultimately, the human development approach to international research illustrates how the basic interests conception of the common good, the egalitarian research imperative, and the integrative approach to risk assessment and management provide a coherent and unified framework for evaluating domestic and international research. This framework provides clear guidance for promoting research that generates social value without abrogating the rights and interests of study participants in the process. It situates research within a larger social context and does a better job of identifying the grounds for holding a wider range of actors accountable for decisions that affect the questions that are asked; the methods that are used to address them; the terms on which studies are carried out; and the prospects for incorporating the resulting knowledge, practices, and interventions into the social systems charged with safeguarding and advancing the basic interests of community members.

2

Fear of the Common Good and the Neglect of Justice

2.1 The Practical and Conceptual Origins of Parochialism

The conceptual foundations of research ethics have been profoundly shaped by a series of problematic commitments (§1.2). These commitments structure its scope and purview, set the terms on which questions in the field can be formulated and addressed, and create a series of fault lines at its conceptual foundations. These fault lines involve important ambiguities and inconsistencies about the relationship between core values—often expressed as the principles of respect for persons, beneficence, and justice—and the requirements they are regarded as justifying. Although these fault lines are latent in domestic research ethics, they are highlighted and stressed when research is sponsored by entities from high-income countries (HICs) and carried out in communities of low- and middle-income countries (LMICs).

This chapter has three goals. The first is to demonstrate how these problematic commitments arise from the cases, policy responses, and intellectual analyses that shaped the birth of research ethics as a distinct field. The second is to illustrate how these views result in a practical and a principled aversion to linking the research enterprise to a larger social purpose that might ground and explain the moral importance of this activity and provide criteria for evaluating its organization and conduct.

The third goal of the chapter is to provide readers who are new to research ethics with some helpful background information about core documents, classic cases, and important regulatory structures. What I offer here is not a proper historical overview, as that is beyond my abilities as a philosopher and unnecessary for our present purposes.[1] Instead, it is intended to reveal

---

[1] Readers interested in a history of medical research and the development of research ethics in the United States should consult Katz et al. (1972), Rothman (1991), Lederer (1995), Washington (2006), and Reverby (2009).

For the Common Good. Alex John London, Oxford University Press. © Oxford University Press 2022.
DOI: 10.1093/oso/9780197534830.003.0002

where the views that I regard as problematic operate in the field and to show how they are bound up with three important influences on the emergence of research ethics as a distinct field of inquiry in the United States.

The first influence derives from features of the particular scandals that gripped the public's attention and created sufficient perception of an unmet social need to spur lawmakers into action. In particular, early scandals often involved the abuse of marginalized groups at the hands of researchers who relied on and exploited the considerable social power they wielded within traditional, Hippocratic medicine. These common features of early scandals created a public perception that oversight was required in order to protect the rights and interests of individuals from the potential for abuse at the hands of researchers in biomedical and behavioral research.

The second influence derives from the institutional mechanisms that were created in the United States to respond to this social need.[2] In 1973 the US Congress initiated hearings that lead to the creation of the National Commission for the Protection of Human Subjects of Biomedical and Behavioral Research (from now on, the "National Commission"). One of its major achievements was a report entitled "Ethical Principles and Guidelines for the Protection of Human Subjects of Research," which would come to be known as the *Belmont Report*. In this report, the National Commission articulated a set of moral principles for regulating research with humans that formed the template for federal guidelines governing research with humans in the United States.

Prior to the creation of the National Commission, scholars from medicine, law, philosophy, theology, sociology, psychology, psychiatry, and other disciplines would periodically turn their attention to ethical issues raised by research with human participants. There was thus intellectual discourse about the ethics of research with humans, but there was not a distinct field with which scholars from different areas could self-identify. The creation of the National Commission, and the body of work that it produced, can be seen as the catalyst for the birth of research ethics as an explicit field of inquiry in which practitioners, advocates, regulators, and scholars from various disciplines could identify as working on a common subject matter. This is the oft-repeated creation story in which research ethics was conceived in postwar

---

[2] I don't claim to know or to chart the influence on these developments outside of the United States, and certainly the history and institutional settings in which research is conducted in Europe and elsewhere are likely very different. For example, see Holm (2020).

scandal and born with the formation of a unified social system for regulating research with humans.

The work of the National Commission gave rise to a series of regulations in the United States, intended to provide a unified set of rules to regulate research with humans. These rules would be applied by independent, local bodies of diverse representation, charged with overseeing the ethical conduct of research with humans. In the United States these bodies are known as Institutional Review Boards (IRBs). Although similar boards existed at various institutions in the United States prior to the work of the National Commission, the rule making that followed the publication of the *Belmont Report* consolidated, standardized, and unified both the rules for regulating research with humans and the institutional systems that were required to review those studies and enforce those rules.

The emergence of research ethics out of a practical policy response to particular revelations of abuse provides part of the explanation for why the conceptual foundations of the field are riven with fault lines. The field emerged with a series of regulations and oversight structures that created the scaffolding for subsequent theorizing. In that sense, research ethics is not like a modern city built from a blueprint that might provide a rationale for its layout and reflect a plan for accommodating future expansion. There was no prior intellectual discipline analogous to urban planning or civil engineering that provided a coherent philosophical framework for the practical policy responses that flowed from the work of the National Commission. Instead, research ethics is more like an ancient city that begins with a central square and grows outward over time as the population expands and local stakeholders have to address particular needs on the ground. In this metaphor, the central square of orthodox research ethics is the IRB and the rules and regulations they consult and apply in evaluating research protocols.

Nevertheless, the work of the National Commission did not take place in an intellectual vacuum and there is an important respect in which contemporary research ethics reflects a third, more intellectual influence. This influence is the victory of a particular perspective on the place of research in a decent political community and the normative force of the claims that it can make on individuals. Undoubtedly, one reason for the ascendancy of this perspective is that it dovetails nicely with, and provides a philosophical justification for, the scope and focus of the field that emerged out of these very practical origins. On a deeper level, however, it reflects the philosophical and conceptual perils that were associated with linking the research enterprise to larger social purposes. For our present purposes it is the structure and relationship of the positions that assert this more intellectual influence that is of particular interest.

In §2.2 I show how efforts to forge a connection between research and larger social purposes have been associated with a social imperative that is seen as licensing the abrogation of the rights and interests of individuals in order to advance the common good. This analysis reveals the pivotal role of one problematic commitment, namely, the idea that research involves an ineliminable moral dilemma, a conflict between the good of the individual and the good of society, and the belief that an imperative to carry out research threatens the rights and welfare of individuals. In §2.3 I show how Hans Jonas (1969) addressed this conflict by denying a link between research and the common good and, in doing so, articulated a philosophical rationale for what I regard as a second problematic commitment, namely, treating research as a largely private activity, severed from the larger social purposes and moral obligations of the state of a just social order.

In §2.4 I show how the structure of early cases of research abuse and the policy responses that followed fostered the third and fourth problematic commitments, namely, the idea that the moral purpose and justification for research ethics is inherently paternalistic and that the moral epicenter of research ethics lies within what I called in the previous chapter the IRB triangle—the discrete interactions of researchers and participants overseen by IRBs. It also reveals how these cases and the regulatory response they generated gave rise to a fifth problematic commitment, namely, the tendency to conceptualize research in functional terms, as a set of goals and purposes that guide individual decision-making and that allow the research activity to be distinguished from treatment and medical practice.

In §2.5 I show how two final problematic commitments follow from those discussed so far. The first is a conception of justice that is severed from social institutions, the division of social labor, and the moral standing of community members. As a result, there is relatively little role for justice, as a distinctly social value, in orthodox research ethics. The second is a related tendency to explicate justice in terms that allow it to effectively be treated as a function of the other pillars of research ethics, namely respect for persons and beneficence.

In §2.6 we see how many of these commitments produced a context in which controversies in international research revealed and exacerbated fault lines running through the foundations of research ethics. In particular, debates over the requirement that research be responsive to host community health needs, that there be provisions for post-trial access to any interventions vindicated in research, and that study participants be provided an ethically appropriate standard of care proved to be divisive and intractable within the conceptual ecosystem described here.

Ultimately, this chapter illustrates several tensions in the foundations of research ethics. One concerns the way that requirements that are supposedly grounded in considerations of justice either appear arbitrary in light of the parochialism of orthodox research ethics or come to be seen as counterproductive. Another concerns an unresolved tension between the pitfalls associated with embracing the idea that research is supported by a moral imperative to advance a set of larger purposes and the perils of neglect that can result from eschewing such social purposes and focusing instead on paternalistic protections of research participants. Chapter 3 then explores how these common commitments can be marshalled in ways that radically undermine core commitments of orthodox research ethics.

2.2 The Peril of Larger Social Purposes

2.2.1 Research as a Progressive Undertaking

The idea that there might be a moral and political imperative to carry out research casts a long shadow over research ethics. On the one hand, this idea reflects a widespread social conception of science as a progressive undertaking. The clinician might inoculate or heal the individual, but the scientist who discovers the vaccine or the therapeutic produces the means of saving countless lives. Pushing forward the boundaries of knowledge creates the means of advancing humanitarian purposes, but on a greater scale than could be achieved by individual compassion alone. Once discovered, new knowledge can be used repeatedly, at different times and in different places, to prevent avoidable suffering and disease, to heal the sick and injured, and to generally improve the conditions of life.

The progressive aspects of science dovetail with and seem to draw especially powerful support from the moral imperative of beneficence and the just ends of society. In the former case, if science holds out the means of advancing not merely the good of a single individual, but the much greater good of many more individuals, then it must be supported by a correspondingly greater moral imperative. Likewise, if the purpose of a just social order is to secure the common good of its members, then science seems to dovetail with and draw support from the legitimate ends of political communities.

Ideas of this kind provide the ground for what has subsequently been referred to as the research imperative.[3] As I will use the term, the research imperative refers to a moral obligation to carry out research for the greater good. The general idea is that advancing social progress by producing the knowledge and the means to avoid premature death and alleviate avoidable suffering is not a morally optional goal. In an influential paper on the ethics of research with children, for example, the theologian Paul Ramsey used this term to describe research of such significant social value that "it is immoral not to do the research" (1976, 21).

On the other hand, Ramsey worried about cases where such research could only be carried out on terms that would themselves represent a moral transgression. Such cases would create a moral dilemma in which "moral agents are under the necessity of doing wrong for the sake of the public good" (1976, 21). It is this potential for conflict, and the challenge of how to mitigate it, that has cast a long shadow over research ethics.

Writing in the immediate wake of the *Belmont Report*, the noted researcher and child psychologist Leon Eisenberg asserted that the recognition of science as a progressive undertaking had been lost in revelations of scandal and that research ethics had lost touch with the moral mission of research to advance morally significant social ends. As a result, he says, "peculiar to this time is the need to restate a proposition that, a decade ago, would have been regarded as self-evident, namely, that fostering excellence in medical research is in the public interest" (1977, 1105).

At the close of his paper, Eisenberg quotes from the speech that Louis Pasteur wrote for the occasion of the founding of the Pasteur Institute. Pasteur writes:

---

[3] Wayne and Glass (2010) claim that Paul Ramsey (1976) was the first to coin this phrase. Ramsey was worried about cases in which it would hinder the public good not to conduct research, yet the requisite studies required the involvement of children who could not consent for themselves. If such research did not hold out the prospect of direct benefit to the children, then he worried that not conducting the research would hinder the public good but conducting it would violate the sanctity of the individual and the prohibition on using individuals in research without their express informed consent. This phrase is also associated with Dan Callahan, who often defined it broadly as the goal of using science to overcome the natural limits imposed on human life including to "overcome death itself" (2000, 654).

Two opposing laws seem to be now in contest. The one, a law of blood and of death, ever imagining new means of destruction, forces nations always to be ready for battle. The other, a law of peace, work and health, ever evolving means of delivering man from the scourges which beset him. The one seeks violent conquest, the other the relief of humanity. The one places a single life above all victories, the other sacrifices hundreds of thousands of lives to the ambition of a single individual. The law of which we are the instruments strives even in the midst of carnage to cure the wounds due to the law of war. Treatment by our antiseptic methods may save the lives of thousands of soldiers. Which of these two laws will ultimately prevail, God alone knows. But this we may assert: that French science will have tried by obeying the law of Humanity, to extend the frontiers of life. (quoted in Eisenberg 1977, 1110)

Pasteur was keenly aware that the methods of science could be yoked to the purposes of war and destruction as easily as to purposes of "peace, work and health." But his identification with the latter invokes the importance of science as an engine of social progress, working to discover the "means of delivering man from the scourges which beset him," including the scourges wrought from the carnage of war.

Eisenberg thinks that this conception of research has been lost in the reforms carried out by the National Commission because the social discourse around research with human participants shifted so heavily toward the protection of participants from abuse and the hands of researchers. To invoke another frequently used metaphor, Eisenberg thinks that the pendulum of public opinion has swung too far, emphasizing protection for individuals but leaving out the social role of research. As he puts it, "I do not deny the necessity for surveillance of the ethics of the research community; the point I stress is that medical research, applied to medical practice, stands alone in its ability to avert unnecessary human suffering and death" (1977, 1106).

2.2.2 Two Sides to the Ledger of Progress

I am interested in Eisenberg's essay, not because of any historical prominence or social impact it may or may not have had, but because it reads like a chart capturing the shifting trajectories of constellations of ideas that stood out in the intellectual firmament of that time. In the ascendency of protectionist norms that emphasize the rights and interests of study participants, it is easy to lose sight of the larger purposes that research rightly advances.

Eisenberg's essay is prescient in that it locates a central part of the social value of research in its unique ability to winnow the wheat of beneficial medical practices from the chaff of harmful and unnecessary theory and practice. It envisions a moral imperative to carry out research that is grounded, in part, in the idea that even when our ability to do good in medicine is not hampered by greed, incompetence, or lack of commitment to the common good, we very often lack adequate knowledge about what practices help and heal and which hurt and harm when we set out with the intention to treat and to aid. The public too often conflates the benevolent intent of medical practitioners with their ability to confer actual medical benefit. As he puts it, the public naively assumes that "what is usual and customary in medical practice" aligns with "what is safe and useful." But this assumption is false, and critics who embrace it are "surprisingly naive about the extent to which medical practice rests on custom rather than on evidence, [and] fail to appreciate the necessity for controlled trials to determine whether what is traditional does harm rather than good" (1977, 1105). Medical research produces information that is necessary to ensure that medical practice is capable of actually bringing about outcomes that are consistent with its therapeutic intention.[4]

If the state has a responsibility to safeguard the rights and welfare of its members, then the work of the National Commission reflects the state's interest in managing the way that research with human participants can put these at risk. At the same time, however, Eisenberg argues that unchecked sickness and disease also fall under the purview of the state and that research is needed to improve the capacity of the state to safeguard the lives and the welfare of its members. Because restrictions on the rate of medical progress also cause harm, Eisenberg argued that the sides of the ledger must be compared. As he emphasizes, "The decision not to do something poses as many ethical quandaries as the decision to do it. Not to act is to act" (1977, 1108).

Although he is not explicit about how the state ought to weigh the concerns on the different sides of this metaphorical ledger, Eisenberg says that "the systematic imposition of impediments to significant therapeutic research is itself unethical because an important benefit is being denied to the community"

---

[4] For an argument to the effect that medical beneficence cannot succeed unless it is accompanied by a duty to learn, see London (2020).

(1977, 1108). Even if he is reluctant to be more explicit, the structure of the reasoning here is clear. First, Eisenberg thinks that research produces an important social good—the knowledge that medicine requires in order to alleviate avoidable suffering and death. Second, he holds that the community has an interest in securing these benefits. Third, because the outcomes of actions that are necessary to secure these benefits must be weighed against the outcomes of actions that protect study participants, the interests of individuals must be weighed against the interests of the community.

Eisenberg may be correct in his assertion that in the decade prior to his writing it would have been regarded as self-evident that "fostering excellence in medical research is in the public interest" (1977, 1105). What he nevertheless fails to grasp, however, is the reason why, by the time of his writing, this idea had come to be seen as dangerous and morally problematic and how his own framing of the research imperative recapitulates some of these problems.

2.2.3 Permission to "Play God"

A decade earlier, others were less guarded in their arguments about what followed from the moral imperative to conduct research. In 1967, at a symposium on the "Changing mores of biomedical research" the influential researcher Walsh McDermott opened the meeting by pronouncing that "When the needs of society come into headlong conflict with the rights of an individual, someone has to play God" (1967, 39). Conveniently, McDermott saw playing God as the prerogative of the expert medical researcher, rightfully entrusted by society to advance its affirmative right to the great benefits of medical progress. Although care should be used to reduce the frequency with which society is presented with such moral dilemmas, McDermott was clear that "there is no escape from the fact that, if the future good of society is to be served, there will be times when the clinical investigator must make an arbitrary judgment with respect to the individual" (41).

McDermott's remarks came only a year after the noted Harvard Medical School professor and physician Henry Beecher published a paper in the *New England Journal of Medicine* detailing twenty-two examples, drawn from a larger sample of research studies published in leading medical journals, in which the rights or welfare of subjects had been violated. In three of

Beecher's examples, established effective therapies were withheld from study participants in the control group of a study. In one case, Beecher notes that, "23 patients died in the course of this study who would not have been expected to succumb if they had received specific therapy" (1966, 1356). In a fourth study, a drug linked to possible liver toxicities was administered to fifty "mental defectives or juvenile delinquents who were inmates of a children's center" (Beecher 1966, 1356). Within four weeks, half of the subjects in the study showed signs of hepatic dysfunction. Yet eight of these patients were selected for further study with half receiving liver biopsies. Once their liver functioning returned to normal, these patients were "challenged" with the drug again until liver dysfunction was observed, with one patient receiving a second challenge with the drug. In the eighteenth study, a melanoma from a terminal patient was transplanted to her mother the day before her death. After 451 days the mother died from metastatic melanoma believed to have derived from the transplant.

Beecher's examples reflect in grim detail the exercise of the authority that McDermott claimed for medical professionals—to make an arbitrary judgment against some unlucky individuals. Individuals were denied established effective treatments for severe medical conditions. They were subjected to invasive, burdensome, painful, and sometimes dangerous medical procedures often to achieve ends that would have been attainable through other means or for durations and to degrees that were unnecessary for strict scientific purposes. Many of the people subjected to these interventions were children, persons with developmental delays or cognitive impairments, as well as demented elderly whose capacity to understand what was being done to them was impacted by dementia or severe chronic illness. Many were also drawn from institutionalized populations, including corrections facilities, children's homes, and long-term care wards. In some cases, it was clear that informed consent for study procedures was not obtained; in many others it was assumed that consent had not been obtained.

Even if some portion of these abuses could have been eliminated with more careful planning or by employing less burdensome study designs or procedures, McDermott argued that in research with humans, the "irreconcilable nature of the conflict" between the individual and society creates a "moral dilemma of clinical investigation" that cannot be fundamentally eliminated. Because the future good of society is so morally weighty, "to ensure the rights of society," clinical researchers must sometimes make an "arbitrary judgment . . . against an individual" (1967, 40–41).

2.2.4 The Arbitrary Judgments of Men

As far back as Aristotle, arbitrary dealings deriving from the rule of individuals rather than the rule of law have been a hallmark of injustice. Yet McDermott insists that "it has been most unwise to try to extend the principle of 'a government of laws and not men' into areas of such great ethical subtlety as clinical investigation" (1967, 41). He is particularly concerned about documents like the *Declaration of Helsinki* (*DoH*), adopted in 1964 after contentious debate by the World Medical Association. This succinct set of ethical statements intended as a guide for physicians who conduct medical research opens with the words, "It is the mission of the doctor to safeguard the health of the people" (World Medical Association 1964). It goes on to say, "The Declaration of Geneva of The World Medical Association binds the doctor with the words: 'The health of my patient will be my first consideration.'" In a later section, dedicated to research in which participants have no reasonable expectation of direct benefit, it states that, "In the purely scientific application of clinical research carried out on a human being, it is the duty of the doctor to remain the protector of the life and health of that person on whom clinical research is being carried out."

McDermott argues that it may have been possible to satisfy this "double ethical charge" in the nineteenth century when researchers were expanding knowledge of health and disease but did not yet have the capacity to intervene in order to "control disease" (1967, 40). But he says "starting, I suppose, with the yellow fever studies in Havana, we have seen large social payoffs from certain experiments in humans, and there is no reason to doubt that the process could continue. . . . Once this demonstration was made, we could no longer maintain, in strict honesty, that in the study of disease the interests of the individual are invariably paramount" (40).

The yellow fever studies in Havana to which McDermott refers occurred in 1900 and were run by the now famous US Army physician Walter Reed.[5] At the time, the source of yellow fever was a matter of dispute. To test the hypothesis that it was transmitted by mosquitoes, a group of subjects were "challenged" with bites from mosquitos fed on the blood of patients known to have the disease. Three members of this group contracted yellow fever and died, including a doctor who had twice challenged himself with infected mosquitoes.

---

[5] For excellent accounts of this case, see Lederer (1995, 2008).

Prior to Reed's studies, more soldiers died from yellow fever in the Spanish-American war than from combat. After the source of the disease was identified and eradication efforts were undertaken, rates of both yellow fever and malaria infection were dramatically reduced. For McDermott, the fact that the information produced from Reed's research could be used to save countless lives was of sufficient moral import that it grounded a right on the part of society to the production of such knowledge. On this view, if that knowledge cannot be procured without the deaths of a few study participants, then it is the moral responsibility of the conscientious researcher to make an arbitrary judgment against a few unlucky souls in order to produce this benefit for society.

Because McDermott thinks that medical research necessarily involves a conflict between the individual and society and because he thinks society has a right to medical progress, he argues that documents that treat the individual as inviolable or sacrosanct, "produce the curious situation in which the only stated public interest is that of the individual. The future interest of society and its sometime conflict with the interest of the individual, in effect, are ignored" (1967, 41). McDermott thus asserts about the *DoH* the claim that Eisenberg would later assert about subsequent reforms more broadly, namely, that the protectionist focus of research ethics leaves out the great social good that research produces, which grounds the moral imperative for its conduct and that McDermott thinks is of sufficient importance to override the rights of the individual.

Because Eisenberg is writing after a long series of scandals and after the work of the National Commission, he is more guarded in his language than his predecessor. For example, where McDermott asserts that individual researchers rightfully bear a mantle of responsibility for advancing the right of the community to social progress, Eisenberg hopes for the creation of a "community of shared responsibility for health research," conceding that in research, like "all professional activity, social controls are necessary" (1977, 1108).

Nevertheless, it is not clear how Eisenberg avoids recapitulating the logic of McDermott's position when asserting that "the systematic imposition of impediments to significant therapeutic research is itself unethical because an important benefit is being denied to the community" (1977, 1108). If the community has a right to the benefits of medical progress, and if regulations that safeguard the rights and welfare of study participants are unethical because they pose an impediment to the provision of this good, then what are the limits to what the community can demand from its members in the production of this information?

Writing after McDermott but before Eisenberg, the eminent physician Louis Lasagna noted his own inability to resolve this question. On the one hand, he asserts that, "In clinical investigation, as in other societal activities, the good of the individual and the good of society are often not identical and sometimes mutually exclusive" (Lasagna 1971, 108). But where McDermott is willing to say that it is the responsibility of the expert researcher to make arbitrary decisions against certain unfortunate individuals, and where Beecher worries about the abuse of this authority, Lasagna is evasive. Instead of stating a normative claim and offering a justification for it, he shifts to a descriptive standpoint in the passive voice, saying, "I believe it is inevitable that the many will continue to benefit on occasion from the contributions—sometimes involuntary—of the few" (109). Lasagna appears unwilling to follow McDermott in his assertion that when the needs of society and the rights of the individual come into conflict, researchers must sometimes play god. Instead, he simply assumes that it is inevitable that someone will do this and his description of the "involuntary contributions" of the few is a thinly veiled euphemism for unlucky souls who are the subject of arbitrary judgments and unwillingly or unknowingly conscripted into service for the greater good.

Lasagna admits that he is "ambivalent" about how to strike a balance between the sides of what he also regards as a deep moral dilemma. He recognizes the importance of medical progress, and he thinks that in the medical context this will require the abrogation of individual rights and that "society frequently tramples on the rights of individuals in the, 'greater interest.'" But, like Beecher, he also realizes that social trust in biomedical and behavioral scientists is not without limits or conditions and that boundaries must be drawn because "we cannot afford to have the cancer of moral decay that comes from frequent and flagrant disregard of human rights gnawing away at the body of science" (1971, 109).

2.2.5 Fear of Moral Decay

The prospect of moral decay from the frequent and flagrant disregard of human rights in science wedded to state purposes had been graphically and dramatically displayed before the world only three decades earlier.

During the Second World War, German scientists had actively and eagerly conducted research in support of the many goals of the Nazi state (Katz et al. 1972; Annas and Grodin 1992). In concentration camps, eminent German physicians and researchers conscripted individuals who the state regarded as morally inferior into often horrific experiments. At Nuremberg, twenty-three Nazi physicians and researchers who had carried out barbaric scientific experiments in concentration camps were tried for crimes against humanity. Of the sixteen defendants who were found guilty, seven were put to death for their crimes, including Dr. Karl Brandt.

In his testimony, Brandt stated that during the time when the Nazi party controlled the German government it imposed a collective system in which "the demands of society are placed above every individual human being as an entity, and this entity, the human being, is completely used in the interests of that society" (Trials of war criminals before the Nuernberg Military Tribunals [Tribunals] 1949, 29). In that period, he argued, "everything was done in the interests of humanity so that the individual person had no meaning whatsoever, and the farther the war progressed, the stronger did this principal thought appear" (30).

Lawyers for the defense argued that, "It would be unjust, however, to conceal the enormous benefit of the human experiment," noting that past discoveries, once made, are often widely adopted and "become the common property of all peoples for the benefit of suffering mankind" (Tribunals 1949, 75). They argued that medical scientists on both sides of the conflict were called on to assist the war effort and that "in nearly all countries experiments have been performed on human beings under conditions which entirely exclude volunteering in a legal sense" (73).

During the cross examination of a witness from the United States, Dr. Andrew Ivy, the defense asked if it was morally permissible to sacrifice the life of a prisoner in a research study if doing so would save the lives of an entire city. When Ivy refused to agree that this was permissible, Brandt's attorney, Dr. Robert Servatius, argued in his closing statement that this response amounted to a view in which "human rights demand the downfall of human beings" (Tribunals 1949, 128).

If the two sides of the moral ledger are in strict conflict, then we appear to be faced with a dire ethical dilemma. If the interest of the community outweighs the sanctity of the individual, then we risk permitting the callous disregard for individual humans in the larger service to humanity. Alternatively, if we regard the individual as inviolable, then we risk elevating concern for human rights over the suffering and preventable death of human beings.

2.3 From Social Imperative to Private Undertaking

2.3.1 Severing Research from the Common Good

This potential for the humanity of the individual to be obliterated under the demands of the greater good, the needs of society, and the goals of progress was the subject of the philosopher Hans Jonas's famous 1969 paper "Philosophical Reflections on Experimenting with Human Subjects." For Jonas, just as for McDermott and others, research reflects in microcosm a larger social conflict between the demands of the state and the rights and welfare of the individual. In research, as in war, Jonas argued, the demands of the collective too easily reduce the individual—a person with a moral worth that merits unconditional respect—to a mere statistic, a data-point no different from hundreds or thousands of others. When persons are made fungible, their identity and individuality are blotted out and individual concern is replaced by a cold algebra of harms inflicted on small groups, necessitated and balanced out by gains to a substantially larger collective (Donagan, 1977, Fried 1974).

For Jonas, close connections between scientific research and the ends of the state or the common good threatened to overshadow the humanity of the individual and, with this, the sanctity and value of the person. The remarkable feature of his response to this threat, however, was not that he sought to constrain or curb the demands of progress—to strike a balance between the sides of the moral ledger—or that he sought to demarcate the just demands of a just state from the unjust demands of various stripes of totalitarianism. Instead, Jonas took the more radical step of challenging the existence of a social imperative to engage in research with humans by severing the connection between research and the common good.

Against intuition and the popular rhetoric of science, Jonas attacked the idea that there is a social imperative to carry out research. Unlike large-scale military conflicts, in which the continued existence of a people might be placed in question, Jonas argued that sickness, injury, and disease are not a threat to society. Societies can survive the normal death rate from such maladies; it is only individuals who cannot. Because disease is a threat to the interests of individual persons and not to society, the quest for progress in medical science is a personal rather than a social goal, an individual rather than a social benefit.

Unlike the proverbial Dutch boy plugging holes in a dyke with tiny and insufficient fingers, Jonas's article is rightly famous and widely influential because it strives to stem the potential for a totalitarian tidal wave at its source. If sickness and disease threaten the individual, there is no social imperative grounded in the rights of society or the common good that can be marshaled to override or justify the abrogation of individual rights or interests.

In slightly different ways, Eisenberg, McDermott, and Servatius had argued that there were two sides to the ledger of social progress—one column for the rights and welfare of study participants and another for society or humanity. As such, they saw the protectionist focus on the human rights of individuals as incomplete, neglecting the rights of society and threatening to undermine the cause of humanity. By arguing that humanity and society are not threatened by suffering and disease, Jonas argued that it is no error to proceed as though "the only stated public interest is that of the individual" (McDermott 1967, 41). On this view, the "future interest of society and its sometime conflict with the interest of the individual" (McDermott 1967, 41) are rightly ignored because the interests of society are not threatened by the maladies that research with humans seeks to ameliorate.

2.3.2 An Optional Goal

If scientific progress is not a right of society, and if there is no moral imperative to carry out research, then it becomes an optional goal. Researchers are at liberty to take up its mantle, but they are not required to do so by any social or moral imperative. As an optional, personal project that particular individuals elect to pursue, the research enterprise is severed from a social context in which the vast needs of the collective can so easily outweigh the interests of a few individuals. The interests that motivate research are not the interests of society, they are merely the morally optional personal interests of individuals.

To draw an analogy, committing one's life to perfecting a musical instrument might be a noble undertaking. But it is not so morally weighty that it can justify the abrogation of the rights and interests of others. If research is similarly a noble personal undertaking, then there may be reasons to patronize science—just as some choose to patronize the arts—but those reasons are not so weighty that they can legitimate the abrogation of the rights or welfare of others.

When Eisenberg laments that research ethics has lost touch with the moral importance of research, his frustration reflects the success of Jonas's gambit. Eisenberg appeals to the value of research in ameliorating the inadequacies of medicine, and in this way he connects the moral significance of medicine to its impact on the lives of individuals. The large-scale delivery of unsafe, ineffective, or positively harmful treatments takes a toll, not on communities, but on individuals. Eisenberg also cautions against seeing death as a part of the human condition and, with this, taking its inevitability as a reason not to recognize an imperative to fight against it. Such an attitude might make sense if we take white, affluent communities of HICs as our reference class. But when we turn to what he calls the "third world," where death from communicable disease is widespread and life expectancies are far lower, the goal of medical progress can readily be seen, not as a quixotic mission to expand the boundaries of long life into some indefinite horizon, but as enlarging the share of humanity that enjoys the life expectancy that has become common in the most fortunate corners of the globe. In these respects, Eisenberg's arguments are prescient.[6]

At the end of the day, however, Eisenberg has no alternative to McDermott's assertion that at the heart of research there is a dilemma in which the rights of society are pitted against the rights of the individual. Without any such alternative, research ethics has found it easier to follow Jonas and to circumscribe the scope of the discipline in a way that forestalls appeals to the common good and the specter of totalitarian science carried with them. Orthodox research ethics reflects Jonas's philosophical reticence about linking research

---

[6] In a prolific body of work, Dan Callahan argued eloquently against the "underlying logic of the research imperative, which is to overcome death itself" (2000, 654; see also Callahan 1990, 2003). One can agree with Callahan that death is an inevitable part of life, and that suffering cannot be entirely extirpated from human life, while still holding that there is a valuable role for medicine to play in helping individuals retain the capacities they need to live out a normal lifespan in which they can form, pursue, and revise a life plan of their own. The research imperative is also sometimes associated with a drive to pathologize an ever-wider range of human differences (Wayne and Glass 2010). Although some may have such an ambition for science, I see no reason why an imperative of the sort I defend in chapter 4 must entail such excesses.

to the common good, to any sort of social imperative for progress, or to the goals and mission of the state or political community.

2.3.3 Frustration without a Viable Alternative

Occasionally, Jonas's position is challenged by scholars who effectively echo concerns that are already voiced in these early critiques. For example, Eisenberg argues that there must be proportionality between "social controls" that we impose on researchers to prevent wrongdoing and the great good that comes from medical research. We must reconcile both sides of the ledger because there is no escaping the fact that "the decision not to do something poses as many ethical quandaries as the decision to do it. Not to act is to act" (1977, 1108). Basically the same idea is expressed nearly thirty years later by John Harris when he writes, "Where our actions will, or may probably prevent serious harm then if we can reasonably (given the balance of risk and burden to ourselves and benefit to others) we clearly should act because to fail to do so is to accept responsibility for the harm that then occurs" (2005, 242).

However, contemporary discussions of the research imperative reflect the reticence of the field to link research to larger social purposes. They tend not to address the question of whether there is a social or moral obligation to carry out research and, if so, how that obligation should shape the goals and priorities of the research enterprise. They emphasize that the failure to recruit sufficient numbers of participants into studies is wasteful, and they focus more narrowly on whether there is a duty on the part of individuals to participate in research (Caplan 1984; Herrera 2003; Harris 2005; Brazier 2008; Rhodes 2008; Chan and Harris 2009; Schaefer, Emanuel, and Wertheimer 2009).

Harris, like Eisenberg, expresses frustration at the deontological bulwarks erected around the rights and interests of study participants and the comparative social indifference toward the loss of life or avoidable disability incurred as a result of the slow pace of medical progress. Although his rhetoric is more temperate, he points out, like McDermott, that society conscripts its members to serve a wide range of roles and purposes, from the military, to jury duty, to mandating vaccination as a condition of public-school attendance.[7] Harris has no sympathy for the idea that researchers should have the unilateral power to conscript participants into research and he sees significant policy reasons to avoid such efforts. Nevertheless, he argues that even if it should not be the first option from the standpoint of policy, the good at stake can be such that it would be "legitimate to make science research compulsory" (2005, 245).

To the extent that thinkers like Harris recapitulate older frustrations with the narrow protectionism of research ethics, the reaction to views of this sort largely reflects a similarly venerable horror at the prospect that the utilitarian calculus on which they are predicated will resurrect the specter of totalitarianism that Jonas sought to exorcise.[8] As a result, whether for philosophical or purely pragmatic purposes, orthodox research ethics tend to avoid discussions of the social mission of research, whether medical research is required as part of a just social order and the extent to which the progress that it offers is genuinely incompatible with respect for individuals as free and equal persons. I suspect that this aversion is less of a reflection of the status of these issues as closed and settled than it is a reflection of wariness about fault lines radiating out from the origins of the field and running through the foundations of the discipline.

In challenging the research imperative, Jonas sought to fortify concern for the rights and interests of individuals against the demands of society for scientific progress. In doing so, however, he provides a philosophical justification for relegating research to the status of a socially optional, private activity, unconnected to larger social purposes. Jonas provides a rationale that transforms the de facto parochialism of nascent research ethics institutions into a de jure conception of the relationship between researchers and the social good. Where the institutional focus on the IRB triangle might be seen as an administrative convenience, Jonas provides the rationale for seeing this focus as the proper lens through which to view the interaction between two parties whose respective interests are on a par.

---

[7] Jones (1993, 86–89) uses the term "soldiers of science" to describe the attitude of Tuskegee researchers toward study subjects. Schaefer et al. (2009, 70) resist the claim that research is sufficiently important to justify compelling people to participate, but they nevertheless say that the duty to serve as a research participant is "in some ways analogous to a wartime call to arms in which not just money but soldiers to fight are needed."

[8] Among others, see Brassington (2007, 2011) and Wayne and Glass (2010).

2.4 Functional Characterization of Research

2.4.1 Practical Influences on Research Ethics

In the previous section I argued that Jonas's arguments provided an explicit philosophical rationale for developments in research ethics that were spurred by much more practical responses to revelations of scandal and abuse. Although this conceptual background is important for the purposes of the present inquiry, the conceptual ecosystem of research ethics was likely shaped more directly by practical responses to revelations of abuse.

In particular, many early cases of abuse involved health care professionals exploiting the discretion and authority that they wielded in virtue of their social role as caregiver to do things that were inconsistent with the duties and obligations of that role. This made it natural to locate the moral epicenter of research ethics in the discrete interactions of researchers with study participants and to conceptualize research in functional terms that would facilitate the ability of IRBs to regulate these interactions.

2.4.2 The Jewish Chronic Disease Hospital Case

Two important cases are worth mentioning in particular. The first, described briefly by Beecher in his 1966 exposé, would come to be known as the Jewish Chronic Disease Hospital Case (Katz et al. 1972, 9–65; Arras 2008). In 1965, the New York State Board of Regents found that researchers at the Jewish Chronic Disease Hospital (JCDH) had carried out a research project on chronically ill residents without properly informing those individuals— many of whom likely lacked the capacity to make decisions for themselves— that they were subjects in an experiment.

Briefly, researchers had learned that it took longer for individuals with cancer to expel foreign cancers cells from their bodies than individuals without cancer. They therefore wanted to know whether this delay was due to the presence of cancer or to the fact that the immune systems of such patients were already compromised. To answer this question, they designed a study in which they would inject foreign cancer cells into the bodies of individuals who were chronically ill but not suffering from cancer. Their hope was that if the delayed rejection time was caused by the presence of cancer, they could use this knowledge in the quest to fight this fatal disease or to devise a test for its presence. They claimed that they were justified in not informing subjects of the nature of this procedure because the word "cancer" was loaded with such significance at the time that many might have refused to participate, despite the researchers' belief that it was highly unlikely that anyone could contract cancer from exposure to foreign cancer cells.

For the Board of Regents, the case was notable because clinicians had used the broad discretion that at that time attended their social role as caregivers to perform procedures on patients that were not for their individual benefit but for the advancement of science. Even if no participant was harmed, the Board of Regents held that participants were wronged when they were denied the right to decide what should happen to their person.

In criticizing this case, Beecher appealed to the *DoH*. This document largely recapitulated moral requirements that had been articulated decades earlier in the trial of the Nazi doctors at Nuremberg. At that trial, the prosecution argued that Nazi research violated a series of requirements that captured the accepted practices and beliefs about the ethical conduct of research. This set of principles would come to be known as the *Nuremberg Code*, and it begins with the bold assertion that, "The voluntary consent of the human subject is absolutely essential" (Tribunals 1949, 181). Even at the trial, however, the defense had shown numerous cases of Allied research in which consent was not obtained or in which it was obtained under conditions that might compromise its moral validity. Although the *Nuremburg Code* would come to be recognized as a prescient document, it had little impact on the conduct of research by American researchers (Moreno 1999). As a result, the twenty years that followed the Nuremberg trials have been described as "a time of vigorous research characterized by a fragmented community of medical researchers who applied inconsistent ethical standards and employed highly variable research practices" (Freidenfelds and Brandt 1996, 239).

The *DoH* repackaged most of the provisions of the Nuremburg Code, now framed as guidance specifically for individual clinicians. In particular, as research had grown more widespread, nurtured by private investment and public funding, physicians grappled with the tension between their fiduciary duty to the individual patient and the researcher's social obligation to generate information that might advance the health of countless future generations of patients.

2.4.3 The Tuskegee Syphilis Study

The second and perhaps the single most important case that came to light during this same period also involved medical practitioners exploiting the social trust they enjoyed in their role as healers for purely research-related purposes. In the early 1960s, an African American epidemiologist in the US Public Health Service (PHS) named Dr. Bill Jenkins heard about a study that had been initiated by the PHS in Macon County, Alabama in 1932. Since the discovery of Salvarsan in 1910, syphilis had been a treatable medical condition. But with the discovery and mass production of penicillin at the end of the Second World War, a highly effective treatment with few side effects became widely available. Nevertheless, the purpose of the study in Macon County was to document the effects of untreated syphilis in a cohort of 400 African American men.[9]

After sifting through the substantial record of publications detailing the study and its decades-long history, Jenkins wrote to other African American physicians and contacted the media in an effort to raise concerns about the ethics of the study.[10] In 1966, another PHS worker, Peter Buxtun, also began voicing serious moral concerns about the study, both within the PHS and more broadly. Ultimately, the PHS convened a blue-ribbon panel of experts to review the project. In 1969 the panel voted, with only a single dissenter, to continue what it saw as important research (Jones 2008).

When news of what would come to be called the Tuskegee syphilis study made headlines in 1972, however, the public's reaction diverged significantly from the response of the blue-ribbon expert panel that had voted to continue the study only three years earlier. PHS researchers had lied to the men in the study about their medical condition, telling them they had "bad blood" rather than revealing a diagnosis of syphilis. They lied about the purpose of their yearly medical examinations and spinal taps, leading the men to believe they were receiving treatment, never disclosing that these purely research-related procedures were part of a study designed to document the effects of untreated syphilis. Researchers had actively prevented the men from receiving medical treatment from public health programs, as a result of examinations that would have been conducted as part of the draft, or in

---

[9] There are numerous excellent historical accounts of this event including Brandt (1978), Jones (1993, 2008), and Reverby (2009). Reverby (2011) discusses parallel studies carried out in Guatemala.
[10] https://www.nytimes.com/2019/02/25/obituaries/bill-jenkins-dead.html

the course of routine medical care. The outrage of a public that was already questioning the traditional distribution of power and social authority in major social institutions was swift and hot.

The Tuskegee syphilis study lasted for forty years. It began before World War II, continued after the trials at Nuremberg, the execution of German physicians for crimes against humanity, the publication of the Nuremberg Code and the *DoH*. Although news of the study shocked the conscience of the lay public, it—like the twenty-two cases of unethical research Beecher had detailed in his 1966 paper—was not a clandestine affair within the PHS. The outrage of the public reflected shock at what could pass for normal behavior in a profession entrusted with significant power and authority. The moral calculus of the researchers who conceived, conducted, and perpetuated these studies was jarringly out of sync with the moral sensibilities of the public in whose name these investigations were ostensibly carried out.

It was public outcry over the Tuskegee study that spurred the US Congress to create the National Commission whose *Belmont Report* would be shaped by these revelations from Alabama. The scandals at Tuskegee and places like the JCDH revealed how easily the deference to clinicians and the discretion to control the agency of patients conferred in the Hippocratic tradition of medicine, still operative at the time, could be coopted for purely research-related purposes.

At Tuskegee, for example, it is unlikely that the study could have been maintained for forty years if members of the PHS had not presented themselves as healers and taken advantage of the social trust that Hippocratic medicine demanded from the recipients of medical care. The men who were unwitting participants in the study believed they were receiving treatment. They believed that medical professionals were acting in their interests. In fact, of course, the activities of those professionals were inconsistent with the best interests of those men. They were directed, not by the goal of curing their disease or preventing its spread, but by the goals of documenting the natural course of untreated disease in African American men.

2.4.4 Research versus Treatment

A natural response to the events at JCDH and Tuskegee was to search for criteria that could be used to determine when the interactions between individuals should be governed by the norms of the doctor-patient relationship and when they fall, instead, into the sphere of research and should be governed instead by the norms of research ethics. The key moral idea is that even if caregivers enjoy some discretion to withhold information or to encourage patients to undertake some course of care, the moral warrant for this discretion would derive from the duty of the caregiver to always act as the fiduciary of the interests of the individual patient. If that same individual professional instead takes up the goals and ends of medical research, then they lay down their sovereign commitment to the medical best interests of patients and, in doing so, can no longer legitimately exercise the discretion of the caregiver. Instead, they must approach patients as researchers and disclose to them the nature of the purposes they are now seeking to advance and conform to the distinct norms of research ethics.

The *Belmont Report* transformed this moral insight into a functional characterization of research as a set of purposes, distinct from the purposes of medical or behavioral health practice. Being able to distinguish "biomedical and behavioral research, on the one hand, and the practice of accepted therapy on the other" allowed these activities to be sorted into their proper sphere of oversight (National Commission 1979).

The *Belmont Report* defines medical practice by the purpose of providing "diagnosis, preventive treatment or therapy to particular individuals" (National Commission 1979). It also is characterized by the use of "interventions that are designed solely to enhance the well-being of an individual patient or client and that have a reasonable expectation of success." The paradigmatic example of practice is when a clinician draws on existing knowledge to deploy established effective interventions for the benefit of the individual patient. In this case, all of the considerations that are relevant to evaluating the use of an intervention relate to its likely impact on the interests of the patient. Few medical treatments are unalloyed goods. They often carry risks and burdens because they involve the administration of toxic and potentially dangerous substances. In administering treatment, therefore, the clinician is required to make the judgment that any risks to the health of a particular patient are outweighed by the prospect of medical benefit for that same patient.

In contrast, the purpose that defines the research activity is to "test an hypothesis, permit conclusions to be drawn, and thereby to develop or contribute to generalizable knowledge (expressed, for example, in theories, principles, and statements of relationships)" (National Commission 1979). To do this, research often involves the delivery of interventions whose likelihood of success is unknown or whose value relative to other options is uncertain. It can also involve practices or procedures that are performed on one person in the hope of generating information or benefits that will only accrue, if they materialize at all, to a different group of persons.

On this approach, research is characterized by a network of justificatory reasons that are fundamentally different from treatment. Treatment is the utilization of current knowledge and established interventions for the singular purpose of advancing the medical best interests of the individual patient. Research is the deployment of interventions whose effects are unknown or uncertain, for the purpose of generating generalizable medical knowledge. This functional account of research serves the practical purposes of IRBs by allowing them to determine when activities fall under the norms of medical practice and when they constitute research and must therefore receive special oversight. It also allows research to be understood in a way that fits entirely within what I called the IRB triangle in the previous chapter—the interactions between researchers and participants that it is the purview of IRBs to oversee.

This way of understanding research, as an activity defined by a distinct set of goals and purposes that can be taken up and pursued by individual researchers, further dissociates research from larger social purposes. Yes, the purpose of research is to generate generalizable knowledge, but the value of generalizable knowledge is left unstated. Conceived of as a set of purposes an individual can adopt, research is severed from any connection to the social institutions that make its conduct possible and that are required to translate generalizable information into practices, procedures, or interventions that actually advance the health interests of patients. Ensconced within the IRB triangle, research is dissociated from any sort of division of social labor and the larger purposes of a just social order that might be relevant to regulating the terms on which that labor is divided and for what purposes it can be justified.

As we will see in more detail in chapter 5, this functional approach to research, with its critical emphasis on the individual decision-maker, reinforces the perception that there is a fundamental moral dilemma at the heart of research with humans. In particular, if research is a set of goals and purposes that guide individual decision-making, and if these goals are inherently distinct from the goals and purposes of clinical medicine, then individual decision-makers will at least sometimes have to compromise one of these sets of objectives in order to advance the other.

2.4.5 The Ecosystem of Paternalism

As the name of the National Commission and its most famous report indicate, the birth of research ethics in a practical policy response to revelations of abuse fundamentally shaped the protectionist stance of the field. Researchers would have to submit to IRBs protocols detailing the nature of their proposed study, its anticipated risks and benefits, and a plan for securing the free and informed consent of participants. Only if this plan meets the approval of this independent oversight body will it be permissible to offer participation to study participants. IRB review would thus mediate the interaction of researchers and study participants with the mandate to protect study participants from abuse. Both conceptually and historically, the protectionism of research ethics is easily seen as a paternalistic effort to safeguard the rights and welfare of people who cannot do this for themselves (Dworkin, 1972; Miller and Wertheimer 2007; Jansen and Wall 2009; Edwards and Wilson 2012).

The paternalism of orthodox research ethics is thus closely connected to the other problematic aspects of the conceptual ecosystem of orthodox research ethics that I have been detailing here. On a practical level, it reflects a concrete policy response to cases of scandal and abuse. On a conceptual level, it reflects the perception that the professional obligations of caregivers and researchers impose conflicting and incompatible goals on the decision-making of individuals that reinforce the larger tendency of the underlying utilitarianism of research to run roughshod over the rights and interests of individuals. Defining research in functional terms facilitates a vision of research oversight in which the most critical ethical issues arise in the interactions of researchers with study participants. A framework that can sort the actions of caregivers and the actions of researchers into different bins, where they can be subject to different moral requirements, facilitates the protectionist goals of IRB review and advances the pragmatic goal of avoiding the types of abuse that set the reforms of the National Commission into motion.

2.5 Justice: The Last Virtue of Research Ethics

2.5.1 Justice Untethered

Severing the research enterprise from larger social purposes and defining research in functional terms that fit neatly within the IRB triangle effectively removes this activity from the sphere that is primarily regulated by considerations of justice. The philosopher John Rawls famously calls justice "the first virtue of social institutions" (1971, 3) because it regulates the operation of social systems that both require social support and create the social order that determines what rights, duties, and opportunities individuals have and their prospects for being free to pursue a life plan of their own on equal terms with their compatriots.

Although the *Belmont Report* lists respect for persons, beneficence, and justice as the three fundamental moral principles to which research must be responsive, justice is arguably the last virtue of research ethics. At the conceptual level, it is the least well defined and clearly grounded. At the operational level its recommendations are the least well translated into explicit, practical requirements. In terms of the volume of scholarship produced in the field it is the least studied, and in the institutional structures that regulate research it has the least influence.

2.5.2 The Consequences of Neglect

The neglect of justice in research ethics has three distinct consequences. First, the justifications for requirements that are linked to this value are often unclear. Second, early discussions of justice in research ethics explicate this value in terms that allow it, implicitly if not explicitly, to be reduced to a function of the other values that constitute the twin pillars of research ethics. Thirdly, considerations of justice that cannot be reduced to applications of respect for persons and beneficence seem to fall outside the scope of the field, to be unwarranted, or in the worst case to be inconsistent with more clearly understood and firmly grounded commitments of the field.

To make the case for these claims, consider how each of these principles is explicated in the *Belmont Report*. Respect for persons, sometimes referred to as respect for autonomy, reflects the importance of being able to make decisions that impact the shape or the quality of one's own life. It is operationalized for persons with decisional capacity through the requirement of free and informed consent. Although informed consent had been elevated to the status of a necessary condition for ethical research in the Nuremberg Code, it was not until the work of the National Commission that this value came to play a dominant role in regulating medical research. Its prominence is grounded, in no small measure, in the fact that if this requirement had been widely adopted after Nuremberg it likely would have been sufficient to avoid most of the scandals that spurred the creation of the National Commission. Because informed consent has been the subject of such voluminous scholarship and discussion, it is almost synonymous with research ethics.

The second core value of research ethics is beneficence, which ranges over the domain of individual welfare or well-being. The *Belmont Report* uses "beneficence" to name the principle that ranges over all considerations that affect individual welfare or well-being. Others sometimes divide this concern for individual welfare or well-being among two values. In the influential terminology of Beauchamp and Childress (2001), for example, beneficence is reserved for an affirmative concern for welfare or well-being while nonmaleficence refers to the negative concern to avoid harm or some other way detracting from well-being. Regardless of how one wants to divide the values that range over this domain, the concern for individual welfare or well-being is operationalized by balancing risks and benefits.

To avoid confusion, I follow the more expansive view of beneficence as including the principle of nonmaleficence. In other words, beneficence ranges over both the avoidance of harm and the provision of benefits.

A key point is that beneficence is not limited to the consideration of whether the risks and burdens of research participation for a given individual are reasonable solely in light of the benefits likely to accrue to that same individual—although satisfying this condition is a clear way of satisfying the requirements of beneficence. Rather, the risks and burdens to one person can be offset by the expectation that benefits will accrue to future beneficiaries of research. Considerations of beneficence thus require judgments in which risks and burdens to some individuals are balanced or traded off against the expectations that benefits will accrue to other individuals. In this sense, beneficence is concerned with the distribution of benefits and burdens both to the same individual and across different individuals.

The *Belmont Report* introduces justice by saying that it addresses the question "Who ought to receive the benefits of research and bear its burdens?"

Understood this way, both justice and beneficence range over the same domain, namely, the distribution of benefits and burdens. Similarly, both deal with judgments about how benefits and burdens are distributed across different individuals or groups.

Justice is also defined as the principle that "equals ought to be treated equally" (National Commission 1979). But this formulation is not very useful without specifying the space of equality—the set of concerns or the domain over which individuals have a right to be treated equally (Sen 1982, Daniels 1990, Korsgaard 1993, Anderson 1999). After all, as consequentialists are fond of observing, beneficence is also grounded in the commitment to giving equal treatment to equals; beneficence involves assigning equal value to the welfare of every individual. Beneficence treats the space of equality as the domain of welfare—individuals have an equal claim to have their welfare be given equal weight to the welfare of everyone else. Because more welfare is better, beneficence requires choosing acts or policies that produce the greatest net welfare. In research ethics, part of the justification for allowing risks to one person to be offset by benefits to others is the prospect that the burdens to the one are outweighed by the benefits to the others. For consequentialists, therefore, giving equal treatment to the welfare of all, impartially considered, is a central feature of the moral point of view. So merely saying that justice requires giving equal treatment to equals is not sufficient to distinguish it from beneficence.

The *Belmont Report* does not indicate the respect in which justice in research requires equals to be treated equally. Instead, we are told that social justice requires that vulnerable groups not be chosen for inclusion in research simply because of their "easy availability, their compromised position, or their manipulability, rather than for reasons directly related to the problem being studied" and that this requirement was widely violated in the nineteenth and early twentieth centuries when "the burdens of serving as research subjects fell largely upon poor ward patients, while the benefits of improved medical care flowed primarily to private patients" (National Commission 1979).

On the surface, beneficence and justice might be distinguished by the specific requirements they place on the distribution of benefits and burdens across different groups. For example, beneficence is operationalized in terms of having a favorable balance of risks and expected benefits. In contrast, justice is operationalized in terms of "fair procedures and outcomes in the selection of research subjects" (National Commission 1979). Whether this surface difference translates into a substantive moral difference depends on the extent to which the considerations that determine the fairness of procedures and outcomes are distinct from considerations that determine the favorability of the balance of risks and expected benefits.

2.5.3 Minimalism about Justice: Reducing It to Beneficence and Autonomy

Part of the problem, however, is that although the *Belmont Report* asserts that fairness requires certain conditions, it does not explain *why* those conditions represent requirements of fairness. For example, we are told that fairness at the procedural level requires not recruiting favored groups for "potentially beneficial research" while selecting "only 'undesirable' persons for risky research" (National Commission 1979). Likewise, "when research is proposed that involves risks and does not include a therapeutic component, other less burdened classes of persons should be called upon first to accept these risks of research, except where the research is directly related to the specific conditions of the class involved."

But both of these restrictions can be explained in terms of beneficence. The *Belmont Report* treats marginalized or disadvantaged groups as already burdened. If research relies disproportionally on members of groups that are already burdened, then it will have a higher risk profile than if it were to rely instead on individuals drawn from groups that are comparatively better off. The reason is that involving a population that is already less burdened is likely to result in fewer harms, or to result in harms of a lesser magnitude. This can be for several reasons.

First, groups that are less marginalized may not be willing to participate in research that is unacceptably risky, and their more stable social position may make it more difficult to force them to participate. Second, to the extent that better-off people experience less stress, fewer physical insults, and suffer from fewer medical problems, they may be less likely to experience some adverse events in the course of research. Third, if they do experience those adverse events, their effects may not be as pronounced either because bearing a lower burden of stress and illness makes them more resilient or because having greater access to social resources enables them to more effectively mitigate harms and cope with their aftermath. As a result, the wrongness of a violation of procedural fairness can be explained in terms of the other core values of research ethics—it is more likely to involve coercion or a form of influence that violates respect for persons or to cause more harm than an approach that relies instead on individuals drawn from better-off groups.

Similar reasoning applies to ensuring that "some classes (e.g., welfare patients, particular racial and ethnic minorities, or persons confined to institutions) are [not] being systematically selected simply because of their easy availability, their compromised position, or their manipulability, rather than for reasons directly related to the problem being studied" (National Commission 1979). Relying on such groups in cases where they do not expect to benefit directly from research participation is more likely to result in a violation of respect for persons or to produce more harm than an approach that relies on less marginalized groups. In contrast, when a study addresses a problem that is experienced by individuals in a group, then their participation is more likely to be voluntary because they are more likely to view the risks as reasonable in light of benefits to themselves or to members of a group with which they identify. And if the research is related to the health needs of the groups included, then it is likely to produce a favorable risk benefit ratio for those groups.

My point is not that the pronouncements in the *Belmont Report* cannot be grounded in justice. It is, rather, that at best the distinct content of justice in the *Belmont Report* is unclear. At worst, the *Belmont Report* is consistent with what I refer to as the minimalist view of justice. On this view, requirements of justice are reduced to a function of beneficence and respect for persons. To ascertain whether a transaction or a social arrangement satisfies the requirements of justice requires a determination of whether it is conducted on terms that satisfy respect for persons and beneficence. Returning to the requirements in the *Belmont Report,* if it is unfair to use deception, force, or fraud to secure the participation of marginalized groups, then it looks like this unfairness can be explained in terms of, and therefore reduced to, respect for persons and informed consent. If it is unfair to conduct research in populations that bear higher risks than less burdened populations, then this seems to reduce fairness to beneficence since fewer harms will result by including less marginalized populations in research. The pressure to frame issues in research ethics in terms that are manageable within the narrow confines of the IRB triangle adds to the tendency to neglect the distinctively social aspects of justice and to explicate it, instead, in terms that derive from the more familiar and central pillars of the field.

2.5.4 Requirements without Grounds

When justice is linked to issues outside of the IRB triangle, stakeholders are left with no justification for the claims that are made. For example, in an important passage the *Belmont Report* says:

> Finally, whenever research supported by public funds leads to the development of therapeutic devices and procedures, justice demands both that these not provide advantages only to those who can afford them and that such research should not unduly involve persons from groups unlikely to be among the beneficiaries of subsequent applications of the research (National Commission 1979).

Although it is clearly stated *that* these requirements are supposed to be grounded in considerations of justice, no clear justification for this claim is offered. However, several features of this claim are puzzling.

First, whether a research discovery provides advantages to people who cannot afford it depends critically on how the larger health system is organized. Even if treatments can be procured at no cost, they often must be administered within health systems that have their own organizational structure and funding model. It may well be the case that a just health system should provide universal access to medical care. But the point for the present purpose is that in the context in which this claim is made, no such position is defended. Since at the time there were no provisions for universal access to health care in the United States (at the time of this writing there still are no such provisions), it is unclear why the use of public funds in one social system (biomedical research) should be sufficient to justify altering entitlements within another social system (the provision of health services).

Second, it is not clear why research that is supported by public funds should be subject to special requirements. If a research group is investigating treatments for a debilitating or fatal disease for which there are currently no effective therapies, would it be ethically permissible for that group to recruit exclusively from populations that are unlikely to benefit from subsequent applications of that research as long as they receive only private funding? On the one hand, even private firms enjoy various forms of social support, from public policies that provide for intellectual property protection to the fact that most research builds on prior findings, a large portion of which are generated from research with federal funding. On the other hand, heaping burdens on already marginalized people in order to generate benefits for people who are already better off seems wrong no matter how that activity is funded.

A major problem with the *Belmont Report* is that it recognizes that aspects of research with humans that fall outside of the IRB triangle can affect the justice of this undertaking, but it lacks the resources to make these connections clear and to provide substantial normative guidance about them. In particular, its focus on the relationship between research and the delivery of health services—on the importance of ensuring access to the applications of knowledge produced in research—reflects a dim recognition that research is one activity that takes place within a larger division of social labor. It is a recognition that issues of social justice are raised by the relationship between systems of knowledge production and the systems that put this knowledge into practice in the form of treatment and preventative services. But the rationale for this focus is left largely unarticulated. As we see in §2.6 similar problems affect requirements in international guidance documents that are ostensibly grounded in justice.

2.5.5 Protectionism and Neglect

As other commentators have noted, the *Belmont Report* emphasizes relationships that must be avoided. For example, marginalized groups must not be recruited because of their "easy availability, their compromised position, or their manipulability, rather than for reasons directly related to the problem being studied" (National Commission 1979). But it does not say that researchers, study sponsors, or anyone else has a responsibility to carry out research that advances the unique health needs of groups that are marginalized, oppressed, or that suffer from excess burdens of morbidity and mortality. As a result, one way to satisfy the protectionism of its recommendations is to avoid carrying out research in such populations altogether.

While such a move avoids a certain kind of wrongful treatment, it leaves some of the most disadvantaged populations subject to the ravages of lethal neglect. As others have pointed out, explicating justice in largely protectionist terms fails to recognize the ways in which groups that are perceived as being vulnerable to exploitation or abuse in research can be harmed when their distinctive medical needs are not the subject of extensive scientific investigation (Dresser 1992; Kahn, Mastroianni, and Sugarman 1998).

Already in 1977, Eisenberg criticized the culture of research regulation for losing sight of the social imperative to carry out research and for being too complacent about the human toll that neglect would produce for those who suffer the highest burden of sickness, injury, and disease. He argued that the importance of this imperative and the toll of neglect was most palpable when one considered "the third world, where infant mortality may be as high as 20 percent and life expectancy no more than 30 years" (1977, 1109). For Eisenberg, "there is a clear moral imperative in developed nations for medical research in tropical diseases to seek to permit two-thirds of the world's population to share in the freedom from pain and untimely death we have achieved for ourselves" (1109).

2.6 International Research Stresses Fault Lines

2.6.1 The Zidovudine Short-Course Controversy

The fault lines outlined previously have been stressed, deepened, and brought into sharp relief in subsequent debates over the ethics of international research. Since the volume of such research began to rapidly increase in the 1990s (Rehnquist 2001; Thiers, Sinskey, and Berndt 2007), international research has been the subject of voluminous and at times acrimonious debate (Angell 1997; Lurie and Wolfe 1997; Annas and Grodin 1998; Benatar 1998; Crouch and Arras 1998; Glantz et al. 1998; Attaran 1999; Benatar and Singer 2000; Macklin 2001; Resnik 2001; Benatar et al. 2003; Flory and Kitcher 2004; London 2005). International ethical guidelines, such as the *DoH* or the *International Ethical Guidelines for Biomedical Research Involving Human Subjects* from the Council for International Organizations of Medical Sciences (from now on, "CIOMS *Guidelines*" for short), stipulate a range of ethical requirements that must be met in order for international research to be ethically acceptable, some of which are explicitly grounded in the value of justice. But these requirements suffer from some of the same problems that arise for the requirements of justice in the *Belmont Report*. Their normative justification is unclear, they often make demands on stakeholders who are outside the IRB triangle, and they are criticized for being inconsistent with some of the core principles of research ethics.

Without a unified moral foundation to anchor their interpretation, the requirements of various international guidance documents have spawned heated and at times divisive debate (Singer and Benatar 2001, Kimmelman, Weijer and Meslin 2009). This was dramatized by early debates about the standard of care in international research.

In 1975 the *DoH* was revised for the first time and two new requirements were added in section II on "Medical Research Combined With Professional Care (Clinical Research)":

II.2.   The potential benefits, hazards and discomfort of a new method should be weighed against the advantages of the best current diagnostic and therapeutic methods.

II.3.   In any medical study, every patient—including those of a control group, if any—should be assured of the best proven diagnostic and therapeutic method. (World Medical Association 1975)

These requirements remained unchanged in the 1983 revision. In 1996 a sentence was added to the end of the text in II.3 to indicate that "this does not exclude the use of inert placebo in studies where no proven diagnostic or therapeutic method exists" (World Medical Association 1996). When the *DoH* was revised in 2000 these distinct statements were combined into a single requirement:

29.   The benefits, risks, burdens and effectiveness of a new method should be tested against those of the best current prophylactic, diagnostic, and therapeutic methods. This does not exclude the use of placebo, or no treatment, in studies where no proven prophylactic, diagnostic or therapeutic method exists. (World Medical Association 2000)

This text was retained in the 2004 revision but, at the last minute, a "note of clarification" was added. That note stated that a "a placebo-controlled trial may be ethically acceptable, even if proven therapy is available," under two circumstances:

—Where for compelling and scientifically sound methodological reasons its use is necessary to determine the efficacy or safety of a prophylactic, diagnostic or therapeutic method; or

—Where a prophylactic, diagnostic or therapeutic method is being investigated for a minor condition and the patients who receive placebo will not be subject to any additional risk of serious or irreversible harm. (World Medical Association 2004)

For many, this note of clarification was a bombshell. For nearly thirty years the *DoH* had been consistent in holding that the prophylactic, diagnostic, or therapeutic merits of a new medical intervention should be tested against those of the best current alternative. But what was presented as a note of clarification appeared to contradict the main requirement of the text. All that was required to justify withholding the best current alternative from study participants was a sound methodological reason. Since vocal proponents of placebo-controlled trials often championed such designs on methodological grounds, many worried that the note of clarification was effectively a free pass for researchers to expand the use of placebo controls.

The inconsistency in the 2004 *DoH* was a major blow to its status. It dramatized the limited value of pithy injunctions untethered from clear normative grounding and exemplified the extent to which that document had become a victim of its own success. In particular, since 1997 the *DoH* had been at the epicenter of a major controversy surrounding the ethics of placebo-controlled trials. That was the year that a pair of editorials published in the *New England Journal of Medicine* decried as unethical a proposal to test a short-course of zidovudine (also known as AZT) for the prevention of maternal-infant HIV infection against a placebo control in sixteen countries in sub-Saharan Africa, Southeast Asia, and the Caribbean (Angel 1997; Lurie and Wolfe 1997). These studies did not originate with industry. They were a collaborative effort among the US National Institutes of Health (NIH), the US Centers for Disease Control and Prevention (CDC), foreign governments, and international public health institutions. Their goal was to find a regimen of zidovudine that might represent a feasible intervention to stem the tide of perinatal HIV transmission in some of the world's poorest countries.

The study was controversial, in part, because a few years earlier a large-scale randomized clinical trial—referred to as the AIDS Clinical Trial Group (ACTG) 076 study—had demonstrated that a long course of zidovudine (from now on, the "076 Protocol") was highly effective at preventing HIV transmission from pregnant mothers to their newborn children, reducing transmission rates by two-thirds. Against this background, the then-editor of the *New England Journal of Medicine*, Dr. Marsha Angell, compared the use of a placebo control in the short-course zidovudine studies to the Tuskegee syphilis study. In her argument in support of this analogy, she quoted the requirements outlined in III.2 from the 1989 *DoH*.

Angell's argument connected the requirements of the *DoH* with the concept of equipoise (this concept is discussed at length in chapters 5 and 6). For now, equipoise can be understood as honest uncertainty among experts about the relative clinical value of a set of interventions for treating a particular medical condition. Angell argued that equipoise between the interventions on offer in the arms of a study is a necessary condition for ethical research and that if there is solid evidence in favor of the superiority of one intervention, then "not only would the trial be scientifically redundant, but the investigators would be guilty of knowingly giving inferior treatment to some participants in the trial" (1997, 847). Extending this logic to placebo-controlled trials, she evoked the language of the *DoH*, holding that "only when there is no known effective treatment is it ethical to compare a potential new treatment with a placebo. When effective treatment exists, a placebo may not be used. Instead, subjects in the control group of the study must receive the best known treatment." The crucial fact for Angell was that "zidovudine has already been clearly shown to cut the rate of vertical transmission greatly and is now recommended in the United States for all HIV-infected pregnant women" (847).

The comparison between the short-course studies and Tuskegee enflamed passions on both sides. For critics, it illustrated the gravity of the transgression involved in denying participants in a clinical trial access to established effective care. Among the initiative's proponents, it sparked outrage since, they argued, the placebo design was necessary to find a method of preventing perinatal HIV transmission that could be implemented in some of the world's poorest countries to stem the tide of a disease that was ravaging their populations.

Ironically, both sides of this debate agreed that finding an alternative to the 076 Protocol that might be feasible for use in LMIC settings was an important and appropriate public health goal. At the time, the zidovudine regimen in the 076 Protocol cost about $800 per mother-child pair. As the heads at the time of the NIH and the CDC, Harold Varmus and David Satcher noted, this was as much as 600 times the per capita health expenditures of some Sub-Saharan countries (Varmus and Satcher 1997).

In addition, the 076 Protocol was resource intensive in other ways. Mothers had to be identified early in pregnancy so that they could begin a lengthy oral regimen of zidovudine. They also had to present at a treatment center for birth so that they could receive intravenous zidovudine. Newborns were then placed on a six-week regimen of oral zidovudine and mothers were required to formula feed their infants because breast feeding is a known rout of HIV transmission. In many cases, however, women in the communities that faced the highest burden of HIV were also underserved by their health systems. As a result, they frequently did not receive prenatal care early in pregnancy and often did not give birth in a healthcare setting. Similarly, while the 076 Protocol required new mothers to avoid breastfeeding, many LMIC communities also suffered from high rates of waterborne diseases which often posed a grave threat to the health of infants. This meant that, in some cases, avoiding breast feeding was untenable.

The widespread support for research that would find an alternative to the 076 Protocol reflects the implicit assessment that it would be more efficient and effective to find an intervention that could be deployed under conditions that were feasible in LMICs than to bridge the economic and infrastructure gaps that made the 076 Protocol an infeasible alternative for LMICs. As a result, the debate in the literature tended to accept the permissibility of pursuing research of this kind and focused, instead, on the choice of control that should be used in such studies.

Nevertheless, it was clear that specific disputes about trial design were being driven by a larger set of issues, often inchoate and unarticulated, with implications that reached far beyond the choice of study control. There was, therefore, an uncanny sense that the debate over the ethics of the placebo control was a kind of proxy war between larger philosophical positions that often remained unarticulated, but which covertly exerted tremendous influence on the judgments of the warring camps.

2.6.2 Two Distinctions and Four Standards of Care

Early attempts to resolve the dispute over the design of the short-course trials focused on explicating the nature of the requirements in the *DoH* and what was meant by the "best current" or "best proven" alternative. Considerable attention focused on what I have called the relevant reference point from which such judgments should be made: were these terms asking about the best alternative in the local population or in some more global center of excellence, such as in the United States or France (London 2000b)?

Proponents of the placebo control argued it did not deny participants care that they would have otherwise received and that it did not impose new or additional health burdens on participants (Grady 1998, 36; Francis 1998; C. Levine 1998, 46; Salim and Abdool 1998, 565).[11] They thus defended using the local reference point for determining the standard of care. But their arguments also tacitly presupposed that the standard of care was to be determined by the actual medical practice in the reference location. This framed questions about the standard of care as largely descriptive questions about the de facto medical practice in the reference community.

In response, some criticized using the local reference point in determining the standard of care. Local practices might reflect what happens as a result of poverty and deprivation rather than the application of sound scientific knowledge. The relevant moral baseline, they countered, referred to a more global reference point where medical practice reflects the current state of medical knowledge. As Angell put it, the recommendation in the United States that all pregnant women with HIV receive zidovudine set the relevant baseline to which the short-course studies should be compared.

But arguments framed as supporting the global reference point were often tacitly rejecting the appeal to de facto practice. In particular, those who appealed to the concept of equipoise often interpreted the standard of care as a normative principle, taking references to "proven" or "established" treatment as indicating practices that are normative. Because they are supported by evidence and reflect the sound clinical judgment of informed experts they are required as the means of discharging a clinician's duty of care. On this de jure interpretation, the standard of care is not set by what actually happens, but by what ought to be provided to study participants given what is known about the safety and effectiveness of the alternative diagnostic, prophylactic, or therapeutic options (London 2000b).

Implicit in this acrimonious debate, therefore, were two distinct sets of issues: Is the relevant reference point local or global? And is the standard of care determined by the de facto practices of some reference community or by a de jure determination based on what is known about the likely safety and effectiveness of alternative practices, policies or interventions? These two

---

[11] During the debate over the *DoH*'s requirement that subjects in clinical trials receive the "best proven diagnostic and therapeutic method," one proposed revision would have required only that subjects "not be denied access to the best proven diagnostic, prophylactic, or therapeutic method that would otherwise be available to him or her" (Brennan 1999, 529). See also Levine (1998, 1999).

axes created the possibility for four distinct interpretations of the standard of care.

For our present purposes one key point is that appeals to the *DoH* were insufficient to surface these alternative interpretations, let alone to adjudicate between then. Without a coherent rationale grounded in a compelling normative foundation, the pronouncements of the *DoH* could be interpreted in different ways. Within the parochialism of orthodox research ethics, two of these interpretations exerted outsized influence.

The first was the *local* de facto interpretation, which holds that the standard of care in a clinical trial is determined by what patients in the host community would actually receive if no trial or research initiative were to take place. In the case of maternal-fetal HIV transmission, this amounted to nothing. The local de facto standard of care was attractive because it takes what happens in the absence of outside intervention as the normatively relevant baseline for assessing alternative actions. If no studies were carried out, women and children in LMIC populations would not receive effective prophylaxis for perinatal HIV transmission.

The second interpretation that received outside attention was the *global* de jure interpretation. This interpretation was embraced by those who rejected the idea that descriptive accounts of the status quo in host communities are normative for determining the care to which participants in clinical trials are entitled. This interpretation holds that the standard of care must be determined by what experts regard as the best means of addressing the problem in question. It combines this de jure interpretation with a global reference point in which the relevant experts are located in global centers of excellence.

Two other interpretations of the standard of care are possible, but these were largely overlooked. One combines the global reference point with the de facto interpretation of the standard of care. This interpretation holds that the standard of care in a clinical trial is determined by the descriptive account of the care that patients receive outside the context of research in global centers of excellence. One reason why the local/global axis was so salient stems from the fact that, in this case at least, both the global de facto interpretation and the global de jure interpretation identify the 076 Protocol as the standard of care. The only difference lies in the rationale for each standard. When Angell appeals to the fact that the 076 Protocol is the standard of care in HIC health systems, it can sound like she is arguing that researchers in LMIC contexts are obligated to provide the 076 Protocol to study participants because this is what would happen (as a descriptive claim) in HICs. But if the standard of care is to be set by the de facto medical practice, then it would be unclear why the actual practice of one community (HIC centers of excellence) should constrain how research is carried out in different communities where patients routinely receive an entirely different level of care. The only morally relevant rationale for appealing to the practices of clinicians in HIC health systems is that those practices reflect the judgments of informed and conscientious experts that the 076 Protocol represents the best way to discharge their duty of care.

A fourth possibility that was also overlooked combines the de jure appeal to the judgments of conscientious and informed experts with the local reference point. The *local de jure* interpretation holds that the standard of care is determined by what conscientious and informed experts judge to be the most effective means of addressing a problem under conditions that are attainable and sustainable in the health systems in which the intervention in question will be deployed (London 2000b). The consensus on all sides of the debate appeared to be that it was morally permissible to search for an alternative to the 076 Protocol that would provide LMIC communities with a meaningful public health tool for reducing perinatal HIV transmission because the 076 Protocol was too resource intensive and logistically demanding to be effectively or equitably deployed on a large-scale basis in those communities. Given this, the local de jure standard of care holds that the short course should be compared against the best proven alternative for preventing maternal-fetal HIV transmission that can be effectively and equitably deployed under conditions that are attainable and sustainable in those communities.

The position that I develop in this book adopts and defends the local de jure standard of care. For our present purposes, however, I want to consider why this position was overlooked in these early debates and why proponents of a de jure standard of care tended to support the global reference point.

2.6.3 The Role-Related Obligations of Clinicians

Angell and others were attracted to what I am calling the *global de jure standard of care* by the basic idea that the existence of equipoise—uncertainty about the relative therapeutic merits of the available medical options—is a necessary condition for ethical research. When this uncertainty exists, it is supposed to create a bridge between the social value of research and the clinician's duty to do her best for each individual before her. The guiding idea is that, in the face of such uncertainty, it does not violate the clinician's fiduciary duty to her individual patient to allow the interventions that they receive to be determined by randomization.

However, if there is no uncertainty about the relative merits of the interventions in a trial, "not only would the trial be scientifically redundant, but the investigators would be guilty of knowingly giving inferior treatment to some participants in the trial" (Angell 1997, 847). Moreover, Angell argued that in order for equipoise to exist between the interventions in a trial that uses a placebo control, it must be the case that there is not already an established effective treatment for the condition in question. "When effective treatment exists, a placebo may not be used. Instead, subjects in the control group of the study must receive the best known treatment" (1997, 847). So Angell rightly recognized that in order for equipoise to exist, it must not only be the case that there is uncertainty about the relative merits of the interventions to which they might be randomized in a trial, but there also must not be an alternative intervention that is known to be superior to one or more of those options (see chapter 5).[12]

Angell argued that a placebo control was unethical in the short-course studies because the safety and efficacy of the 076 Protocol was established on the basis of substantial evidence. Its adoption in the United States and other HICs reflected consensus in the expert medical community about its status

---

[12] Here it seems like Angell is replicating a common mistake about equipoise because she initially frames the question as uncertainty regarding only the interventions that are compared within a trial. This would be a problem because a researcher could design a study to test the relative merits of interventions A and B when in fact there is an option C that is known to be superior to both A and B. If equipoise only referred to the arms of a trial, then a comparison of A and B would be ethically permissible, but it would violate both of Angell's desiderata. That is, the scientific value of such a study would be questionable—given that C is known to be superior to both—and an investigator randomizing participants to A or B would be guilty of knowingly giving inferior treatment since C is known to be the superior option. But this is not the case, as demonstrated by her assertion that if an effective intervention exists a placebo is not morally permissible. Kukla (2007) asserts that debates over the standard of care reveal fundamental problems with the concept of equipoise since that concept deals only with interventions being tested in a clinical trial. Kukla formulated the principle of equipoise (PE) as follows: "In order to begin or to continue an experiment on human subjects, one must be in a state of equipoise with respect to the relative expected health outcomes for participants in different trial arms" (179). However, prior discussions of equipoise in precisely this context were explicit that such a formulation would be unacceptable. London explicitly formulated the principle of equipoise to require a comparison between interventions on offer in the trial and those outside the study:

> Equipoise exists between interventions I1 and I2 relative to problem P in a treatment setting S, just in case credible doubts exist about the relative net therapeutic advantage of I1 and I2 for treating P in S and there is no intervention I3 that is preferable to either or both I1 and I2 for treating P in S. (2001, 324)

as the best method for preventing maternal-fetal HIV transmission. In light of this knowledge, she contended, testing the short-course zidovudine regimen against a placebo would violate equipoise and, with this, the clinician's duty not to deny study participants access to interventions that are known to be safe and effective.

The traditional conception of equipoise thus seemed to entail what I referred to as the global de jure interpretation of the standard of care. When considering whether a study begins in equipoise, it must not be the case (in this view) that there is an intervention that is regarded as preferable to one or more of the study arms anywhere in the world. Because the 076 Protocol was recognized as superior to placebo in centers of excellence in HICs, a study that would randomize participants to the short course of zidovudine or a placebo would violate this standard.

2.6.4 Problems for the Global De Jure Standard of Care

What I have called the global de jure standard of care appears to gain considerable support from an idea that is so widespread and intuitive that it functions as what I describe in §5.1.1 as the first dogma of research ethics. This is the idea that the fundamental moral norms governing the interactions between the parties within the IRB triangle derive from the role-related obligations of medical professionals. The global de jure standard of care is required in order to ensure that there is sufficient uncertainty at the beginning of a study to reconcile the researcher's duty of personal care with the requirements of sound science.

One important problem with the global de jure standard of care, however, is that it undermines the position it is supposed to support. It not only rules out comparing the short-course of zidovudine to a placebo, it rules out comparing it to the 076 Protocol as well (London 2001, 318–319). Those who opposed the placebo-controlled trial design as unethical did not oppose the larger project of finding an alternative to the 076 Protocol that might represent a feasible public health intervention for LMICs. Rather, they argued that the short course regimen should be tested against the 076 Protocol, since it was clearly the best proven alternative. However, although proponents of this design pointed to evidence suggesting that a short-course would likely be preferable to a placebo (Lurie and Wolfe 1997), it was unlikely that the short-course would be as effective as the full 076 Protocol. If it was unethical to compare the short course to a placebo because the latter was known to be inferior to the 076 Protocol, then it would be similarly unethical to compare the short-course to the 076 Protocol since there was widespread agreement that the short-course was likely to be inferior to this alternative.

Stated in more general terms, the global de jure standard of care rules out as morally impermissible efforts to find interventions that might have a meaningful impact on public health in the context of LMIC health systems if those interventions are not expected to be at least as effective as available alternatives—even if those alternatives require a background infrastructure and social and economic conditions that are unobtainable or unsustainable in LMIC settings. Setting out to look for interventions that would produce widespread health benefits in LMIC settings but that are unlikely to be as effective as the strategies that can be implemented in the most advanced infrastructure of the most resource-rich countries simply cannot be reconciled with the goal of ensuring that no study participant is denied a level of care that falls below the global de jure standard.

Another implication of the global de jure view is that open questions of science only arise in global centers of excellence. The reason is that global centers of excellence possess sufficient resources to turn existing knowledge into the most effective clinical practices. This is why their practices are treated as the standard of care, on this view. In such contexts, if a medical goal cannot be achieved, then this inability reflects a lack of knowledge, rather than a lack of personnel, proficiency, infrastructure, technology, or some other social or material resource. As a result, on this view, knowledge gaps that are the appropriate targets for clinical research only arise in such high-resource contexts because it is only in such contexts that we clearly see the limits of existing knowledge.

From this standpoint, the 076 Protocol represents a prime example of such a best practice. In global centers of excellence in the United States and France, the 076 Protocol could be effectively implemented, cutting maternal-fetal transmission rates by two-thirds. Health systems in LMICs fell short of the financial, human or institutional resources that typify these global centers of excellence. As a result, they experienced a gap between the health needs of the populations they serve and their ability to meet those needs as effectively and efficiently as they can be met in global centers of excellence.

Embracing the global de jure standard of care entails that health systems that fall short of the financial, human, or institutional resources that typify global centers of excellence have two options for closing this gap: *trickle down* or *develop up*. The first option is to wait for the benefits of new knowledge to trickle down to them. In other words, wait until the various costs of implementing gold-standard practices fall to the point where they are within the reach of less well-off health systems. The second option is to increase the resources devoted to their health systems to develop up to the point where gold-standard interventions are no longer out of reach.

What health systems that fall short of the abilities of global centers of excellence cannot do, on this view, is undertake research initiatives that seek to identify alternatives to the global de jure standard of care that might enable less robust health systems to more effectively, efficiently, or equitably address the health needs of the people they serve. If we accept the global de jure standard of care, then anyone looking for a less efficacious but more affordable and easier to deliver alternative to the 076 Protocol would be acting unethically.

The argument against the use of placebo controls in the short-course zidovudine trials that Angell presents deploys a package of values that are the bread and butter of orthodox research ethics and that were, therefore, widely shared in the research ethics community. But it has the embarrassing implication that it rules out as unethical the alternative approach to international research that Angell and others endorse. This inconsistency reflects deeper problems in orthodox research ethics that arise when the research activity is evaluated in isolation from its relationship to background social institutions and larger considerations of justice.

2.6.5 Not Just a Problem for International Research

Arguments about international research challenged orthodox research ethics because its narrow focus on interactions within the IRB triangle rested on unstated presumptions about the relationship between research and a wide range of background conditions. Disconnected from the larger purposes of a just society, research is evaluated relative to role-related obligations of professionals without a clear sense of how those obligations relate to background considerations of justice within health systems, let alone justice across national boundaries. But the positions that were defended in the international context would also have unexpected consequences on domestic research initiated and conducted in LMIC settings.

If research must be consistent with the global de jure standard of care, that would rule out a wide range of domestic research that might be conducted in LMICs by LMIC health authorities. Although the controversy over internationally sponsored research was the *occasion* on which these arguments were formulated, the arguments themselves are perfectly general. If there is uncertainty about the merits of interventions A and B for a particular medical condition but it is known that in a global center of excellence C is superior to both, then it follows that participants cannot be randomized to A or B, no matter who is doing the randomization.

The awareness that parochial debates about trial design had such far-reaching implications was illustrated powerfully by a memorable exchange from the short-course debates. In their defense of the short-course trials, Varmus and Satcher (1997) concluded by quoting from a letter to the NIH written by Edward K. Mbidde, chairman of the AIDS Research Committee of the Uganda Cancer Institute. The quote read:

> These are Ugandan studies conducted by Ugandan investigators on Ugandans. Due to lack of resources we have been sponsored by organizations like yours. We are grateful that you have been able to do so. . . . There is a mix up of issues here which needs to be clarified. It is not NIH conducting the studies in Uganda but Ugandans conducting their study on their people for the good of their people.

In a letter to the editor of the NEJM, Carel IJsselmuiden argued, "Since the Tuskegee study was conducted by Americans on Americans, this argument obviously does not stand" (IJsselmuiden 1998, 838).

For Angell, IJsselmuiden, and others in their camp, withholding treatment that is known to be effective (in global centers of excellence) that results in serious harm to study participants is wrong, no matter whether the study is conducted across national borders by international sponsors or within national borders by domestic health authorities—whether American (Tuskegee) or Ugandan (as in the short-course zidovudine studies).

Despite the logic of the argument just outlined, IJsselmuiden's letter goes on to focus again on the use of placebo controls. It says that "it violates the principle of justice that a continent impoverished through colonialism, and forced to continue to be unable to provide gold-standard treatment because of debt traps, will continue to provide the human laboratory where placebo-controlled trials can be conducted because locally affordable care is often no more than placebo treatment" (IJsselmuiden 1998, 838). Gold-standard treatment is identified with the practices of HICs and so reflects what I'm calling the global de jure standard of care. It is contrasted with the de facto state of affairs in LMICs where actual medical practice often reflects deprivation. Given the history of extractive relationships between northern sponsors and host countries of the global south, IJsselmuiden sees the short-course studies as unjustly taking advantage of deprivation to run placebo-controlled trials.

In a subsequent letter to the editor in the NEJM, Mbidde rejects the charge that the short-course studies are designed to take advantage of circumstances of deprivation. In doing so he argues that the design of the studies reflects the health needs and priorities of Uganda and the importance of conducting research that addresses the health needs of Ugandans:

> Ugandan studies are responsive to the health needs and the priorities of the nation. Research subjects have been selected in such a way that the burdens and benefits of the research will be equitably distributed, and the appropriate authorities, including the national ethics review committee, have satisfied themselves that the research meets their own ethical requirements. With these requirements met, if Ugandans cannot carry out research on their people for the good of their nation, applying ethical standards in their local circumstances, then who will?

Mbidde's reply is emblematic of the frustrations experienced by both sides of this debate. The global de jure standard of care seems to follow from core commitments of research ethics. If it is correct, then it would not be permissible for Ugandans to conduct research on their own people, in response to their own health needs and priorities, if that research entails a deviation from the best practices for treating or preventing a disease that have been established to be effective in the most resource rich centers of excellence. However, everyone involved in this debate wants to endorse the moral permissibility of conducting research that is aimed at enhancing the ability of LMIC health systems to meet their own health needs and priorities. But if it is morally permissible for nations to conduct research of this kind in order to address the health needs and priorities of their people, then the global de jure standard of care must be rejected.

This exchange illustrates how the debate about placebo controls had the feel of a kind of proxy war in which narrow issues of clinical trial design were being asked to do the bidding of larger positions that remained covert and hidden. The arguments being offered in support of particular trial designs had implications that reached far beyond the choice of control, but orthodox research ethics lacked the resources to foreground those larger issues and to engage them in a way that might resolve the resulting dilemma.

This exchange also illustrates frustrations generated from a failure to clarify all of the possible formulations for the standard of care and the justifications that might support them. Proponents of the local de facto standard of care argued that this baseline does not deny study participants access to care they would otherwise receive and, in turn, allows research to generate evidence about whether new interventions are superior to the status quo. But when the status quo reflects poverty, deprivation, indifference, or exclusion, the level of care that individuals from marginalized groups actually receive can fall below the level of care to which they are entitled. In those cases, gaps in care may not represent knowledge gaps at all. In other words, there can be cases where individuals are routinely denied a level of care that is attainable and sustainable in their own community. When that occurs, the local de facto standard of care doesn't track circumstances where new knowledge is needed. Angell, IJsselmuiden, and others were correct that this standard of care licenses powerful parties, whether local or domestic, to exploit the most disadvantaged members of the most disadvantaged communities without thoughtful concern for whether such research represents the most effective or efficient way of responding to their needs.

In contrast, the global de jure standard of care prohibits any use of research to generate the knowledge that less-advantaged communities might need in order to address important health needs under the unique social, political, and economic constraints that could realistically be achieved in their community. In order to avoid extractive relationships, it closes off research as an avenue for social progress and requires LMIC populations to wait for innovations to trickle down or until they can develop up to the capacity needed to support the global best practices.

The language in Mbidde's reply can be seen as an attempt to escape a dilemma created from envisioning only these two possibilities. Invoking a nation's "own ethical requirements" raises the possibility that different moral standards might govern research in different communities. But the prospect that ethical standards for research might be lower in LMIC communities raises the specter of an ethical relativism that devalues the lives of people in LMICs. The desire to avoid double standards in international research

(Macklin 2004) reflects the idea that there should not be one set of norms to evaluate research in HICs and a different set of norms to evaluate research in LMICs.

It was in this context that the World Medical Association became the epicenter for political lobbying that ultimately resulted in the note of clarification in the 2004 revision of the *DoH*. Its inclusion was a serious blow to the document's credibility not just because of the contradiction it introduced into the text, but because its inclusion seemed to confirm that its pronouncements rested on a foundation of arbitrary institutional authority. If lobbying the organization could change the rules, then those rules must reflect institutional power rather than sound moral reasoning.

2.6.6 Research Unmoored from a Just Social Order

In the conceptual ecosystem of orthodox research ethics, the local de jure standard of care was not a salient option. That standard of care requires that study participants be provided with what experts judge to be the most effective strategy for preventing or addressing the problem in question under conditions that are attainable and sustainable in the local health systems where the intervention in question will be deployed (London 2000b). But a defense of this standard depends on there being a morally significant relationship between research and health systems such that falling below this standard is unjust while providing more than this standard might be permissible, but not a strict moral duty. Moreover, any such defense would have to explain how to apply this same standard coherently and consistently to domestic research in HICs and LMICs as well as to international or cross-national research (see chapter 9).

Orthodox research ethics had no account of the relationship between research and the social structures or institutions of a community that might motivate or make the local de jure standard salient. Kukla (2007) argues that this problem reflects the fact that some concepts in orthodox research ethics presuppose highly idealized background conditions. In particular, Kukla says that the concept of equipoise presupposes an "an idealized research context of unlimited resources and access to care that rarely is incarnated" (173). However, if the concept of equipoise assumed a background of unlimited resources then it would be surprising that it has been regarded for so long as a valuable guide to reconciling social value with the rights and welfare of study participants in the context of domestic research in HICs. After all, as Kukla is well aware, there is no community in which medical resources are unlimited.

The problem, rather, is that concepts like equipoise, fiduciary duty, and optimal care have been deployed in orthodox research ethics unmoored from explicit connections to more general requirements of a just social order that shape and limit the obligations and entitlements of community members. There was no explicit guidance about how to link questions about the standard of care and equipoise to the background social and economic conditions of the communities in which research takes place. Because such background questions fall outside the narrow boundaries of orthodox research ethics, stakeholders were left to fill in these details for themselves.

Orthodox research ethics relied on the tacit presumption that researchers and research ethics committees would share the same set of implicit background assumptions about the significance of various health needs and the economic, social, and material conditions under which those needs are to be met. When researchers in New York consider whether equipoise obtains between a set of interventions, for example, they may tacitly frame this question against the background of infrastructure and resources that are typical of the health contexts in the United States. When they submit research protocols to a research ethics committee, the latter would be more likely to evaluate them under a similar set of expectations. Likewise, researchers in Uganda, conducting domestic research in Uganda, might implicitly frame the question of equipoise against the background of the infrastructure and resources that are typical of health contexts in Uganda. When they submit their protocols to a Ugandan research ethics committee, the latter would likely evaluate it under a similar set of background presumptions.

Research ethics was unprepared for cases in which disagreements turned on these larger questions. In that sense, international research was the occasion to consider these issues, but the issues that were raised were more general and would have implications for research ethics, regardless of where research would be conducted or who would conduct it.

2.6.7 Responsiveness and Reasonable Availability

Despite the controversy that they generated, the short-course zidovudine trials were aimed at developing interventions that might make a meaningful public health impact on perinatal HIV transmission in LMICs.

Proponents of these studies argued that they were broadly in line with additional requirements found in international guidelines that are grounded in considerations of justice. Subsequent controversies challenged these additional requirements, in part because they clashed with more straightforward applications of beneficence and respect for autonomy.

The claim that collaborative international research should be responsive to the health needs of the host community was first enunciated in the CIOMS *Guidelines*.[5] In the discussion of justice in the opening section on "general ethical principles," we are told that "in general, the research project should leave low-resource countries or communities better off than previously or, at least, no worse off." Here again we see justice equated with the distribution of benefits and burdens. This line is followed with the claim that such research "should be responsive to their health needs and priorities in that any product developed is made reasonably available to them, and as far as possible leave the population in a better position to obtain effective health care and protect its own health" (2002, 18).

The statement that research should be responsive "in that any product developed is made reasonably available" blurs the distinction between the requirement of responsiveness and the requirement of post-trial access. This may reflect a more general lack of clarity at that time about the relationship between these requirements. For example, as late as 2004, the *DoH* did not explicitly state that medical research must be responsive to the health needs of the host population although it contained a statement about post-trial benefit. Paragraph 10 of the 2004 version said that "Medical research is only justified if there is a reasonable likelihood that the populations in which the research is carried out stand to benefit from the results of the research." This statement, however, was often cited by commentators as an instance of the requirement that research be responsive to the health needs of the host community (Annas and Grodin 1998; Macklin 2001).

The relationship between these two requirements has been clarified in subsequent versions of these guidelines. Guideline 10 of the 2002 text on "research in populations and communities with limited resources" states that:

> Before undertaking research in a population or community with limited resources, the sponsor and the investigator must make every effort to ensure that:
> - the research is responsive to the health needs and the priorities of the population or community in which it is to be carried out; and

- any intervention or product developed, or knowledge generated, will be made reasonably available for the benefit of that population or community.

I will refer to the first condition as the "responsiveness requirement" and the second condition as the requirement of "reasonable availability."[13]

For someone like Eisenberg, these requirements might be seen as reasonable consequences of a moral imperative to carry out research that staves off preventable suffering and premature death. In order to carry this imperative to fruition, research must focus on unmet health needs that produce the largest burden of avoidable morbidity and mortality, and its fruits must then be made available to the populations suffering under these burdens of sickness, injury, and disease. In chapter 4 I will defend the existence of such an imperative and then in chapter 9 I will provide a defense of these requirements on roughly these terms.

However, in a conceptual ecosystem in which research is effectively treated as an optional undertaking, severed from the larger social purposes of a just social order, the focus on ensuring that research leaves host communities better off, and no worse off, grounds these requirements on a foundation that provides compelling reasons for rejecting these very requirements. Arguments to this effect are the subject of chapters 3 and 8. For our present purposes it is sufficient to note that if the underlying moral value that motivates these requirements is that host populations not be made worse off and be made better off by research participation, then these requirements appear arbitrary at best and affirmatively harmful at worst (e.g., see Wolitz et al. 2009). We can illustrate these concerns with the Surfaxin case.

2.6.8 The Surfaxin Case

Surfactants are naturally produced substances that are essential to the lungs' ability to maintain proper airflow and oxygen absorption. Extremely premature infants often do not produce enough surfactant to maintain adequate airflow and gas exchange in their lungs, a potentially life-threatening

---

[13] A similar clarification was made in the 2008 *DoH* in paragraph 17 which states, "Medical research involving a disadvantaged or vulnerable population or community is only justified if the research is responsive to the health needs and priorities of this population or community and if there is a reasonable likelihood that this population or community stands to benefit from the results of the research." A survey of other documents that articulate similar requirements can be found in London and Kimmelman 2008. On requirements of post-trial access see Sofaer and Strech (2011).

condition known as respiratory distress syndrome. Respiratory distress syndrome can be successfully treated with the use of surfactant replacement therapy, in which artificial or naturally derived surfactants are used to increase the surface area of the lungs that can absorb oxygen and facilitate gas exchange. By 2001 roughly half a dozen surfactant agents were commonly used to save the lives of desperately ill newborns in HIC health systems.

In 2001, the pharmaceutical firm Discovery Laboratories proposed a double-blind, randomized, placebo-controlled clinical trial of their new surfactant agent, Surfaxin, in impoverished Latin American communities where neonatal intensive care units are often poorly equipped and where children did not have access to surfactant replacement therapy. Discovery Laboratories proposed to upgrade and modernize the intensive care units in the host countries so that all of the children in the clinical trial would receive improved medical care. Children in the trial would then be randomized so that half would receive Surfaxin and the other half would receive a placebo.

Critics argued that the study was in conflict with established guidelines for international research ethics. Whereas the zidovudine short-course studies were motivated by the health needs of host communities, this study seemed to be motivated by the pecuniary interests of a firm from a HIC. Surfactant replacement therapy was not widely available in the settings where the study was planned but there was nothing about Surfaxin that made it particularly attractive for LMIC settings. If this was not a violation of the requirement that research in LMICs should be responsive to host community health needs, it was at least a deep tension.

Second, Discovery Laboratories was looking to LMIC health systems as a way to quickly generate the evidence needed to secure regulatory approval from the FDA so that it could tap the lucrative drug markets of HICs. As such, there was no pre-trial agreement that Surfaxin would be made reasonably available in the LMIC settings where it was being tested if its efficacy was established in the proposed studies. This bolstered concerns about the responsiveness of the trial to host community health needs and represented a transgression of the requirement that study sponsors, researchers, and host communities establish before the initiation of a trial a plan to make any product vindicated in the research reasonably available in the host community.[14] Without such an agreement, numerous commentators argued that

---

[14] CIOMS Guideline 15 from 1993 reads "As a general rule, the sponsoring agency should agree in advance of the research that any product developed through such research will be made reasonably available to the inhabitants of the host community or country at the completion of successful testing.

researchers and their sponsors exploit participants and host communities (Annas and Grodin 1998). As such, critics charged that the study represented the unfair use of LMIC populations for the profit of a private firm whose product would primarily benefit patients in HICs.

Finally, critics of this study argued that a placebo control would not have been permissible in the United States and that its use in an LMIC constituted an unfair double standard (Lurie and Wolf 2007). Randomizing roughly 325 dangerously ill newborns to placebo violated the requirement to ensure that every participant in the trial would receive an adequate standard of care. Given the availability of established effective surfactant agents, critics argued, the study should have tested Surfaxin against a known effective alternative. Although the use of a placebo control might generate information about the efficacy of Surfaxin relative to a baseline of not administering surfactant replacement therapy, that baseline was only relevant to health systems in which such treatment was not a feasible option. Because Discovery Laboratories was looking to market their product primarily in HICs, where surfactant replacement therapy was the standard of care, the placebo design seemed to address the wrong scientific question.

In response to these objections, proponents of the trial argued that conducting the trial in LMIC settings represented a win-win solution to a bad problem. As Robert Temple of the US Food and Drug Administration put it, "If they did the trial, half of the people would get surfactant and better perinatal care, and the other half would get better perinatal care. It seems to me that all the people in the trial would have been better off" (Shah 2002, 28). If the trial had to be redesigned and Discovery Laboratories decided to locate the more expensive active-controlled trial to a HIC, then nobody in the host community would receive any of the benefits the study promised. As a result, everyone would be made worse off. Discovery would have to spend more money and take a longer time to generate the information needed to gain access to the market. This in turn would delay the availability of a new therapeutic agent for patients who might need it and it would not improve the welfare of anyone in the LMIC host communities who might otherwise have had access to the benefits of this study.

Exceptions to this general requirement should be justified and agreed to by all concerned parties before the research begins" (CIOMS 1993).

2.6.9 Minimalism about Justice

Temple's position is a straightforward application of the traditional values of established frameworks for research ethics and represents the core of what I am calling the minimalist approach to questions of justice (§2.5.3). The minimalist approach seeks to avoid becoming bogged down in long-standing and protracted debates about thick or substantive conceptions of justice. Instead, it adopts a thin or minimal view that focuses narrowly on whether discrete interactions are mutually beneficial and freely undertaken. In this respect, issues of justice are effectively reduced to a function of principles that play a more familiar and well worked-out role in research ethics, namely, beneficence and respect for persons.

Temple's position was that randomizing roughly 325 dangerously ill newborns to placebo does not violate the nonmaleficence requirement because newborns in these communities did not otherwise have access to surfactants. The roughly 325 participants who received Surfaxin would likely be made better off since the expectation was that Surfaxin was likely to confer a net therapeutic advantage over the baseline of not receiving surfactant replacement therapy. If the trial were not conducted, newborns in the host community would not receive surfactant replacement therapy. So, participating in the trial would not make them worse off than they otherwise would have been and would likely make at least some of the participants better off.[15]

Nothing in these requirements specifies how significant the improvement over the status quo must be for a research initiative to be permissible, or how the host community must benefit from the research initiative. There are principled reasons, however, that make the minimalist reluctant to specify further substantive constraints on research. According to the minimalist, these details about the level and type of benefit require value judgments that are best left to the discretion of those in the host community. From this point of view, in fact, imposing stronger restrictions on international medical research appears misguided at best, and positively malevolent at worst, because they might prevent host communities from participating in research that could provide them with *some* net benefit. Stronger restrictions on

---

[15] The minimalist takes the placebo to be consistent with the relevant "standard of care," because that is defined as the treatment that participants would have received had there been no clinical trial. The study participants randomized to placebo are therefore not made worse off. For a similar statement in the context of perinatal HIV intervention trials, see Grady (1998, 36). For critical assessment of such views, see London (2000b). This issue is discussed in chapter 9.

international medical research are therefore viewed as working against the autonomy of LMIC populations and, with this, their ability to look after their own interests as they see fit. Stronger restrictions are unjustifiably paternalistic, on this view, because they limit the autonomy of LMIC populations to decide for themselves which benefits make research activities worth participating in.

In effect, the minimalist position derives the content of justice from the accepted pillars of contemporary bioethics, and of research ethics in particular. A just research initiative is one that faithfully adheres to the standard principles of nonmaleficence, beneficence, and respect for autonomy. Put in slightly different terms, the minimalist holds that any research initiative that satisfies the conditions of nonmaleficence, beneficence, and respect for autonomy is morally permissible because it offers *fair terms of cooperation* to the host community.

The minimalist's requirements are intended to ensure that the benefits of research do not accrue solely to the sponsoring party while the host community bears all of the burdens. They leave room for host communities to bargain for the best terms of cooperation that they can get, and they prohibit agreements that do not in some way serve the interests of the disadvantaged party. Initiatives that meet these conditions are viewed as fair because they provide mutually beneficial terms of cooperation that each party can freely accept. From the perspective of the minimalist, there may be many reasons that researchers and their sponsors should be as generous as possible when carrying out international research initiatives, but *requiring* more than the minimalist's conditions risks creating scenarios in which *everyone is worse off*.[16]

Without a justification for giving special weight to the knowledge and information that research produces, two considerations weigh in favor of rejecting responsiveness and reasonable availability and broadening the

---

[16] There may be cases, however, where the minimalist will require that researchers or their funding agencies make the fruits of a research initiative available in a stronger sense. If, for instance, the host population itself must allocate significant resources to carry out a clinical trial—whether in terms of money, personnel, or something else—then a stronger guarantee might be needed in order to ensure that the research initiative as a whole does not violate the beneficence requirement. That is, guarantees of free access, or price reductions, may be required in order to ensure that the host community receives a net benefit from the research initiative. Such guarantees, therefore, compensate for the burdens assumed by the community in facilitating the particular research initiative. Here again, though, the reasons for requiring such an agreement derive from the more fundamental need to ensure that the nonmaleficence and the beneficence conditions are met, and respect for the autonomy of the host community requires that it be the judge of whether the compensations repay the costs.

range of goods that should be relevant to evaluating the fairness of research transactions.

One consideration is that different stakeholders can reasonably support research for different reasons. Some support it in pursuit of profits from intellectual property and the sale of medical interventions. Others might seek smaller benefits in the form of compensation or incentives offered for study participation. Some support it as a means to publication, promotion, tenure and perhaps also reputation and fame. Others might seek the medical benefits that come from access to care, or from access to investigational interventions that might offer a chance of relief or cure where existing methods have failed. Still others may want to contribute to the fight against a disease that they have experienced, that someone in their family has experienced, or that takes a significant toll in their community. Respect for autonomy seems to press in favor of respecting the judgments of individuals about the reasons that they might be willing to participate in research.

A second consideration is that research itself can be an avenue for the provision of a wide range of benefits. Researchers or study sponsors can provide medical services, food, access to transportation, or provide money directly to study participants. Research can provide employment to people in host communities, increase economic activity, and be a conduit for improving laboratories, hospital facilities, or other aspects of the infrastructure in a community.

If the goal is to ensure that research does not make LMIC communities and participants worse off, and to ensure that it leaves them better off, then it has been argued that this can be more reliably and effectively achieved by embracing the plurality of motives that may lead stakeholders to want to support research and the plurality of ways in which research can produce benefits for those stakeholders. On this view, what matters when assessing the fairness of research transactions is not the distribution of specific kinds of goods, but whether the various parties to the transaction receive a sufficient amount of benefit to render the transaction non-exploitative (Participants 2002, 2004; Wertheimer 2010, chapter 8).

The responsiveness and reasonable availability requirements presuppose something special about the relationship between the social systems that produce new knowledge and the social systems that apply that knowledge for the benefit of individuals and communities. But orthodox research ethics has been profoundly shaped by a conceptual ecosystem that either resists connecting research with the larger social purposes of a just social order or, at best, treats such connections as falling outside the purview of the field. Against the background assumption that research is a morally optional private undertaking, the requirements of responsiveness and reasonable availability appear arbitrary to the extent that they prohibit research in which host communities do not receive access to the fruits of that research (if there are any) but in which they would receive an assortment of other benefits that they regard as meaningful and sufficient to make research participation reasonable. If these requirements prevent research from taking place, then burdened communities are harmed to the extent that they are prevented from accessing benefits that they regard as sufficient to offset the burdens of research participation.

In the face of these criticisms, the requirements of responsiveness and reasonable availability seem not just paternalistic, but unjustifiably paternalistic. They appear to limit the autonomy of burdened populations by reducing the range of research in which they can participate even when that research can be presented as satisfying the underlying moral requirements that supposedly justify and motivate those very moral restrictions.

2.7 Conclusion

Recent debates about the ethics of international research expose some of the fault lines running through the foundations of orthodox research ethics. Unmoored from a clear account of justice that links the research enterprise to the larger purposes of a just social order, requirements that are ostensibly grounded in justice appear arbitrary at best and self-defeating at worst. Given the tendency to explicate justice in terms of access to benefits and ensuring that host communities are not made worse off, orthodox research ethics appears to assert requirements that frustrate this goal and can be challenged in terms of both beneficence and respect for autonomy.

As we see in the next chapter, the consequences of reducing justice and fairness in research ethics to the maintenance of mutually beneficial agreements between free and informed persons has the potential to undermine a broad set of commitments in orthodox research ethics. It undermines not only the field's paternalistic focus, but also widespread commitments to protecting participants from unfairness, injustice, exploitation, commodification, and even threatens the status of informed consent. The goal of the next chapter, therefore, is to illustrate these far-reaching consequences and to motivate the search for an alternative that recovers the connection between research and the larger purposes of a just social order without licensing the denigration of persons or the abrogation of their rights and interests in the process.

3

The Anvil of Neglect and the Hammer of Exploitation

Fault Lines in Research Ethics

> Given the nonideal background conditions under which people find
> themselves, there should be a very strong presumption in favor of
> principles that would allow people to improve their situations if they
> give appropriately robust consent, if doing so has no negative effects
> on others, and this even if the transaction is unfair, unjust, or ex-
> ploitative. (Wertheimer 2008, 84)

3.1 Three Moral Pitfalls

If research ethics is to provide sound normative guidance to decision makers
constrained to act in our non-ideal world, it must help them navigate three
moral pitfalls: sanctioning neglect of the most vulnerable (sanctioning neglect), saddling those who seek to be ethical with an overly demanding set
of moral requirements (demandingness), and justifying widespread wrongdoing as the lesser of the available evils (sanctioning wrongdoing).

In chapter 2 we saw how early defenders of the research imperative
viewed research with humans as a way to advance the common good by
creating the knowledge and means necessary to avert human suffering and
premature mortality. We also saw how these same proponents understood
this social imperative as inconsistent with equal regard and the sanctity of
the individual within the domain of research with human participants. If
embracing the research imperative avoided the pitfall of sanctioning neglect, it purchased this at the price of sanctioning wrongdoing. Given the
moral dilemma perceived as lying at the heart of medical research, this

For the Common Good. Alex John London, Oxford University Press. © Oxford University Press 2022.
DOI: 10.1093/oso/9780197534830.003.0003

social imperative placed hefty demands on a few study participants against whom researchers would be permitted to make arbitrary judgments to meet the needs of the many.

In reaction, orthodox research ethics has practically defined its moral mission as constraining the extent to which social demands for medical progress can be used to justify perpetrating wrongs or harms on research participants. Influenced by Jonas's bold argument that the normal burden of suffering and disease is not a threat to the community, orthodox research ethics has tended to deny that there is a social imperative to advance the common good through research. If research is a morally optional undertaking, then the motivations that lead researchers or sponsors to conduct research are beyond the scope of the field.

From a certain practical standpoint, this approach makes a fair amount of sense. If researchers and sponsors have powerful pecuniary motives to undertake research, then one might think that research ethics does not need to articulate a moral imperative to conduct such inquiry. If the scientific enterprise contains within it the inherent potential for overreach and abuse, however, then research ethics can leave grand questions about the goals of science to others and focus instead on upholding strong constraints on the way that individual researchers can interact with study participants inside the IRB triangle.

The current equilibrium in research ethics emphasizes protecting study participants from wrongdoing, but these protections should not be purchased at the cost of sanctioning neglect. If research is an optional social undertaking and there is no moral impetus for powerful parties outside of the IRB triangle to carry out certain kinds of research, then erecting protectionist fortifications around the rights and interests of study participants ensures that the poor and the marginalized are not subject to exploitation, commodification, or other forms of injustice or abuse. But it does nothing to protect those same groups from the ravages of indifference.

Faced with this problematic tradeoff, a group of critics have recently challenged the protectionist stance of orthodox research ethics. They are concerned that the strong moral constraints at the heart of orthodox research ethics disadvantage study participants who would be willing to accept forms of study participation that are excluded by current protectionist norms. As a remedy, these critics question whether a research ethics that is suited to the non-ideal world in which we live should instead try to avert the harms of widespread neglect by weakening some of the demands of morality and permitting the violation of norms against exploitation, unfairness, and injustice.[1] Perhaps the most rigorous and compelling of these is Alan Wertheimer's defense of what he refers to as the principle of permissible exploitation (PPE), which is glossed in the quote with which this chapter begins.

PPE is so heterodox that many in research ethics may have difficulty taking it seriously. As a policy proposal, this skepticism is warranted. As I argue in a moment, PPE permits more wrongdoing than its proponents recognize; rather than making morality less demanding, it shifts those demands onto the shoulders of the worst off; it represents a highly asymmetric concern for the status of different moral agents; and, from a policy standpoint, these problems are likely to lead to consequences that even proponents of PPE want to avoid.

However, reflecting on PPE as a piece of philosophical reasoning is a valuable diagnostic exercise. Part of what makes this proposal so fascinating is the way that it draws on and repurposes premises that are woven into the foundations of contemporary research ethics. This makes it surprisingly easy to defend this view by drawing on familiar claims in the conceptual ecosystem of orthodox research ethics. As a result, I hope to show that many of the problems with PPE are not merely problems with this heterodox view; they reflect a larger instability in fault lines that run through the foundations of research ethics.

3.2 The Targets of PPE

3.2.1 Norms of Respect

Although PPE focuses on exploitation, Wertheimer is clear that the argument for this claim generalizes to other forms of unfair or unjust treatment. In fact, the logic of this position is sufficient that it would apply to any instance of what I will call "norms of respect." This is a class of norms that deal with a person or people's interest in being treated as having a certain moral status, such as being recognized as the moral equal of others or as an agent whose worth is not solely a function of the goals and projects of others. Norms in this class include prohibitions on exploitation, domination, manipulation, commodification, unfairness, and injustice.

[1] The clearest example is Wertheimer (2008). See also Cooley (2001).

Norms of respect can implicate welfare in various ways. For example, being coerced into performing a demeaning act can both reduce a person's welfare and represent a violation of their status as a person whose rights and interests should be respected. But particular circumstances, social arrangements, or offers might pit these aspects against one another. For example, if performing a demeaning act represents a way for the agent to secure a net increase in welfare, then welfare-oriented considerations might conflict with the fact that the demeaning act continues to be problematic insofar as it represents a diminution or transgression of a norm of respect.

Similarly, distributive justice and fairness may require that in addition to being mutually beneficial, agreements or social arrangements must reflect the moral status of individuals. If, in a given case, fair wages require equal pay for equal work then a fair arrangement of wages must not simply provide workers with a net benefit, but that benefit would have to reflect the background status of equality among workers who perform the same tasks. Imagine now a toy case in which a firm could hire a new worker but only if it paid that worker half the salary of those already doing the same job. The proposal might be advantageous to both the firm and to the worker in terms of its impact on welfare, but it would be objectionable on the grounds that it violates the stipulated requirement of fairness.

Even if forms of disrespectful treatment do not result in a net reduction in a person's welfare, they might be wrong because they involve treating a person as lesser, as inferior, as subservient, or as an object whose value derives from its usefulness to others. PPE does not deny that such treatment is wrong. Instead, it holds that whether norms of respect should be upheld, or their violations should be permitted, depends on the effect that such permission or prohibition will have on the welfare of the individual in question.

3.2.2 Responsiveness, Reasonable Availability, and the Standard of Care

As pharmaceutical research has grown into one of the most profitable industries on earth it has also become an increasingly international endeavor (Glickman et al. 2009). Entities from high-income countries (HICs) now routinely sponsor clinical trials of new medical interventions in low- and middle-income countries (LMICs; Rehnquist 2001; Thiers et al. 2008).

LMIC populations are often attractive to researchers because they include large numbers of people with specific medical conditions, many of whom are "treatment naïve," meaning that they have not had access to effective medical care in the past (Petryna 2009).

The disparity between sponsors and host communities in wealth, medical and public health infrastructure, access to medicine, and other social determinants of health has generated concern that individuals and populations in LMICs not only will be harmed and abused, but also subject to forms of treatment that violate norms of respect. At the end of the last chapter, we saw how several guidance documents enumerate moral standards that are grounded in justice or fairness, with the goal of averting these problems. Three requirements common to such documents are in the crosshairs of PPE.

One is the requirement that all members of a trial, including members of the control group, should receive a "standard of care" that is consistent with the current best practices for the treatment or prevention of the condition in question. People in resource-poor communities often lack access to a wide range of established, effective treatments for health problems. This requirement is meant to prohibit studies that randomize some participants to a placebo, or to some other form of care that is less effective than an available alternative that could be made available to participants in the host community.[2]

Insofar as this requirement holds that the standard of care must go beyond what is necessary to ensure that study participants are not made worse off and also receive some positive benefit from study participation, it is in the sights of PPE. Even if the placebo control used in the Surfaxin study was unethical because it violated the standard of care, PPE asserts that such a study should not be prohibited if doing so would leave vulnerable participants worse off.

The "responsiveness" requirement holds that studies in low-resource communities should be responsive to the health needs and priorities of those communities and the requirement of "reasonable availability" states that, prior to the initiation of a study, there must be an agreement in place that would make any intervention vindicated in the trial available to members of the host community. To the extent that these requirements are grounded in justice they may reflect important ideals

---

[2] This requirement is discussed at length in chapter 9.

of equal partnership, respect between individuals in communities that are separated by disparities in wealth and power, and requirements on the fairness of agreements.

PPE holds that studies that are not responsive to host community health needs and priorities and that are conducted without assurances of posttrial access may be morally wrong but that we should nevertheless permit them as long as study participants or host communities would voluntarily agree to them because they offer benefits that will avert worse outcomes.

PPE is thus distinct from the view we examine in chapter 8, the so-called fair benefits view, which challenges some of these same requirements on different grounds. In particular, the fair benefits view holds that if exploitation is about ensuring that less advantaged parties receive a fair *amount* of benefit, rather than a particular *kind* of benefit, then we should dispense with the responsiveness and reasonable availability requirements in favor of a process that allows host communities to negotiate for a larger share of a wider range of benefits (Participants 2002, 2004; Wolitz et al. 2009). This view holds that exploitation and unfairness are wrong and that exploitative and unfair agreements should be prohibited, but it challenges the criteria that have been articulated for these requirements and proposes an alternative set of criteria for these requirements. In contrast, PPE holds that agreements that are exploitative, unfair, and so on, are wrong but that we should sometimes permit these moral wrongs if doing so represents a way of respecting the decisions of disadvantaged parties about the best way to improve their circumstances.

Additionally, PPE must not be confused with skeptical views that deny that violations of respect are actual moral wrongs. PPE does not deny that exploitation, unfairness, injustice, and the like are moral wrongs. Nor does it hold that these norms are not violated if people voluntarily consent to be treated in ways that would otherwise transgress these norms. For Wertheimer, someone in a sufficiently dire situation can freely and knowingly consent to a deal that is exploitative, and the moral wrongness of that exploitation is not eliminated by the presence of voluntary consent.

What makes PPE distinctive is its focus on the *moral force*, weight, or significance that should be assigned to violations of norms of respect. It holds that mutually beneficial transactions, freely entered by informed parties, should not be prohibited, even if they involve exploitation, unfairness, or injustice and are therefore morally objectionable or wrong.

3.3 The Justification for Permitting Violations of Respect

Here is the argument in favor of PPE, altered to reflect its general application to norms of respect.[3]

1. Afflicted is in sufficiently dire circumstances that neglect will result in Afflicted suffering significant harm or disadvantage.
2. Better-off has the resources and ability to interact with Afflicted in a variety of ways, including ways that would make Afflicted significantly better off.
3. Better-off has "no obligation to transact with A [Afflicted] on any terms" (Wertheimer 2008, 82).
4. Better-off is only willing to engage in an exchange with Afflicted that would be regarded as morally wrong in that it involves a violation of respect (it is exploitative, commodifies Afflicted, involves the domination of Afflicted, treats Afflicted unfairly or unjustly . . .).
5. If Better-off cannot engage in an exchange with Afflicted on the above terms, Better-off will opt not to transact with Afflicted at all.
6. Afflicted would, with full knowledge of the relevant facts, freely engage in such a transaction with Better-off in order to receive what Afflicted judges to be a worthwhile benefit, even though the exchange subjects Afflicted to a violation of respect.
7. Neglect is therefore worse for Afflicted than being morally wronged.
8. Prohibiting violations of respect makes Afflicted worse off than permitting them.
9. Therefore, prohibiting violations of respect works to the disadvantage of the person whose interests protectionist norms against violations of respect are supposed to safeguard.
10. Therefore, Better-off ought to be permitted to perpetrate a violation of respect against Afflicted, so long as the following "proviso" is met: permitting this conduct has no negative effects on others.

Perhaps paradoxically, the upshot of PPE is that enforcing norms of respect leads to a situation where Afflicted would have been better off if those moral requirements were not enforced and both Afflicted and Better-off were permitted to engage in a voluntary transaction that violates a norm of respect.

---

[3] For example, see Wertheimer (2008, 82).

In effect, the claim is that constraints against violations of respect are self-defeating in the sense defined by Applebaum (1999, 38–152). They are supposed to protect individuals from unfair, degrading, or abusive treatment but merely ensuring that individuals are not so treated does not entail that a better deal is available to them. Because we are stipulating that Afflicted faces bleak alternatives that will result in significant harms (premise 1), enforcing norms of respect impedes, rather than advances, the interests of the very persons these norms are supposed to protect.

When the enforcement of moral norms is self-defeating, the proponents of those norms can be decried for frustrating the cause of the downtrodden and those who seek to act immorally can claim the righteous mantle of assisting those in need (Zwolinski 2007). What is perhaps worse is that there is a kernel of truth in this perversity. Those who never venture out among the poor may not treat them unfairly or treat them with disrespect, but their high-minded neglect may also be disastrously lethal. Otherwise, premise 6 would not be true and people like Afflicted would not vote with their feet and agree to be exploited, commodified, or treated unjustly.

PPE is thus most charitably read as a reaction to the concern that orthodox research ethics leaves the most vulnerable prey to lethal neglect by placing fairly demanding moral requirements in the way of agents like Better-off who might actually interact with the vulnerable and advance their welfare. If the responsiveness requirement prevents Better-off from conducting a clinical trial in some population because the knowledge it will generate is only relevant to HICs, then Better-off cannot offer Afflicted the chance to participate and possibly receive benefits that Afflicted would like to enjoy. These benefits might include access to medical care that Afflicted would not otherwise have received, or the provision of food, transportation, or direct remuneration.

So, too, if Better-off is required to provide members of the control group with the standard of care that is available in HICs, or to provide the study intervention after the completion of the trial to host-community members at steep discounts, Better-off may not conduct the trial. This may prevent unfair treatment, but it also deprives some people of potentially significant benefits that they may have been willing to accept. Unlike proposals to revise the content of requirements regarding the standard of care or posttrial access (see chapters 8 and 9), PPE assumes the content of these norms as stated in guidance documents and argues that even if they are morally sound, they should not be enforced because they are morally self-defeating.

In effect, PPE views norms of respect as creating an inefficiency in a market—individuals who would freely engage in mutually beneficial transactions are prohibited from doing so. To solve this problem, PPE reduces the demandingness of moral requirements grounded in norms of respect by permitting some wrongdoing if doing so enables those who are worst off to advance their welfare interests and avoid the ravages of neglect.[4]

3.4 Repurposing Shared Values

3.4.1 Beneficence

Although the conclusion of the argument for PPE is a radical departure from orthodox research ethics, the argument in support of that conclusion draws heavily on one implicit and two explicit aspects of the conceptual ecosystem of orthodox research ethics. The explicit aspects are the centrality of the twin pillars of research ethics: beneficence, operationalized as concern for welfare, and respect for autonomy, operationalized as informed consent. The implicit aspect is the idea that researchers and participants are in a private relationship and engage in private transactions, unfettered by larger duties of obligations.[5] Recognizing that PPE draws from the same well of concerns and the same structure of values used in orthodox research ethics is necessary to appreciate how PPE reveals a larger tension in the field. Because there is something unsettling about the different ways in which orthodox research ethics and PPE seek to resolve this tension, it is important to understand the structure of the values that create it in order to motivate the search for a better way forward.

First, although the argument for PPE is about the force of certain moral wrongs, and not about whether violations of respect are actually moral wrongs, the considerations it uses to establish the relative weight of the wrongs in question reflect a welfare consequentialist conception of beneficence. They are *consequentialist* because premises 7, 8, and 9 each focuses on the consequences associated with the salient alternatives. The central reason

---

[4] Strictly speaking, PPE rests on an empirical assumption regarding the extent to which enforcing norms against exploitation would raise the price of carrying out research in LMICs to a point where it is no longer attractive to firms from HICs. If the cost savings to firms from relocating research to LMIC settings is great enough, then enforcing norms against exploitation might not deter such research. For a defense of this possibility, see Wenner (2016) and Ballantyne (2010).

[5] Wenner (2016) explores this point in greater detail.

that Better-off's unethical conduct should be permitted, in this view, is that permitting it brings about better consequences for Afflicted than prohibiting it. They are *welfarist* because PPE focuses on, and assigns overriding importance to, the welfare of Afflicted. Exploitation may be worse than neglect in terms of the respect that is shown to Afflicted as a moral agent, but PPE treats the diminution in welfare that derives from neglect as worse than the loss of status that might attend violations of respect.[6]

The appeal to consequences and welfare in PPE is not an appeal to an exogenous value that has to be imported into research ethics from the outside. It is, rather, an appeal to one of the core principles of orthodox research ethics: beneficence. PPE hinges on the fundamental idea that the welfare of others represents a moral reason in favor or against actions that will help that person or harm them, respectively. Its conclusion hinges on the idea that, as long as the proviso is satisfied, those reasons should be decisive in determining the conduct of agents who can help, including the relative weight that regulators or other outsiders assign to violations of respect.

3.4.2 Respect for Persons and Consent

Second, because PPE requires that violations of respect be permitted only when transactions are voluntary and informed, its proponents can claim, at the very least, that their position is consistent with a very basic but fundamental commitment to respect for persons. Those who find themselves in difficult circumstances are often faced with difficult decisions, but the proponents of PPE hold that we should not deny them meaningful avenues

---

[6] In order to avoid begging thorny questions about the relationship between welfare and Afflicted's status interests, premises 7–9 would have to be reformulated and an additional premise added:

7*. Neglect is therefore worse for Afflicted (with respect to welfare) than being morally wronged.

8*. Prohibiting the moral wrong would make Afflicted worse off (with respect to welfare) than not prohibiting it.

9*. Therefore prohibiting the moral wrong works to the disadvantage of the person whose interests moral protections are supposed to safeguard (with respect to welfare).

9.5. In the presence of free and informed consent, violations of respect should not trump or prohibit benefits to welfare.

There is a serious concern that such claims simply assert what is at issue—namely, that serious threats to welfare are worse, all things considered, than serious threats to the status of a person. On this question, see Athanasiou et al. (2015).

for advancing their own welfare if they view those avenues, once all things are considered, as their best available alternative.

A more extreme position holds that PPE alone shows adequate respect for the autonomy of people like Afflicted because the ultimate purpose of rights is to protect a person's interests and it should be up to that person to decide whether their interest in respect is more important than securing some possible benefit. Taking this choice from Afflicted, in other words, not only deprives Afflicted of possible benefits, but it unduly restricts Afflicted's autonomy.[7]

The force of PPE thus derives from values that constitute the twin pillars of orthodox research ethics: respect for autonomy and beneficence or concern for welfare. But these values are repurposed to make an antipaternalistic argument against norms that are traditionally grounded in the value of justice and norms of respect. If the norms of research ethics are fundamentally grounded in, and intended for, the protection of individuals like Afflicted, pointing out that people in Afflicted's position may prefer exploitation or injustice to lethal neglect challenges the paternalism of protectionist norms on their own ground—their impact on the interests of the very people they are supposed to protect.

3.4.3 Options and the Private Sphere

The third commonality between the argument for PPE and the commitments of orthodox research ethics is less explicit. To see it, consider how odd it is that both accept the truth of premise 3, namely, that Better-off does not have a prior obligation to provide assistance to Afflicted, given the centrality of beneficence in both orthodox research ethics and the argument for PPE.

If a framework for moral decision-making includes beneficence, then, if all else is equal, that framework would seem to be committed to what I will call "weak consequentialism."

Weak Consequentialism: There is a standing duty to benefit those in need (like Afflicted), as long as it imposes only minor costs to the welfare of agents

---

[7] On the role of respect for autonomy in PPE, including the extent to which PPE is intended to be anti-paternalistic, see Wenner (2016).

who incur the duty (such as Better-off) or to their ability to pursue their (otherwise) morally permissible projects and plans.[8]

If weak consequentialism is the only principle in a moral theory, then the theory itself is consequentialist. More commonly, a claim like this is likely to figure in a broad range of theories that are pluralistic in the sense that they include a consequentialist component (such as a commitment to beneficence) while also embracing constraints on its reach (in the form of rights, for example).[9]

In orthodox research ethics, both justice and respect for persons give rise to prohibitions that serve as constraints on the pursuit of beneficence. If justice requires that groups that are already marginalized or burdened in some way must not be involved in research that does not address their specific health needs, then recruiting such participants is forbidden, even if doing so would be a way to produce more good in the long run. Likewise, if respect for persons requires that no participant be recruited into research without having first given their free and informed consent (or having a proxy decision maker do so if they lack capacity to make that decision for themselves) then it is impermissible to conscript participants into research without their free and informed consent, even if doing so would produce important social benefits.

Although constraints fence in and limit the extent to which beneficence can require acts that are morally problematic in some other regard, constraints do not limit the demands of beneficence when it does not come into conflict with some other value. As a result, even though orthodox research ethics contains a number of constraints on the reach of beneficence, its commitment to beneficence should entail that considerations like those in weak consequentialism require the rejection of premise 3. Better-off would be obligated to interact with Afflicted, and to advance Afflicted's interests as much as possible, so long as there is not another action available to Better-off that would bring about a greater good and the costs to Better-off do not exceed the relevant threshold.[10]

---

[8] Compare this to Singer's strong altruistic claim: "if it is in our power to prevent something bad from happening, without thereby sacrificing anything morally significant, we ought, morally, to do it." And to Singer's weak altruistic claim: "if it is in our power to prevent something very bad from happening, without thereby sacrificing anything of comparable moral importance, we ought, morally, to do it" (Singer 1972).

[9] For a useful primer on consequentialism and constraints, see Kagan (1997).

[10] If there is some way that Better-off could bring about more good by not interacting with Afflicted, then Better-off would be obligated to adopt *that* course of action, and 3 would still be false. Strictly speaking, weak consequentialism supports a duty to aid people like Afflicted in most cases,

However, both PPE and orthodox research ethics reject the claim that Better-off has a duty to assist Afflicted. As such, they must share a further commitment that tempers the reach of principles of beneficence in cases where Afflicted and Better-off could transact without any violation of a norm of respect. The only way for such theories to reject the stronger claim of a duty to aid in this circumstance is to recognize what are sometimes called "options."[11]

An option is basically a permission or a liberty right to act in ways that bring about less good than the agent could bring about through another feasible course of action. Frequently the existence of options is grounded in the idea that it is morally permissible for agents to avoid acts that require that they take on morally significant burdens. To be morally significant, burdens to the agent, understood in terms of her own interests or her ability to advance those interests, must be sufficient to outweigh, override, or otherwise mitigate the claims that the interests of others place on the agent.

There are significant disagreements about where to locate the threshold on the costs that an agent can be required to bear in the service of morality.[12] In part, these disagreements reflect deeper divisions over the role of morality in human life, and the force of moral reasons. But the proponents of options argue that there is in fact such a threshold and that it is necessary to preserve a "zone of moral indifference" within which the conduct of agents is not subject to the demanding assessment of morality (Fishkin 1982, chapter 4).

A different way of stating this idea is that options protect a sphere of "moral autonomy" within which agents have the permission or the liberty to shape their own life and conduct according to their own values, goals, and aspirations, free from demands that would be placed on them by a fully impartial responsiveness to the interests of others (Kagan 1997, 236). Options

---

because instead of a single best or optimal option, Better-off might be faced with a set of alternatives that are "maximal" in the sense that there are several actions that are not dominated by a better act but which are superior to all other possibilities open to Better-off. If interacting with Afflicted is a member of this maximal set, but so are alternatives that involve not interacting with Afflicted, then Better-off would be at liberty to choose not to interact with Afflicted in the sense that Better-off could choose another act from the maximal set. If Better-off chooses to interact with Afflicted, however, then Better-off would then be obligated to help advance the welfare of Afflicted as much as possible.

[11] My use of the terms "option" and "constraint" follows that of Kagan (1997, chapter 3).
[12] See Cullity (2004).

are sometimes referred to as "agent-centered prerogatives" to reflect the idea that they grant the agent the prerogative to give disproportionate weight to her own interests (Scheffler 1994). In each case, the salient question concerns the point at which the agent can no longer remain indifferent to others or at what point those interests can legitimately restrict or intrude upon her sphere of moral autonomy.

If both orthodox research ethics and PPE treat agents like Better-off as having no duty to aid or assist people like Afflicted, then the interactions between researchers and participants fall into a private sphere of moral discretion. In other words, they reflect the widely accepted idea that research with humans is a morally optional undertaking, unconstrained by larger social purposes, in which the primary ethical considerations are limited solely to the terms of the discrete transactions between the parties within the IRB triangle.

The idea that the interactions between researchers and participants fall into a private sphere of moral discretion is bolstered by the proviso in premise 10. PPE holds that conduct that violates norms of respect should be permitted so long as it remains confined to the discrete interactions of researchers and study participants. If permitting such violations were to have a larger social effect of making other parties worse off, then the proviso would kick in and violations of respect would be prohibited.

There is thus an important sense in which PPE challenges orthodox research ethics for not being sufficiently responsive to its own values.[13] In the private transactions between researchers and study participants, the welfare consequentialist concerns of beneficence provide the moral force for permitting violations of respect and define the limits on their permissibility. If individuals like Afflicted freely choose to be wronged in order to advance their welfare interests, then the paternalistic prohibition of such interactions is self-defeating.

---

[13] In this regard, the critique involved in PPE is simply a variant of the more general critique that consequentialists make against deontological rights or constraints of any kind: they are suboptimal. That is, constraints against violations of respect prevent people like Afflicted from enjoying gains in welfare that people like Better-off could bring about by violating such norms. Sophisticated welfare consequentialists agree that often we should respect the rights of agents, not because such rights have intrinsic moral value, but because such rights function as heuristics that mark out as salient courses of action that tend not be optimific over the long run. In cases where we can be confident that violating a right will produce more good than respecting it, however, the welfare consequentialist will claim that respecting the right makes no sense.

3.5 Permitting Too Much

3.5.1 Undermining Consent

The analysis of the previous sections represents PPE as reorganizing core commitments of orthodox research ethics in a way that strikes a different (and, according to its proponents, a better) balance between the demandingness of morality and the perils of neglect. Because it is built out of many of the underlying commitments of orthodox research ethics, this proposal is more of a challenge to the status quo than it might first appear.

In particular, without a clear and explicit account of justice to ground prohibitions on unfair and unjust relationships, those practical requirements dangle in the moral wind. They appear arbitrary at best and misguided at worst precisely because the neglect of their grounding or justification or the location of that justification in the distribution of benefits and burdens create a conceptual ecosystem in which the other commitments of the field can be marshalled to support permitting their violation.

Nevertheless, there are a number of grounds for concern over the way PPE tries to reconcile the pitfalls of sanctioning neglect, justifying wrongdoing, and the demandingness of morality. To begin with, the logic of the PPE justifies more wrongdoing than its proponents want to permit. For example, proponents of PPE want to ensure that violations of respect are limited to cases in which agents like Afflicted give their free and informed consent. But since informed consent is itself grounded in a norm of respect, the logic of PPE seems to extend to violations of this requirement as well.

First, recall that PPE presupposes options of sufficient weight that even minor burdens to Better-off are capable of outweighing or trumping Afflicted's welfare interests. We are committed to this by the supposition that Better-off has an option not to interact with Afflicted, if doing so is burdensome to Better-off, even if this would provide Afflicted with significant welfare benefits. If Better-off did not have an option of this kind, then premise 3 would be false.

Second, the requirement to seek informed consent imposes costs on Better-off. Consent forms have to be created. They have to be translated at an accessible educational level, in the local dialect, and then work has to be done to overcome various barriers to communication including educational gaps and cultural differences. During the consent process, people sometimes say, "no." Perhaps Afflicted doesn't fully understand the extent to which study participation would be an avenue to improving Afflicted's situation. Perhaps Afflicted doesn't want to be a participant in research, or doesn't want to be a subject in exploitative research. Whatever the reason, when potential participants refuse to participate, Better-off faces the extra costs and work of having to seek out and approach additional people and seek their consent.

Third, informed consent is itself a requirement that is grounded in a norm of respect—respect for the status of a person as morally sovereign over decisions that impact the shape and course of their life. PPE views constraints against violations of respect as inefficient to the extent that they prevent Afflicted from securing welfare benefits. Constraints against transgressing norms of respect can be outweighed by Afflicted's welfare interests. If Better-off could involve Afflicted in research without Afflicted's knowledge—perhaps by hiding the fact that Afflicted is participating in research—and if Afflicted is likely to receive a net welfare benefit from the interaction, then by transitivity Better-off should have the option to violate the constraint against exploiting Afflicted without Afflicted's consent. Doing so may be wrong—just as exploitation with Afflicted's consent is wrong—but PPE seems committed to the conclusion that it should not be prohibited.

3.5.2 The Participant-Centered Version

To be clear, there are at least two versions of this argument. The "participant-centered" version focuses on the impact of being exploited without consent on Afflicted's well-being. It holds that Better-off should not be required to secure the informed consent of Afflicted to be exploited or treated unfairly if seeking that consent would impose a cost on Better-off and if Better-off's exploitation of Afflicted would still leave Afflicted better off than would be the case if there were no interaction. After all, recall that Afflicted faces the prospect of serious harm outside of any transaction with Better-off and in the world of non-ideal agents, many in Afflicted's situation may not recognize that they would be better off being wronged than being neglected. The recipient-centered version of the argument thus allows Better-off to exploit Afflicted without Afflicted's permission so long as Afflicted receives a net benefit from the interaction.

If the participant-centered version of this argument sounds familiar, that's because it shares common features with traditional arguments in favor of medical paternalism—with some notable differences, however. In medical paternalism, the clinician had a strong duty to act in the best interests of the patient grounded partly in the patient's dependence on the specialized medical knowledge the clinician possesses and the patient lacks. Consent was regarded as unnecessary because it might cause distress or lead the patient to deviate from the clinician's recommendations about how best to promote the patient's medical best interests (Goldman 1980).

In the patient-centered extension of PPE, the more powerful party need only have a strategic commitment to Afflicted's best interests. This commitment is strategic in that it is necessary for Better-off to achieve Better-off's ultimate goals. Similarly, permission to violate the requirement for informed consent is grounded in the importance of the benefits Afflicted stands to receive from the transaction and the fact that Better-off might deny those benefits to Afflicted if Better-off is required to incur the costs of securing Afflicted's informed consent. Ironically, in both Hippocratic paternalism and the patient-centered extension of PPE, it is concern for the welfare of Afflicted that underwrites the permission to violate a key requirement of respect for persons.

3.5.3 The Impartial Version

The impartial variant of the previous argument shifts its focus from the welfare of Afflicted to the welfare of some larger group. This transition is facilitated by noting that, in research ethics, risks to particular participants do not need to be offset by benefits to those same participants in order to be permissible. Rather, risks and burdens to study participants can be justified by the prospect of future benefits to other people.

With this premise in place, the impartial variant permits Better-off to exploit, wrong, or commodify Afflicted without consent, so long as this imposes fewer costs on Better-off than the alternatives and creates social benefits sufficient to outweigh the burdens to Afflicted. The impartial version of this argument looks very similar to justifications for conscripting participants into research that are grounded in some larger research imperative. In particular, both arguments entail that researchers should be permitted to involve participants in research without their informed consent.

Nevertheless, these arguments differ significantly in their structure. The argument that attempts to justify conscription on the basis of a larger social obligation to facilitate research is inconsistent with the claim that Better-off is free to interact with Afflicted on whatever terms Better-off wants. In other words, that argument does not recognize a robust sphere of moral autonomy for Better-off. As a medical researcher, Better-off would not be free to determine whether and how to interact with Afflicted by consulting her personal interests, and the justification for abrogating informed consent is not grounded in costs to Better-off. Rather, Better-off is only justified in abrogating informed consent, on this model, to the extent that doing so is necessary to discharge the researcher's prior obligation to advance the common good.

In contrast, Better-off is able to dictate the terms on which Better-off is willing to interact with Afflicted within the argument for PPE because that position recognizes a robust sphere of moral autonomy on the part of Better-off. The impartial extension of PPE allows Better-off to abrogate the requirement of informed consent if doing so produces a large enough social benefit, *but there is no independent obligation to bring about this social benefit.* Better-off happens to pursue a private project in which Better-off takes on the personal goal of producing a social benefit. But Better-off has ultimate discretion over when, whether, and how to pursue Better-off's personal goals. This includes the moral discretion to determine when the costs to Better-off of pursuing this goal are sufficiently high that Better-off does not want to transact with someone like Afflicted. Enforcing the requirement of informed consent imposes a burden on Better-off's ability to advance Better-off's personal projects. If increasing the welfare of others is capable of justifying violations of norms of respect, then that justification would appear to extend to the abrogation of informed consent.

Interestingly, Wertheimer and colleagues have argued that because research is an activity that produces an important public good, there is a general duty to participate in research (Schaefer et al. 2009). They explicitly reject arguments that would ground this obligation in beneficence because, on their view, beneficence is too demanding. Instead, they argue that the generalizable medical information that research produces is a public good and it remains a public good even if it is produced by private companies or private individuals (2009, 68). This produces a kind of moral asymmetry. Private entities are at liberty to decide which projects to undertake—they are not fettered by obligations of justice or beneficence—but there is a duty to participate in research that flows from the status of this information as an important public good.

Wertheimer and colleagues argue that this duty to participate is not so strong that individuals can be compelled to participate in research. But PPE is not about whether, in this case, compulsion is morally permissible. It is about whether, given that compulsion would represent a moral transgression of an individual's interests in retaining sovereignty over their person and autonomy over their various life choices, we ought to enforce that moral prohibition. My point is that the same argument that justifies permitting the moral wrong of exploitation in research would also permit the moral wrong of conscripting individuals into research in which the information they help to generate contributes to the public good of generalizable medical information.

The impartial variant of PPE is constructed from premises that are shared by orthodox research ethics and by PPE. It recognizes a strong sphere of moral autonomy that protects individuals in their private pursuits while recognizing the fundamental moral importance of individual welfare. But there is also a sense in which the robust sphere of personal autonomy serves as a shield to Better-off against the claims that people in Afflicted's position might make against them for assistance and for fair, non-exploitative, non-demeaning treatment. When Better-off has as a personal project advancing the welfare of large numbers of future patients, this allows Better-off to both remain indifferent to Afflicted's plight (this follows from the claim that Better-off enjoys a sphere of autonomous choice protected by an option and is required in order for premise 3 to be true) and to justify exploiting, dominating, commodifying, or demeaning Afflicted for the benefit of future people.[14]

The arguments I just presented challenge PPE on its own terms because they use the concern about inefficiencies associated with norms of respect that motivate PPE to show that those concerns also justify adopting an even less demanding morality that permits more wrongdoing than even proponents of PPE want to allow. The welfare consequentialist elements of

---

[14] Wenner (2016, 43) raises a distinct argument that is worth noting in this context as well. Suppose that with the cost structure imposed by fair agreements, Better-off could conduct one research study with Afflicted but that if we permit Better-off to exploit Afflicted then Better-off would have the resources to conduct an additional study involving a second population, so long as we permit this second study to also be conducted on exploitative terms. In this case, although welfare consequentialist concerns are not strong enough to create a moral obligation for Better-off to interact with afflicted on fair terms, it would support a moral obligation on regulators not just to permit, but to maximize, the frequency of mutually beneficial and voluntary exploitation. Proponents of PPE might respond that they can resist this implication because it violates the proviso in premise 10. I consider the problematic implications of this response in §3.7.

PPE also facilitate the transition from the participant centered to the impartial variant of the position. In both cases, Better-off's decision about who to interact with, and on what terms, remains a private matter, shielded from outside interference by a fairly strong agent-centered prerogative. Given the logic of PPE, preventing research that imposes burdens on people who are already in a terrible situation doesn't improve the lot of those people, but it does deprive both researchers and future populations of people of potentially valuable medical resources.[15]

It might be objected that my critique is faulty because it misrepresents the role of consent in PPE. The claim would be that PPE is not committed to holding that Afflicted's welfare interests outweigh Afflicted's interests in respect, but only that we should respect Afflicted's determination, as expressed through informed consent or refusal, as to the relative importance of Afflicted's welfare and Afflicted's interest in respect.

This is a plausible objection, but it misses a key point. PPE is a position about the moral force of violations of respect and not about whether or not such a violation has occurred. As such, PPE is itself predicated on the claim that even if Afflicted consents to being exploited or degraded, Afflicted is still wronged by the subsequent exploitation and degradation. This is why PPE is committed to the idea that Afflicted's welfare interests should be allowed to trump Afflicted's interests in respect and why PPE is distinct from positions that hold that the agent's consent has the morally transformative effect of rendering what would be exploitative or morally degrading conduct non-exploitative or non-degrading. The point of my critique is that exploiting Afflicted without Afflicted's consent is wrong, but the logic of PPE justifies permitting this wrong as long as the resulting act provides Afflicted with benefits that leave Afflicted better off than Afflicted would otherwise have been (the patient-centered extension of PPE) or if the benefits that Better-off can produce for others are sufficient to outweigh the costs to Afflicted (the impartial extension of PPE).

---

[15] The impartial position comes exceedingly close to embracing a full-blown consequentialist position, but it falls short of that in a critical respect that relates to the demandingness of the position. That is, consequentialism is more demanding in that it imposes a duty on agents to promote the welfare of others, and if it were the case that the only way to do that was to exploit a certain population of people in clinical research then, as long as all else was equal, researchers would be obligated to do that. The impartial position considered above is less demanding in that it does not endorse such a duty. So it does not *require* anyone to exploit others. It simply says that if large numbers of people can benefit from such research and there are agents like Better-off who are willing to conscript vulnerable people as "soldiers of science" to do it, then we should not stand in their way.

3.6 (Un)Equal Respect

3.6.1 Threats to Autonomy and the Integrity of a Life

Although it permits certain transgressions against Afflicted, PPE appears to do so against a more fundamental background of equal moral regard: Afflicted and Better-off are each moral agents who should be seen as sovereign over their own life and whose free and informed decisions should be respected. Limiting violations of respect to cases in which Afflicted consents to the violation might thus be seen as affirming this more fundamental value of equal respect.

The appearance of a strong commitment to equal regard, however, is misleading. Any concern for the autonomy of agents like Afflicted that grounds the requirement of informed consent in PPE is at best a dim simulacrum of the profound regard PPE shows for the autonomy and integrity of the life of agents like Better-off. Recall that we began this section by noting a tension in PPE between the welfare consequentialist elements of the argument on which it rests and the fact that weak consequentialism would provide grounds to reject the claim that Better-off has no prior obligation to transact with Afflicted. We noted that the permission in premise 3 might reflect the common view that weak consequentialism is an implausibly high moral standard because it forces agents like Better-off to compromise the integrity of their lives in order to help those like Afflicted. As such, we suggested that premise 3 might be grounded in an option or agent-centered prerogative whose moral importance is grounded in preserving the integrity of Better-off's life and Better-off's sovereignty over it.

But if we are genuinely concerned about autonomy and the integrity of an individual's life then we should question the grounds on which this concern is applied to the demands that morality and policy might make on the life of Better-off without being applied with equal force to the demands that such a weaker moral framework places on Afflicted. As David Sobel has argued, "costs that a moral theory permits but does not require are sometimes relevant to the demandingness of that theory" (Sobel 2007, 13).[16] Afflicted's autonomy and the integrity of Afflicted's life are threatened by moral frameworks (such as those common to orthodox research ethics and PPE) that sanction the indifference of others to Afflicted's basic needs and by the

---

[16] Similar ideas are elaborated at length in Nagel (1991) especially chapter five.

proposal embodied in PPE to empower others to breach norms of respect in order to further advance their own personal projects.

From the standpoint of agents like Better-off, PPE is less demanding than consequentialist views that would entail the rejection of premise 3 and current ethical frameworks that include options but that enforce norms of respect. From the standpoint of agents like Afflicted, however, PPE is an incredibly demanding theory. In this case, however, the objectionable burdens come not from what morality requires agents like Better-off to do in order to help others, but for what it requires agents like Afflicted to suffer and to lose in order to ensure that agents like Better-off are not fettered in *their* life plans by duties to help others.

The point is that in order for Better-off to have an option of the force we have been considering here—one that outweighs or trumps significant and avertable threats to the welfare of others—there has to be a strong moral ground of respect for Better-off's autonomy and the integrity of Better-off's life. But a symmetrical application of this concern for the autonomy and integrity of Afflicted's life undermines such a strong option and entails the negation of premise 3—that is, it entails a duty on the part of parties like Better-off to aid or assist parties like Afflicted precisely because parties in Afflicted's position are in dire circumstances that threaten their ability to pursue their life plans. If we want our moral frameworks to be responsive to the autonomy of agents and their ability to maintain the integrity of their life, then in situations where that ability is threatened for agents like Afflicted, and agents like Better-off can help to avert such a loss at little personal cost, we should require more from agents like Better-off than either PPE or orthodox research ethics recognize. Since norms of respect are tied closely to the value of autonomy and concern for the integrity of each individual's life, there is a strong case for requiring Better-off to interact with Afflicted on terms that advance Afflicted's interests in both welfare and respect.

If this is correct, then PPE is not entitled to the defense that the permission to wrong takes place against a deeper recognition of moral equality. Rather, PPE shows asymmetric concern for the interests of Afflicted and Better-off in that it is more sensitive to the way that moral constraints and consequentialist requirements to provide aid to people like Afflicted threaten Better-off's autonomy and sovereignty over Better-off's life than it is to the way that taking this very position threatens those same interests on the part of Afflicted.

At this point, it is important to remember that the main reason for focusing on PPE is for what it reveals about fault lines running through orthodox research ethics. The argument examined in this section holds that PPE should be palatable because it is limited in its scope, sequestering violations of respect to contexts in which individuals autonomously accept such treatment. The problem with this move is that it obscures the way that the agency of some parties is protected and advanced at the expense of others. This asymmetric concern belies the idea that PPE preserves something like a baseline of moral equality against which a standard contractual relationship plays out. This asymmetric concern for autonomy, respect, and moral equality is not unique to PPE, in that this asymmetric concern is grounded in premises and features that it shares with orthodox research ethics.

3.6.2 Providing Assistance and the Fair Division of Moral Labor

It might be objected that even if we grant that sickness, injury, or disease can undermine Afflicted's autonomy and that Afflicted therefore has a claim to assistance, it doesn't follow that Afflicted would have that claim specifically against Better-off. This is probably correct, as far as it goes. In other words, we need to know more about the relevant division of social labor and about Better-off's role in it, before we could make such a determination. But I take this point to reinforce the poverty of the parochialism of orthodox research ethics. If, for example, there is a social obligation to promote the common good through medical research and if this places Better-off under a moral obligation to conduct research that advances this goal, then there may well be circumstances under which premise 3 is false; Better-off has a duty to carry out research that involves parties like Afflicted; and those parties have an enforceable claim to conditions that satisfy norms of fairness, justice, and respect.

In the next chapter, I make the case for just this position. There is a moral imperative to advance the common good through research and this imperative includes an obligation to adhere to strong norms of respect. The point of the analysis presented so far is not to identify the values that will provide the foundation for the positive view I will develop in this book. It is, instead, to illustrate that PPE repurposes the core values of orthodox research ethics in ways that reveal fault lines in the field. These fault lines concern the way that research is treated as a private undertaking of individuals with no explicitly defined and well-delineated social obligations whose interactions are to be regulated primarily by the values of beneficence and respect for persons. PPE marshals these commitments to undermine not just the paternalism of orthodox research ethics but the moral force of its already anemic commitment to justice.

3.7 Violating the Proviso

In the previous section I argued that PPE tells us something important about the status of the conceptual foundations of research ethics. There is another respect in which a flaw with PPE reveals a problem with orthodox research ethics: namely, both tend to portray research as a largely private interaction between two parties—researchers and participants. There is no sense that this interaction takes place within a larger social division of labor, that this division of labor is structured by social aims and constrained by rules that must govern similar interactions for a range of different parties in different contexts, times, and places. This decontextualized view is illustrated most dramatically in the inclusion of the harm proviso in the argument for PPE.

In contrast to what is portrayed as the self-defeating character of theories that prohibit violations of respect, PPE is supposed to represent a way of empowering the downtrodden to advance their welfare interests in the limited context of mutually beneficial and voluntary interactions. The hope is that benefits that would not have materialized under a strong prohibition of violations of respect will materialize if those prohibitions are weakened and the harm proviso is obeyed—namely, "if doing so has no negative effects on others."

How likely is it that the proviso would be violated? Here we face a tension between the context in which PPE is enunciated and the nature of the specific examples used to motivate the principle. That is, PPE is enunciated in the context of a longstanding debate within research ethics about the rules, principles, and requirements that ought to govern research that is sponsored by entities from HICs and carried out in LMIC populations. This longstanding debate is fundamentally a dispute over institutional design. At issue are the norms, goals and constraints that should govern the interactions between a range of stakeholders—from researchers, participants, and host communities, to funding agencies of various sorts including national and local governments, non-governmental organizations, and corporations—across time and different places.

In contrast to the debate over institutional design, the argument in favor of PPE outlined above depicts the discrete interaction of two seemingly isolated individuals. To some degree, this also reflects the traditional focus of orthodox research ethics. Orthodox research ethics is overwhelmingly concerned with the ethics of the researcher-participant relationship.[17] Similarly, the central mechanism for putting the norms of research ethics into practice is the IRB, an oversight body that reviews individual protocols. But the situation of a private individual conducting an isolated private transaction with another private individual is very different from policy questions about how the institutions of scientific research ought to be designed and regulated. These norms and institutions govern the interactions of a wide range of parties, some of which are repeated interactions over time. The probability that the proviso will be violated differs substantially between these two situations.

In particular, it is difficult to see how an institutional design that incorporated PPE as an explicit policy would not violate the harm proviso. The reason is that the system in which violations of respect are officially prohibited effectively places a floor on the "price" that researchers and sponsors have to "pay" in order to secure the cooperation of host communities without wronging them. From the standpoint of PPE, this price is too high because there may be some agents, such as Better-off above, who are "priced out" of the market—they choose not to interact rather than to pay a nonexploitative price.

Adopting PPE as a principle, however, would remove this floor on prices and destabilize the current price equilibrium. Those who are currently paying, or who would have paid in the future, the higher, respectful, price would face competitive pressures not to "overpay" as prohibitions are removed against either demanding a lower price to carry out the same transaction or simply finding someone else to transact with at the lower price. As a result, those communities currently hosting clinical trials on fair, nonexploitative, or respectful terms would stand either to lose out on hosting future studies that they would otherwise have hosted, or to be pressured to accept less than they would otherwise have received. I elaborate these arguments in detail in chapter 8.

[17] As we will see in chapter 5, this is the central focus of Fried's (1974) classic work on equipoise, and the entire debate over the requirement of clinical equipoise has revolved around reconciling the clinician-researcher's obligations to safeguard the welfare of individual participants with the demands of scientific research. See for example Marquis (1983), Miller and Weijer (2003), and Miller and Brody (2003).

These concerns are particularly relevant to the case of international research since this is a highly dynamic enterprise that is driven in large part by the potential for cost savings. Research sponsors are continually seeking ways to reduce costs so that they can minimize expenses and maximize profits. So-called "contract research organizations" (CROs) are corporations that have emerged with the explicit goal of making a profit by more efficiently matching research with host communities. Their emergence has made international research highly mobile, increasing competition between potential host communities and giving CROs the leverage to lower the costs of conducting research in order to capture profits for themselves.

In this context, endorsing PPE as a rule would put those who operate on fair terms of cooperation at a strategic disadvantage (see also Wenner 2016). Given the imbalance in supply and demand between the vast pools of sickness and disease in LMICs and the comparatively small number of clinical trials, market forces would drive research sponsors to make more exploitative offers in order to remain competitive.

Because implementing PPE as a principle that defines the permissible operation of the institutions of international research would result in some research participants being worse off than they otherwise would have been, such a use of PPE would violate the harm proviso. At best, therefore, PPE would have to be interpreted as a principle of individual morality that governs the conduct of researchers as private individuals. Whether this interpretation of the principle avoids violating the harm proviso will depend on a variety of factors including the degree of publicity associated with such choices and the willingness of third parties to enforce a division of labor and social norms that encourage or discourage it. In this regard, the motives of efficiency and competitive advantage would provide powerful incentives for sponsors and CROs to "encourage" researchers (through incentives such as profit sharing or punitive measures such as negative evaluation or reductions in funding for researchers whose activities are viewed as unnecessarily costly) to alter existing or future conduct in ways that are currently regarded as impermissible but that would be sanctioned under PPE. The same shift in equilibrium that would result from adoption of PPE at the level of policy could easily be replicated at the level of individual behavior via the application of employer incentives, market forces, and social norms.

Even if regarding PPE as a principle for regulating the conduct of researchers as private individuals can avoid violating the harm proviso, this way of "saving" the principle comes at a steep price. Namely, it renders PPE largely irrelevant to the fundamental questions in research ethics concerning the policies and norms that should regulate the institutional design of research and govern the conduct of the myriad stakeholders that contribute to its proper functioning.

I have been arguing that PPE offers important insight into a fault line running through the foundations of orthodox research ethics. PPE shows that when the requirements of responsiveness, the standard of care, and post-trial access are viewed as constraints on the discrete interactions of private individuals, they look like gargantuan protectionist fences intended to protect vulnerable individuals that wind up subverting that goal by "protecting" those very individuals from the only interactions that might enable them to improve their desperate condition.

3.8 Taking Stock: Testing the Health of Conceptual Foundations

Environmentalists are sometimes chided for caring a great deal about little things—the health of streams in a watershed, the plight of this or that species of toad—that seem inconsequential to outsiders. PPE might seem like an inconsequential anomaly not worth the attention that I have paid to it here. But one reason that environmentalists care about streams and toads is that they are indicators of the health of watersheds and ecosystems, larger interconnected systems that create the niche for a diversity of life. So, too, my claim has been that PPE reveals something about the health of orthodox research ethics, the state of its conceptual foundations.

PPE exploits the myopic focus of orthodox research ethics on the narrow interactions of researchers and participants. The irrelevance of PPE to the large-scale questions of institutional design in research ethics reveals the importance of stepping back from the myopic focus of orthodox research ethics and considering questions of fairness and justice from the standpoint of research as a larger social system in which the activities of diverse parties are knit together in a web of cooperation. In part, PPE founders because it misconstrues the extent to which the system of medical research and its oversight and regulation involves the design and regulation of institutions and practices involving the cooperation of different parties over an extended period of time. But this shortcoming is not unique to PPE. It is a shortcoming of the system of research ethics that PPE uses and repurposes for its own ends.

Similarly, PPE is likely to be dismissed for its willingness to permit the exploitation of the vulnerable. But PPE is a reaction to the willingness of orthodox research ethics to uphold strong moral prohibitions against disrespectful treatment while treating research that would advance the interests of those who suffer from the most significant burdens of sickness and disease as morally optional. Repugnance at the way PPE strives to solve this problem does not ameliorate the underlying dilemma. It still leaves some populations trapped between the anvil of neglect and the hammer of exploitation.

The view of research as a morally optional undertaking was motivated, in part, by a fear of what would happen if research ethics embraced a more demanding duty to advance the common good. In the next chapter I revisit the question of whether there is a social imperative to carry out research. I argue that Jonas (1969) was correct to reject such an imperative as grounded in a certain conception of the common good, but mistaken in thinking that the view of the common good that he rejects is the only or the best way of thinking about that concept. Equipped with a better conception of the common good, I argue that there is a social imperative to carry out a certain kind of research but that this imperative, contrary to the assertion of McDermott (1967), requires extending the rule of law into the realm of research with humans.

PART II
RESEARCH AMONG EQUALS

4

The Common Good and the Egalitarian Research Imperative

4.1 Revisiting the Common Good

Orthodox research ethics has largely rejected the idea that there is a social imperative to support and carry out research with human participants. We canvassed some of the practical and philosophical reasons for this in chapter 2, including Hans Jonas's influential argument that the ordinary toll of sickness, injury, and disease is not a threat to society, but to the interests of individuals and that, as such, medical research is not grounded in a social imperative (Jonas 1969). As a result, orthodox research ethics tends to treat research as an optional activity that stakeholders are free to undertake, if they choose, as part of their personal, private projects. Appeals to the common good as a ground for a social imperative to carry out research are now rare and are likely to be greeted with skepticism as rhetorical excess or as an ambiguous façade obscuring less meritorious motives.[1]

In this chapter I argue that both proponents and critics of a research imperative have presumed a particular conception of the common good, which I call the *corporate conception*. Jonas was correct in his assertion that there is no moral imperative to undertake medical research as a way of securing the corporate conception of the common good. However, both sides of this debate were mistaken in thinking that this is the only or the best way to understand the common good.

---

[1] Arendt expresses this skepticism succinctly when she says, "the liberals' political philosophy, according to which the mere sum of individual interests adds up to the miracle of the common good, appeared to be only a rationalization of the recklessness with which private interests were pressed regardless of the common good" (1973, 336). See also Nozick (1974, 33) for the idea that talk of a social good "covers up" the fact that something is done to one person for the sake of a benefit to another.

For the Common Good. Alex John London, Oxford University Press. © Oxford University Press 2022.
DOI: 10.1093/oso/9780197534830.003.0004

As an alternative, I describe and defend what I call the *basic* or *generic interest* conception of the common good and argue that this grounds what I refer to as the *egalitarian research imperative*. In contrast to the parochialism of orthodox research ethics, the egalitarian research imperative recognizes that various forms of research with human participants are part of a larger division of social labor. Because this division of labor draws on and influences the capacity of institutions that impact the basic interests of community members, there is a social imperative to carry out research that generates the evidence needed to enable a community's basic social systems, such as a community's medical and public health systems, to effectively, efficiently, and equitably safeguard and advance the basic interests of that community's members. This imperative is grounded in a fundamental concern for the status of each community member as free and equal, and this grounding shapes both the goals and purposes of the research enterprise as well as the terms on which it is to be organized and conducted.

To make this argument, in §4.2 I elaborate the pragmatic value of appeals to the common good and explicate the way that the implicit structure of such appeals shapes moral decision-making. In §4.3 I describe the corporate conception of the common good and show how this is the focus of Jonas's famous critique, and I bolster criticisms of this view in §4.4. In §4.5 I describe the basic or generic interests conception of the common good and in §4.6 demonstrate how it can be formulated within a diverse range of ethical and political frameworks.

In §4.7 I argue for the egalitarian research imperative and show how it grounds both the purpose of research, and the terms on which it can be carried out, in respect for the status of individuals as free and equal. In §4.8 I show how the resulting position expands the scope and purview of research ethics with some illustrative examples provided in §4.9.

4.2 The Structure of Appeals to the Common Good

4.2.1 Pragmatic Value

Normative appeals to the common good have a pragmatic value that derives, at least in part, from their implicit moral logic or structure. In particular, appeals to the common good often play a special role in securing individual and collective action. If some action, policy or other instrument can be successfully portrayed as necessary to support or preserve the common good, then this constitutes a strong, prima facie reason for individuals and groups to support it. Moreover, appeals to the common good can build on and marshal prior commitments and shared understandings, or they can function as a conduit through which such understandings can be forged or built.

Appeals to the common good that are invoked within communities that share a history or identity often portray some action or undertaking as having special importance in relation to the shared purposes of this common identity. In contrast, appeals to the common good can also secure collective action in the face of moral and political pluralism. When individuals or groups are not part of a discrete community or do not share a common comprehensive conception of the good, appeals to the common good highlight an action or undertaking as important relative to some underlying, shared interest. For example, prior to the Persian Wars around 492–449 BCE, ancient Greek city states shared a common language but no national identity. They were, instead, divided by rivalries and sharp cultural differences. However, they were able to unite in response to the threat from Persian forces because they could see external invasion as a threat to interests they shared in common—political sovereignty and territorial integrity—even if those interests were not connected to membership in some prior political community.

This pragmatic flexibility reflects a logic to such appeals that is independent of substantive conceptions of the good or comprehensive moral or political doctrines that might provide the content to such claims. As a result, competing substantive political or ethical doctrines can each use appeals to the common good to package their key commitments in an effort to support collective action among their adherents. At the same time, successful appeals to the common good can also indicate that some value or interest is of sufficient importance that it must be explained or accounted for within the framework of a particular comprehensive doctrine. For example, if security is recognized as a sufficiently widespread interest that it can support collective action, then different moral or political theories might seek to account for and explain the moral or political significance of this interest. As a result, appeals to the common good can reflect explicit tenets of widely held comprehensive doctrines or they can enjoy a kind of pre-theoretical intuitive force that different comprehensive theories might try to capture and to formulate more precisely.

4.2.2 The Implicit Structure of Appeals to the Common Good

Although the implicit structure of appeals to the common good is rarely explicated, it plays an important role in organizing moral decision-making. For our present purposes, we can begin with a common normative claim involved in appeals to the common good:

Normative Claim (NC): There are circumstances in which the interests of individuals may permissibly be subordinated to the common good.[2]

For example, McDermott's claim that "to ensure the rights of society, an arbitrary judgment must be made against an individual" (1967, 40) can be read as asserting that the greater good of society outweighs and legitimates the subordination or abrogation of individual rights and welfare.

Second, we require some specification of the circumstances under which this normative claim applies. The weakest, and therefore least controversial, specification simply asserts that the normative claim is most likely to be operative in cases where there is a clear and present threat to the common good itself.

Triggering Condition (TC): The presence of a clear and present threat to the common good constitutes a circumstance in which it may be permissible to subordinate the interests of individuals to the common good.[3]

Finally, these two claims together entail that efforts to promote the common good must remain within certain boundaries.

Practical Constraint (PC): The means used to pursue or secure the common good must not themselves conflict with or subvert the common good.

---

[2] Jonas's argument clearly presupposes this claim. Pettit is committed to this view when he asserts, "there is a big difference between constrained interference that is designed for a common good—say, the interference of a law that no one contests—and arbitrary interference" (1997, vii, see also 68). Aquinas articulates this claim when he says, "the common good should be put before the good of an individual" (2005, 213). See also Harris, for example, who says "It is widely recognized that there is clearly sometimes an obligation to make sacrifices for the community or an entitlement of the community to go so far as to deny autonomy and even violate bodily integrity in the public interests and this obligation is recognized in a number of ways" (2015, 244).

[3] This condition is explicitly discussed by Jonas. Harris appeals to this condition when he says, "medical research is a public good, that may *in extremis* justify compulsory participation" (2015, 245).

Although this is only a schematic representation, it enables us to clarify two points. First, appeals to the value of certain individual rights, such as civil liberties, may not be an appropriate response to arguments of this type because the NC does not deny that individual rights or civil liberties are important to the interest of individuals. It claims only that it is sometimes acceptable to limit or otherwise subordinate individual interests to something of equal or greater importance. If individual rights or civil liberties are in the class of individual interests, then an appeal to the common good represents an intuitive way to formulate a permission to override or abrogate them. Unless one is prepared to argue that such rights or liberties are absolute and inviolable, the case for overriding or breaching them becomes more compelling as the perceived threat to the common good becomes more severe.

The second point is that, as we will see in a moment, different substantive accounts of what constitutes the common good will license different actions in the NC, determine what sort of concrete threats are sufficient to meet the TC, and what substantive PC limit the means that may be used in pursuing the common good in practice. In order to avoid equivocation, one must ensure that each of these claims is explicated in terms of the same substantive account of the common good. Formulating the NC in terms of one conception of the common good and grounding the TC or the PC in a different conception would break the justificatory link between these claims. To evaluate the soundness of arguments of this type, we require detailed information about what the common good is in defense of which it may sometimes be permissible to subordinate or curtail individual interests.

4.3 The Corporate Conception of the Common Good

4.3.1 Interests Distinct from Individuals

The NC draws a contrast between the interests of individuals, on the one hand, and the common good, on the other. However, there are at least two ways of drawing this contrast that yield importantly different conceptions of the common good.

One fairly natural way to draw this contrast is to identify the common good with the good of the community conceived of as an entity that exists in its own right, persisting through time, with interests that are in some meaningful sense distinct from those of its individual members. On this view, the

NC draws a fairly blunt distinction between the good of two different parties. One party is monadic—the individual agent—and the other is corporate— the collective agent or the body politic.[4]

Aquinas appears to have this conception of the common good in mind when he says, "There is also a common good that relates to one person or another qua part of a whole; for example, to a soldier qua part of the army, or to a citizen qua part of the city" (Aquinas 2005, 131).[5] Similarly, in his testimony before the tribunal at Nuremberg, the defendant Dr. Karl Brandt seems to have this view in mind when he says that the Nazi party imposed a system in which "the demands of society are placed above every individual human being as an entity, and this entity, the human being, is completely used in the interests of that society" (Tribunals 1949, 29).

When Jonas asserts the normative claim that it is sometimes permissible to subordinate the interests of individuals to the common good, he notes correctly that "the common or public good" represents an unknown element in this equation. He then goes on to assume, at least for the sake of the argument, that the common good represents the good of society as something "distinct from any plurality of individuals" (1969, 221).

It is against the backdrop of this assumption that Jonas argues that most common illnesses, such as "cancer, heart disease, and other organic, noncontagious ills," do not pose a threat to the common good because the normal death rate from these causes does not prevent society from "flourishing in every way." As he puts it, "a permanent death rate from heart failure or cancer does not threaten society" (1969, 228). These are not threats to the common good—to society as a corporate entity—but to the lives of individuals. From the standpoint of society, as a body politic that persists as different individuals are born, live, and die, the goal of finding treatments to ameliorate sickness, injury, and disease does not benefit the corporate entity, but only the parts from which it is composed. Because the whole can survive the normal death rate from these causes, medical progress is an individual rather than a common good and is therefore morally optional.

---

[4] This is what Brennan and Lomasky describe as a strongly irreducible social good, which they define as, "G counts as a common good for society S if (1) G is good for S and (2a) G is not good for all or most of the citizens of S or (2b) G is good for S irrespective of whether G is good for the citizens of S" (2006, 223).

[5] As Thomas Williams explains, for Aquinas "Human beings are parts of a whole; that whole is the community. And parts exist for the sake of the whole. Just as you should not impair the body's integrity for just any old reason (chop off your hand just because you feel like it), but you should amputate if that is the only way to save the body, so also you should excise dangerous people if that is necessary for the safeguarding of the community" (Aquinas 2005, xviii).

The argumentative strategy that Jonas adopts reveals the logic of appeals to the common good. Given the corporate conception, in order to pose a threat to the common good (to meet the TC) something must endanger the continued existence, proper functioning, or collective welfare of society as a whole. Jonas's strategy is to argue that under "ordinary" circumstances, most common diseases and ills threaten the lives and interests of individuals, not of the community as a whole. Without a threat to the common good, the TC has not been met. Without meeting the TC, the NC has not been grounded or justified. Absent such a justification, researchers are not empowered to ignore, override, or subordinate the rights and welfare of individuals to the larger social goal of advancing the common good.

Notice, however, that if something *is* deemed to constitute a threat to the common good, this view yields only the weakest possible PC on the steps that can be taken in response. That is, if the common good is identified with the continued existence or collective welfare of society as a whole, then the PC states that the means that are used to pursue or secure the common good must not themselves conflict with or subvert the continued existence or collective welfare of the community as a whole.

Something that poses a threat to "the whole condition, present and future, of the community" may create a state of emergency "thereby suspending certain otherwise inviolable prohibitions and taboos" (Jonas 1969, 229). Once the TC has been met, violations of civil liberties and harms to individuals would have to be egregious in scope and deleterious in their direct and indirect effects before they would threaten to undermine this view of the common good. After all, just as ordinary sickness and disease are not a threat to the community before the TC has been met, the violation of individual rights and liberties and a loss in individual well-being do not threaten the existence of the community after the TC has been met.

What Jonas seems to recognize so keenly is that the corporate conception yields a surprisingly broad permission for authorities to subordinate the interests of individuals to the common good once the TC has been met. Notice too that concealing harms to individuals that are justified by appeal to this conception of the common good makes it less likely that the PC will be violated. As such, this conception of the common good seems to underwrite less than transparent and perhaps overtly deceptive social practices in order to ensure that public scrutiny does not threaten to destabilize the community.

This last point explains why McDermott, Lasagna, and others who saw researchers as empowered to make "arbitrary judgments" against specific

unlucky individuals also argued that this sacred trust must remain sufficiently private or discrete as not to threaten or undermine the ability of
researchers to produce these social benefits. If sickness and disease threaten
society, then society can take whatever steps are necessary to secure its preservation, as long as those steps remain with the bounds of the PC.

Because the corporate conception of the common good yields such a weak
PC, this framework tends to focus debate on whether or not the triggering
conditions for the normative claim have been met. As a result, this conception
of the common good makes it difficult to locate a middle ground between the
following two extreme interpretations of the TC).

4.3.2 Strict Triggering Conditions

Jonas endorses what we might call "strict conditions" on when the TC has
been met. On this view, common and pervasive threats to the welfare of individual agents such as most major diseases and illnesses, most criminal activities, and fairly steep social and economic inequalities, do not pose a threat to
the common good. It is only in the most extreme cases—cases in which plague,
famine, anarchy, or revolution threaten health and safety on a grand scale—that
such conditions threaten the persistence, proper functioning, or aggregate welfare of the community as a whole.

On the view that Jonas adopts, efforts to ameliorate or address the ordinary,
common causes of avoidable suffering, loss of functioning, or death for individuals cannot draw their support from an appeal to the common good. They are
not sufficient to activate the TC and justify the NC. If efforts to address these
conditions require concessions from individual agents, then the strict position
Jonas adopts either prohibits them, or requires that the justification for seeking
them be drawn from an appeal to something other than the common good.

By adopting the strict position on when the TC is met, Jonas shields individual interests against the potential for overreach and abuse latent in appeals
to the common good and the NC. In doing so, he also rebuts the claim that
there is a social imperative to carry out research with human participants.
This shifts the justification for this activity outside the public sphere and into
the private sphere of individual interest.[6]

---

[6] The logic of the move Jonas makes is recognized even by critics who seek to revive the idea that
the status of medical knowledge as a public good is sufficient to ground a research imperative. In the

4.3.3   Lenient Triggering Conditions

In contrast, what I will call the "lenient position" on the TC is more willing to view "ordinary" sources of individual morbidity and mortality as threats to the common good as defined by the corporate conception.[7] This position is lenient in the sense that it sets a lower bar for the triggering condition. To do this from within the corporate conception of the common good, it has to focus less on the persistence through time of the community and more on its aggregate welfare or, as Arendt phrases it, "the sum total of individual interests" (1973, 152).[8]

Certain forms of utilitarianism support a view in which the sum total or aggregate social welfare is created by combining the gains and losses to individual welfare at a particular time without keeping track of how those changes in welfare affect the life of individual agents across time. For example, Parfit describes a view that rejects the idea that there is a deep metaphysical or moral truth to the personal identity of individuals over time. On this view, what matters are the quality of the experiences that occur in the lives of persons at a given time, not how those experiences are connected to past or future experiences. As Parfit puts it, "If we cease to believe that persons are separately existing entities, and come to believe that the unity of a life involves no more than the various relations between the experiences in this life, it becomes more plausible to be more concerned about the quality

---

hands of these critics, the research imperative is no longer a social imperative to carry out research of a certain sort. Rather, it is framed as a moral imperative that individuals participate in research. Nevertheless, as one group puts it, "If it turned out that biomedical research with human participants was not that important after all—that society would not be much worse off if all research on humans were to cease—there would be no obligation to participate" (Schaefer et al. 2009, 68).

[7] Harris notes that communities sometimes have "an entitlement to go so far as to deny autonomy and even violate bodily integrity in the public interest," (2005, 244), and although he seems to think that this should be reserved for cases of "extremis," he seems to have a lower threshold for appeals to the common good to override individual interests than Jonas. Similarly, in 1997, the Secretary of Health and Human Services, Donna Shalala, testified before congress that the traditional requirement of patient consent for disclosure of medical information must give way to "our public responsibility to support national priorities—public health, research, quality care, and our fight against health care fraud and abuse." Critics of this proposal saw it as an instance of the subordination of human subject protections to the "interests of science and society" (2005, 244) pointing to what they saw as "Shalala's willingness to use bureaucratically designated 'national priorities' as a rationale for overriding a traditional patient right and, potentially, patients' civil rights as well" (Woodward 1999).

[8] Arendt argues that imperial powers saw economic and political expansion as a way to serve the common good because, although different individuals have different interests, they share common economic interests that were advanced by expanding economic opportunities. Such powers thus saw expansion as a way to increase the sum total of individual interests in their community (Arendt 1973, 152).

of experiences, and less concerned about whose experiences they are" (1984, 346).

On such a view, "the impersonality of Utilitarianism is therefore less implausible than most of us believe" (Parfit 1984, 346). The view is impersonal in the sense that it assigns value to the net utility of states of affairs regardless of how the underlying utilities (pleasures and pains or whatever metric is used to define the good) are distributed across specific individuals. This creates a corporate conception of the common good because the community's welfare is an aggregation of the pleasures and pains of its constituent members at a given time, without concern for how those pleasures and pains are distributed across its members.

On this view, the TC can be more lenient, as anything that avoidably reduces aggregate welfare might trigger the NC. To the extent that preventing, curing, or ameliorating sickness, injury, or disease on a large scale increases aggregate welfare, then the means of effectuating these gains can be viewed as helping society to avoid a collective threat—the loss of social utility that avoidable morbidity and mortality bring.

When Eisenberg asserts that "the decision not to do something poses as many ethical quandaries as the decision to do it," he appears to be making a clearly consequentialist claim. This underwrites his assertion that, "the systematic imposition of impediments to significant therapeutic research is itself unethical because an important benefit is being denied to the community" (1977, 1108). Here it is unlikely that he is referring to the community in the corporate sense. When he says that "there is a clear moral imperative in developed nations for medical research in tropical diseases, to seek to permit two-thirds of the world's population to share in the freedom from pain and untimely death we have achieved for ourselves" (1977, 1109), it is the magnitude of the benefits to the welfare of large numbers of people that seem to underwrite the moral imperative.

Adopting a more lenient TC has the potentially attractive feature of grounding a social imperative to support the research enterprise. But because the corporate conception of the common good yields such a weak PC, the willingness to exact even the most profound sacrifices from the individual, or a minority of individuals, in order to secure the good of the majority may turn out not to be a moral failing, but a requirement of civic virtue in such a view. When the aggregate welfare is impersonal, there is no constraint against increasing it in ways that exact a heavy toll from individual agents. The only practical constraint on exacting sacrifices from individuals in the name of the common good is that any harms or wrongs must be compensated for sufficiently by the increase in aggregate well-being.

Some utilitarians were at pains to prevent this kind of conflict between the interest of the individual and the demands of the collective by stressing that the way welfare is distributed across the life of a particular individual matters morally.[9] These theorists are thus sensitive to the potential for utilitarian theories to run roughshod over what most political liberals regard as a foundational requirement of morality, namely, the need to respect the sanctity or dignity of the individual person, what Rawls calls the "separateness of persons" (Rawls 1971, 22–33).

It is not surprising that those with a more utilitarian bent are likely to be unpersuaded by Jonas's argument. Jonas mounts his defense of individual rights and welfare with an argument in defense of the strict position on when the NC is triggered. That position was motivated by a conception of the community, as an enduring entity, reflected in Nazi ideology, and represents a natural interpretation of claims about the right of humanity or the state to medical progress. But that view requires a strict interpretation of the TC and it is this view that Jonas exploits. In contrast, a more permissive view of the triggering condition is likely to be adopted by utilitarians who think that they have sufficient information to make interpersonally comparable assessments of aggregate social utility of a fine enough grain to determine when social policies that adversely impact the rights or welfare of individuals generate a sufficient amount of welfare to offset those losses.[10]

[9] Sidgwick says, "It would be contrary to Common Sense to deny that the distinction between any one individual and any other is real and fundamental, and that consequently I am concerned with the quality of my existence as an individual in a sense, fundamentally important, in which I am not concerned with the quality of the existence of other individuals: and this being so, I do not see how it can be proved that this distinction is not to be taken as fundamental in determining the ultimate end of rational action for an individual" (1930, 498). Parfit frames his discussion of the separateness of persons as a response to Sidgwick: "Sidgwick held this view because he believed the separateness of persons to be a deep truth. He believed that an appeal to this truth gives a Self-interest Theorist a sufficient defense against the claims of morality. And he suggested that, if we took a different view about personal identity, we could refute the Self-interest Theory. I have claimed that this is true" (1984, 329).

[10] See Hardin (1998) for an insightful discussion of the way that the presence or absence of information about interpersonal comparisons of utility alters the norms that can be grounded in a consequentialist framework.

4.3.4 Diversity and (Spurious) Consensus

I suggested previously that arguments about the common good are some-what independent of comprehensive moral and political theories. It is worth reiterating, therefore, that communitarians who are comfortable treating the state or the community as a distinct entity that persists through time, and utilitarians who hold that communities are nothing more than collections of individuals, may disagree about strict and lenient interpretations of the TC. But such disagreements can take place against the shared background assumption of the corporate conception of the common good.

During times of relative peace or security, disagreement over strict and lenient positions may flourish between proponents of such different comprehensive views. In a time of social crisis, however, these divisions are more likely to collapse. The larger the social threat, the more difficult it will be to resist the claim that the TC has been met. Proponents of different comprehensive moral and political theories may suddenly find themselves in agreement because the fact that they share the corporate conception of the common good is obscured by the more salient or prominent division over the stringency of the TC. As a result, in times of national crisis, both communitarians and liberals may find themselves embracing the same NC and therefore willing to tolerate fairly high demands on some, so long as those demands do not violate the same fairly weak PC).

Understanding the logic behind such a convergence is particularly important for two reasons. To begin with, if proponents of different comprehensive views find themselves converging in the way I just described, they may perceive this as an overlapping consensus that therefore takes on special epistemic, or at least political, credence. Additionally, if the role of embracing a corporate conception of the common good in forging this consensus is not subjected to explicit reflection, it may become increasingly difficult to see dissenters as rational or reasonable. Without seeing the possibility of an alternative conception of the common good, the only way to interpret continued dissent within this framework is to see it as a claim that the (TC) has not been met. As fear of calamitous consequences render such a position more difficult to make, however, it also becomes harder to see dissenters as rational.

The corporate conception of the common good, however, is only one possible way of construing the relationship between individual interests and the common good. In §4.5 I will outline an alternative way of construing this relationship that yields very different normative conclusions. First, however,

I want to note some of the reasons why we ought to be skeptical of the corporate conception of the common good.

4.4 Problems with the Corporate Conception

To begin with, the corporate conception of the common good is overly broad in what it recognizes as threats. For example, it would include as threats to the common good cases where the persistence of a community is threatened by causes that do not endanger the moral rights or welfare of its individual members. Such cases might include the dissolution of the community through mass emigration, peaceful succession, or pervasive civil reforms in which central social and cultural structures are dissolved and replaced by alternatives. In such a case, the threat of the dissolution of the community could activate the TC and justify state action that would adversely impact the rights or welfare of community members, even though the threat the state is facing would not adversely affect the rights or welfare of *any* of its constituent members.

Similarly, if the focus is the aggregate welfare of the community, this conception of the common good can still be overly broad in what it recognizes as a threat. For instance, imagine a large population of people, each of whom has a relatively low level of individual welfare. Reducing the size of the population through emigration or lower fertility rates will reduce the overall aggregate welfare of the community simply by reducing the number of people. Policies that reduce population size threaten the common good by lowering aggregate welfare, even though it is possible to reduce aggregate welfare in ways that harm no one and lead to a state of affairs in which the welfare of every remaining individual increases.[11]

On the other hand, this conception of the common good also appears to be overly narrow in what it recognizes as potential threats. On the corporate conception of the common good, the preservation of features that constitute

[11] As a simple example, consider 100 people, each of whom has a utility of 60. If emigration and lower fertility rates reduced the population by half and increased the welfare of the remaining 50 people by a positive amount that is less than 30, the aggregate population level will decrease while the welfare of every individual will increase. This is a strong result because every remaining individual is strictly better off than they previously were. A weaker version would hold as long as some people are made no worse off and others are made better off as a result of a decrease in population. In this way, exceedingly large populations might decline in ways that reduce overall, aggregate welfare without making anyone worse off but also making some people strictly better off. Nevertheless, such trends would constitute threats to the common good and so be targets for state action.

the identity of the community as a whole can justify acts or policies that reduce the rights and welfare of community members. This can happen, for example, when a culturally, politically, and economically dominant class exacts heavy sacrifices from individuals in marginalized groups to secure the transmission of culture and the maintenance of social order that perpetuates the exclusion or subjugation of marginalized groups. Worries of this kind likely motivated Jonas's critique.

Likewise, policies that increase overall utility may have a deleterious effect on the welfare of the individuals who comprise the relevant community. The clearest example of this occurs from absorbing or adding new members, either through population increase or immigration, in a way that increases aggregate welfare while diminishing individual welfare. Here again it is possible to increase the total social welfare while making every individual in the community worse off.[12]

In these cases, the corporate conception of the common good can accept, and may even require, significant compromises to the rights or welfare of fairly sizable portions of the population, so long as those compromises do not threaten the persistence of the community as a whole or the aggregate welfare of its members.

The corporate conception faces these problems because it treats the community as something whose perfection or proper function is in a meaningful sense distinct or uncoupled from the flourishing or proper functioning of its members. Given this divergence, however, it becomes unclear why the perfection, proper function or flourishing of this corporate entity should take normative precedence over that of the individuals that comprise it.[13]

Such worries are exacerbated by the tendency for the pursuit of such non-personal ideals to require significant personal sacrifice, often from

[12] For instance, adding n people with a total utility of y to a population of size m will increase the aggregate utility of the population while making every individual worse off as long as the decrease to each individual's utility is greater than zero and strictly less than $(n + m)/y$. These objections are an instance of what Parfit refers to as the "repugnant conclusion" (1984, 381–390).

[13] Brennan and Lomasky make a similar argument when they argue that strongly irreducible social goods are "irrelevant to rational political activity" because the community and the individual are each treated as separate entities that can fare well or fare badly and there is "no special connection between their farings" (2006, 224). They point out that such a special connection cannot be established by appealing to the fact that individuals can value the fact that their community embodies some irreducible social good because this grounds the importance of the common good in the prior value of individual preferences or commitments. It is also worth mentioning that Jonas (1969, 221) raises related concerns about what I am calling the corporate conception. It is therefore appropriate to read Jonas's argument as dialectical in nature. That is, he is claiming that even if we assume the corporate conception of the common good we can still provide a sturdy foundation for informed consent for most peacetime circumstances.

members of the most vulnerable classes. They are also exacerbated by the convenient congruence between the needs of these ideals and the protection, enrichment, entertainment, and general aggrandizement of a powerful, prosperous few.[14]

For these reasons, the corporate conception of the common good provides a poor framework within which to evaluate important normative questions. It is insufficiently responsive to the interests of individual community members and it places inordinate emphasis on establishing that the TC has been met. Within this framework, for example, debate will focus on whether a public health emergency represents a clear and present danger to the common good. Establishing that this is the case allows us to treat basic rights and liberties and the traditional principles of research ethics as peacetime luxuries that can be abrogated in this time of crisis. What this framework does not provide is any sense of a principled way to make specific decisions about when or to what extent such traditional protections may be modified. It simply enunciates the permissibility of setting them aside.

The potential for abuse that is latent in this position can therefore lead reasonable people to avoid acknowledging a health emergency as a threat to the common good, even when such a threat adversely affects the health and welfare of potentially sizable groups of individuals. This fosters zero-sum thinking and can therefore exacerbate conflicts over controversial cases. It is also extremely difficult within this framework to draw support from a concern for the common good for specific, substantive limits on permissible means in a way that is sensitive to the interests of the individuals involved. This adds to the difficulty of finding integrative or win-win solutions to conflicts that do arise within this framework.

4.5 The Basic or Generic Interests Conception of the Common Good

4.5.1 Personal Interests

It is crucial, therefore, to consider another way of distinguishing individual interests from the common good. What I call the "basic or generic

14 See note 1 in this chapter.

interests" view draws a distinction, not between the interests of individuals, on one side, and groups or communities on the other, but between two sets of interests that can be attributed to every individual.

One set of interests is individual or personal. These include the goals and ends that derive from the particular life plan an individual has adopted, as well as interests that derive from the various ways that a person's life can go better or worse relative to that plan. These are first-order interests in the sense that they are interests that one has in virtue of the particular life plan one has adopted, including a conception of a good or flourishing life.

Talk of "adopting a life plan" is likely to be misleading to the extent that it gives the impression of a single moment in which an agent performs a self-conscious act of deciding to pursue a discretely formulated and clearly articulated plan or script for a life. In reality, this process is often inchoate, extended across time, and undertaken tacitly and implicitly. Children are often raised to have certain values and aspirations that structure their ac-tivities and pursuits, along with their conceptions of success and failure, without questioning the values they have effectively inherited from their parents, friends, and community. At other times in life—after a traumatic event or a major transition such as graduating or ending a relationship— individuals sometimes do reflect on the values and ideals after which they strive: whether those values and ideals are defective or wanting, whether they would be better served, in some meaningful sense, by editing and revising some aspect of their goals, values, ambitions or criteria for success and failure.

Regardless of the extent to which a life plan is explicit or implicit, such a plan represents a set of values and a conception of the human good or human flourishing that provides a structure for evaluating opportunities and deter-mining the magnitude of a benefit or a harm. For example, a person who organizes her life around hiking and mountain climbing may value striving for excellence in physical strength and endurance, cultivating the mental toughness necessary to resist fatigue and the desire to quit, and appreci-ating the beauty and grandeur of nature. For such a person, sitting inside at a desk all day, typing at a computer, might seem like a hellish existence, even if it came with lucrative remuneration. In contrast, the novelist or aca-demic who enjoys reading and writing for long hours may view the hardships and inconveniences of camping and hiking as precisely the kind of drudgery that modern conveniences were invented to obviate. They would prefer to sit at a computer, exploring new ideas, crafting elegant prose, or insightful arguments to trudging up a muddy hillside and sleeping on wet grass without a shower.

The point of these stereotypical examples is merely to illustrate how the values, aspirations, goals, and ideals that a person embraces can shape a life in which activities that would be of low value to one person can be deeply meaningful and valued by another. The interest that these parties have in spending long hours on the trail or at a desk, in having a membership at a gym or a subscription to a literary magazine, are all personal interests in the sense that they derive their value from their place in a particular life plan.

4.5.2 Basic or Generic Interests

Personal interests are distinguished from basic or generic in this sense: although individuals may differ widely in their particular tastes, preferences, career choices, and personal ideals—their individual or personal conception of the good—they each share a general interest in being able to pursue whatever life plan they have adopted. Rawls refers to this as a higher-order interest in the sense that it takes a person's first-order interests as its object (1982, 164–165). At an even more general level, this shared higher-order interest is the subject of what Rawls refers to as a person's highest-order interest (164–165). This is their basic or generic interest in being able to develop and exercise their basic intellectual, affective, social, and physical capacities in order to be able to formulate, pursue, and revise a meaningful life plan, including forming and maintaining relationships of significance with others.

During periods of growth or change, people sometimes adopt this kind of higher-order perspective or they seek the help of a counselor or advisor who provides assistance in assuming this perspective. In such cases, people consider what their talents and aptitudes are; what activities draw on those aptitudes in a way that might create a sense of fulfillment and accomplishment; and how those aptitudes or activities might align with career plans and vocational options, hobbies and avocational opportunities, social movements and volunteer opportunities, or other forms of association that are available in their society. At such a time it would not be uncommon for such a person to say that they are looking for the same thing as everyone else—a life plan that fits their personality, gifts, proclivities, and limitations that they might inhabit and within which they might grow and find a sense of meaning and belonging.[15]

The stockbroker, the triathlete, the chemist, the sculptor, the musician, and the soldier may have radically different conceptions of what activities and accomplishments are worthwhile, of the prospects that are to be feared or avoided, of the resources that are valuable for advancing their ends, and of the criteria for success and failure. Nevertheless, with reflection each can see the others as fundamentally the same as them in this basic respect, namely, that each shares the generic interest in being able to develop a life plan of their own, to be able to revise it in light of reflection and experience, and to be free from arbitrary interference so that they can undertake these pursuits on terms that are consistent with the equal ability of their compatriots to do the same.

4.5.3 Justice and the Space of Equality

What I call the basic or generic interests view identifies the common good with this set of basic or generic interests. One of the goals of a just political order is to secure the common good in the sense that a just political order is one in which the basic institutions of society are designed and function to create and maintain social conditions in which every one of its members can develop and exercise their basic intellectual, affective,

---

[15] As Mill puts it:

There is no reason that all human existences should be constructed on some one, or some small number of patterns. If a person possesses any tolerable amount of common sense and experience, his own mode of laying out his existence is the best, not because it is the best in itself, but because it is his own mode. Human beings are not like sheep; and even sheep are not undistinguishably alike. A man cannot get a coat or a pair of boots to fit him, unless they are either made to his measure, or he has a whole warehouseful to choose from: and is it easier to fit him with a life than with a coat, or are human beings more like one another in their whole physical and spiritual conformation than in the shape of their feet? If it were only that people have diversities of taste that is reason enough for not attempting to shape them all after one model. But different persons also require different conditions for their spiritual development; and can no more exist healthily in the same moral, than all the variety of plants can in the same physical atmosphere and climate. The same things which are helps to one person towards the cultivation of his higher nature, are hindrances to another. The same mode of life is a healthy excitement to one, keeping all his faculties of action and enjoyment in their best order, while to another it is a distracting burden, which suspends or crushes all internal life. Such are the differences among human beings in their sources of pleasure, their susceptibilities of pain, and the operation on them of different physical and moral agencies, that unless there is a corresponding diversity in their modes of life, they neither obtain their fair share of happiness, nor grow up to the mental, moral, and aesthetic stature of which their nature is capable. (1880, 39–40)

and social capacities in order to form, pursue, and revise a reasonable life plan.[16]

Basic interests help to define the sense in which a just social order treats people as free and equal. A just social order treats people as morally free when it recognizes their status as individuals "who exist for their own sake and not for the sake of someone else" (Aristotle 982b25–27). This status is reflected in the interest that individuals share in being able not only to form and pursue, but also to revise, a life plan. Individuals can take on a wide range of commitments within their personal projects, and those projects can entail differences in rank or standing or accomplishment relative to the criteria within those shared projects. But those distinctions must not compromise the deep interest that individuals retain in being able to reassess their commitments and projects and memberships and to act on those revised assessments. Honoring or respecting moral freedom requires concrete social action to secure for all community members, across a complete lifespan, the personal and social conditions necessary to realize this interest in practice.[17]

Basic interests define the sphere of moral equality because they represent the common, highest-order interest that all persons share in being able to forge and pursue a life of personal meaning and interpersonal connection and importance. Relative to these interests, there are no grounds for discriminating or favoring individuals. Whether a life plan is reasonable or not is to be judged from this highest-order standpoint and hinges on the extent to which it is consistent with a social order that recognizes all other individuals as having the same generic interests, and therefore as having the same moral and political standing. A life plan of patriotic service to one's particular country may be reasonable, in this sense, because it is consistent with the equal status of others to develop and pursue a life plan of their own. In contrast, a life plan that involves pursuing the supremacy of one racial or ethnic cast and the domination or systematic oppression of other racial or ethnic

---

[16] This point about the relationship between basic interests and the basic social structures of a community is taken up again in chapter 9.

[17] It is noteworthy that Pettit identifies freedom as non-domination with the common good (1997, 120–126; see also 2004). In other words, the purpose of a republic is to provide a social order that protects individuals from arbitrary interference from others and in which their dignity and status as the moral equal of their compatriots is recognized in law and in practice. This is a common good, for Pettit, both in the sense that being free from arbitrary interference is an interest shared by all persons and in the sense that this good can only be realized by action taken at the community level. This notion of community level action—embodied in the rule of law and checks and balances of institutions—is captured here in the idea that the basic structures of a society must function so as to preserve for individuals the real freedom to formulate, pursue, and revise a life plan.

casts is not reasonable because it denies to others the ability to develop and exercise the basic interests that all people share.

Given the generic interest conception of the common good, the NC that the interests of individuals may permissibly be subordinated to the common good is to be understood as holding that an individual's pursuit of his or her individual or personal good must sometimes be subordinated to, or constrained by, the basic interests that individuals need in order to form, pursue, and revise a life plan. In this regard, the claim that a White supremacist ideology is unreasonable and therefore should not be tolerated in a just society represents an instance of the NC—the ability of a person to identify with and to promote personal projects, including the formation of relationships and identities of interpersonal meaning and significance, must be constrained by the legitimate interests of others in being free to develop and exercise the very intellectual, social, and emotional capacities that are presupposed in that person's pursuit of his or her own particular ends. Because the White supremacist embraces an identity that denies the equal moral status of others—their generic interest in being free to develop and pursue a life plan of their own without arbitrary social interference—a just social order can use social authority to deter the dissemination, cultivation, and pursuit of this identity.

4.5.4 Threats to Basic Interests

Many more things pose a threat to the common good on this view than on the corporate conception. Premature mortality and severe morbidity threaten the integrity of a life by shortening its duration or reducing the extent to which a person can develop and exercise their particular talents and abilities. To formulate, pursue, and revise a life plan, individuals draw on a network of intellectual and affective capacities. These capacities can be hindered or undermined by injury and disease including various forms of physical and mental illness. A person's ability to pursue a reasonable life plan can also be frustrated by impediments to or restrictions on the capabilities they use to navigate the physical world, to engage in social life, to enter public and private spaces, and to convert resources into the functionings necessary to take advantage of social opportunity (Sen 1999b; Nussbaum 2000).

The ability to formulate, pursue, and revise a life plan of one's own is not solely a function of an individual's physical or mental condition. Individuals can be prevented from exercising those capacities in practice if the laws or social norms to which they are subject prohibit their participation in society on equal terms with their compatriots. Racism, sexism, ableism, and other forms of discrimination frustrate the generic interests of individuals by preventing their development or preventing their exercise in practice. Restrictions on access to education, for example, prevent individuals in targeted classes from developing their basic intellectual, affective, and social capabilities and also deprive them of access to a social space in which the exercise of those abilities is a gateway to additional social, economic, and political opportunity.

The basic or generic interest of individuals in being able to formulate, pursue, and revise a life plan can thus be set back by a range of factors that detract from the fair value of this interest. To enjoy the fair value of this interest, it is not sufficient to recognize individuals as free and equal on paper. Rather, to enjoy the fair value of their basic interests, individuals require the freedom to exercise the intellectual, affective, and social abilities necessary to advance those interests; they also require social protections for that exercise and access to the opportunities in which those capacities can be deployed (Sen 1999; Nussbaum 2000). When individuals have the resources, protections, and opportunities to realize the fair value of their basic human capacities then we can say that they have the real freedom to exercise these capacities in the service of a meaningful life plan.[18] Given the diversity of individual capability sets, this can include access to equipment (e.g., braces, wheel chairs, Braille text) or supports (e.g., translation or transcription services) that enable persons with disabilities to function in ways that are necessary to take advantage of opportunities that would be open to them in light of their various talents, abilities, and interests.

Because the way that social systems are ordered has such a profound impact on the basic interests of persons, the common good should be understood as a set of shared interests that encompass both the ability of individuals to develop and exercise their basic intellectual, affective and physical abilities and their shared interest in being subject to social arrangements that foster and promote their capacity to translate these abilities into the functionings needed to formulate, pursue, or revise a life plan of their own. The members of a community have a claim on the basic structures of their community that

---

[18] On this idea in the political theories of Locke, Kant, and Mill, see Korsgaard (1993) and Anderson (1999). For the link between the concept of "fair value" applied to basic liberties and human capabilities, see Korsgaard (1993), Rawls (2001, 175), Nussbaum (2000), and Sen (1999a and 1999b).

they function on terms that give each person an effective opportunity to cultivate and use their basic intellectual, affective, and social capacities to pursue a meaningful life plan.

The generic interest conception of the common good thus yields a TC that is easier to meet because many more things threaten the common good, so conceived. This means that social undertakings aimed at ameliorating or addressing a much wider range of social and biological ills draw their normative support from safeguarding and advancing the common good.

4.5.5 Internal Constraints

However, the generic interests conception also yields a PC that provides much more substantive and robust limits on the way that efforts to address these conditions may permissibly be carried out. In particular, efforts to safeguard and secure the generic interests of people must not themselves violate or trample on the basic interests of individuals.

Just as the effects of disease, for example, do not need to be widespread to pose a threat to the common good so conceived, neither does a contemplated abrogation of individual rights or basic liberties. Just as all individuals have an interest in being free from or protected against the possible ravages of injury and oppression, so too do they have a generic interest in knowing that their control over their person will be safeguarded and respected as the community strives to provide such protections. As a result, efforts to provide the social, material, environmental, and medical conditions necessary for individuals to enjoy the fair value of their basic interests must be designed and carried out in ways that respect the basic interests of the people who carry out this effort.

One key means of advancing the common good within these constraints is to encourage a division of labor in which different tasks associated with advancing the common good can be formulated in terms that are attractive to community members as arenas in which they can pursue goods, ideals, or values that are salient within their personal conception of the good. For example, in a decent society, children require education. To advance this basic interest, educational careers should be formulated on terms that attract individuals who can see in this form of public service an arena in which to develop and exercise their love of learning, their enjoyment of performing, or numerous other traits or commitments.

The goal of such a division of social labor is to create opportunities for individuals to take up, as part of their first-order life plan, activities, and roles that are necessary to secure the basic interests of community members. In some cases, these activities and roles take the form of career opportunities, as when individuals become teachers, adopting as part of their first-order life plan the project of providing a service and a good (teaching and knowledge) that students require in order to be able to develop and exercise their basic interests in being able to formulate, pursue, and revise a life plan of their own.

In the case of medical research, being a researcher has long been seen as a pathway for advancing the common good. The view I defend in the rest of this and the next chapter is that there is an imperative to treat study participation in a parallel fashion, not as a career but as a social opportunity open to community members through which they can contribute to the common good with credible public assurance that, in doing so, their own basic interests will not be knowingly compromised in the process.[19]

This way of distinguishing individual interests from the common good avoids the zero-sum thinking of the corporate conception which distinguished all of an individual's interests from the distinct interests of the community. When individuals come into conflict over the pursuit of their individual goods, the goal is to resolve the conflict in a way that is maximally responsive to the common good—that is, to the shared basic interests of each in being able to develop and exercise the basic intellectual, social, and affective capacities they need to formulate, pursue, and revise a life plan and to pursue relationships of meaning and significance. In other words, the goal is to resolve conflicts at the level of the individual good by searching for *integrative solutions*—modifications in individual goals and ends that enable each party to pursue and exercise their shared basic capacities for agency and welfare. When goals or ends conflict, an integrative solution is one that modifies those goals and ends so as to meet or satisfy the underlying legitimate interests that provide the rationale or motivation behind those goals or ends.[20] In the next two chapters, when we explore how it is possible to

---

[19] Whether research participants should be treated like volunteers, similar to volunteer fire fighters or paramedics, or paid as professionals is the subject of vigorous debate. In this work I lean toward the view that they should be treated as volunteers. To make this the case, a range of steps should be taken to relieve any burdens, hardships, and expenses that participants might incur through research participation. For the debate about whether research should be treated as a paid profession see Dickert and Grady (1999), Lemmens and Elliott (1999), Anderson and Weijer (2002), Lynch (2014), Różyńska (2018), and Malmqvist (2019).

[20] For a more detailed discussion, including types of integrative solutions, see Rubin, Pruitt, and Kim (1994, 168–195).

implement such requirements in practice, I develop what I call the integrative approach to risk assessment and management. That approach is integrative in this sense: it resolves conflicts over the reasonableness of risks in research by distinguishing these two sets of interests and allowing individuals greater discretion over the risks they face to their personal interests while requiring that research respect a principle of equal concern when it comes to their basic interests.

4.6 Multiple Instances of the Generic Interests View

4.6.1 A Communitarian Formulation

Like the corporate conception, the generic interests view can be formulated within a variety of theoretical frameworks that are separated by some of the most commonly disputed issues in moral and political philosophy. For philosophically minded readers, it can help clarify the content of the generic interest view to see how it can be formulated within different traditions of social and political justice that begin from different starting points and appeal to a range of different moral considerations. Readers who are less interested in the way this view can be formulated in different philosophical traditions should feel free to skip this section.

For instance, Charles Taylor is a communitarian in the sense that he thinks community membership and social obligation have a certain kind of priority over individual rights. As a result, he has argued that individualist or atomistic political theories that postulate pre-societal or pre-political rights rest on a mistaken view of the basic capacities of agents (Taylor 1979). Granting a certain priority to the community and to obligations of membership does not rule out the generic interests view of the common good, however.

On Taylor's view, what makes some social arrangements preferable to others is the extent to which they create the conditions in which individuals can develop the deliberative and social capacities necessary to entertain alternative forms of living, to engage in a vigorous public debate, and the extent to which they ensure participation in the ongoing development and improvement of the community. The perfection of the community is therefore defined by its responsiveness to the generic interests that its members share in being able to develop and exercise their basic deliberative and social capabilities.

The social obligations that have priority over individual rights are obligations to respect in others the same set of generic interests that are presupposed in one's pursuit of one's own particular projects and relationships. For Taylor, this means that some of one's particular ends (accumulating a vast personal fortune, for example) may have to be modified to accommodate a commitment to sustain the social institutions that create the conditions in which members of the community enjoy the freedom to develop and exercise the very capacities that make the pursuit of these particular ends possible.

Taylor is also a communitarian in the sense that he thinks the development of our individual human potential cannot be achieved outside of some social matrix, some prior set of social structures and practices that countenance certain identities and certain possibilities for self-development as practical possibilities. There is a sense in which this social matrix precedes each of us—we are born into it and our development is shaped by it—and makes a claim on our allegiance.

But, on Taylor's view, we have a duty to belong to a certain sort of society only because it is within such social arrangements that we can develop the fundamental capacities for reflection and agency that we exercise in formulating and carrying out a life plan. Taylor rejects the contractualist idea that a just state derives its moral authority from the voluntary consent of the governed, arguing instead that its moral authority derives from its justice. Nevertheless, he holds that the justice of a social order, on this view, consists in its being organized around creating and supporting citizens who enjoy the fair value of their ability to formulate and carry out a reasonable life plan of their own.

Although the norms and institutions of society precede us, Taylor argues that their purpose does not lie in the impersonal perfection of the state or the community per se. Rather, the fundamental purpose of the state and the community lies in cultivating and supporting the basic interests of the individual human persons who constitute its constituent members. Taylor emphasizes that one of the reasons that individuals need the capacities that a just state cultivates is to be able to engage in the civic life of the community and preserve the justice of the state. But the capacities that individuals require to engage in public deliberation and the civil life of the community are the same capacities we use to contemplate our personal projects and plans and to communicate and form bonds of intimacy with our friends and loved ones.

Taylor's communitarianism is a form of perfectionism—a view that morality and justice are ultimately grounded in a certain conception of human nature. As such, it is what Rawls refers to as a comprehensive doctrine, an account of human nature and the human good that competes on the same level with all other such comprehensive views. But this comprehensive, communitarian view locates the common good of community members in the basic intellectual, affective, and associative capacities that citizens exercise in the public life of the state and that free and equal individuals employ to formulate, pursue, and revise a life plan of their own.

4.6.2 A Purely Political Contractarian Formulation

In contrast, John Rawls rejects Taylor's perfectionism and his communitarianism. Rawls offers, instead, a contractarian theory of justice in which the generic interests conception of the common good is presented as a purely political conception of persons that is used to define the constraints on constitutional essentials that can be supported in a democratic society by an overlapping consensus of reasonable comprehensive theories. On Rawls's view, members of society may differ in their comprehensive theories of the good—they identify with different groups, support diverse causes, value competing goals, and endorse different standards for honor, success, beauty, achievement, and other thick aesthetic and moral concepts. Despite this diversity in their first-order conceptions of the good, Rawls argues that these individuals can see themselves as sharing the common higher-order project of formulating and pursuing a life plan. As such, they can recognize a shared, highest-order interest in being able to develop and exercise what Rawls refers to as their two moral powers: their capacity to form a substantive conception of the good and their capacity to regulate their conduct by principles of right (1971, 19, 504–510).

Unlike Taylor's perfectionism, Rawls grounds what I am calling the generic interests conception of the common good in a purely political standpoint. This is a standpoint that is available to members of a pluralistic modern society from which they can see themselves as sharing in a common project—developing and exercising their basic moral powers in the pursuit of a personal, first-order conception of the good life. This highest-order standpoint doesn't compete with the comprehensive views that individuals formulate and embrace as their first-order conception of the good.

Rather, the interest in being able to formulate, pursue, and revise a life plan is presupposed in the pursuit of any first-order life plan and, with this, the interest in having the basic or generic capacities that are presupposed in the formulation and pursuit of any such first-order conception.

In Rawls's political theory, these generic interests set the terms for the just operation of the "basic structure" of society, a term that Rawls uses for "the way in which the major social institutions distribute fundamental rights and duties and determine the division of advantages from social coopera-tion" (1971, 7). These interests ground the constraints that members of a lib-eral democratic community can accept for determining the constitutional essentials of society (Freeman 2000). Within what Rawls calls "justice as fairness," securing the generic interests conception of the common good for all citizens is given strict priority over the pursuit of the particular, personal goals that constitute each individual's personal conception of the good. In other words, the basic interests of some individuals cannot be compromised or traded in order to achieve greater personal good for other members of the community.

4.6.3 A Natural Law Formulation

The claim that frameworks can share a commitment to a particular concep-tion of the common good while differing in their background commitments is further illustrated by the defense that natural law theorist John Finnis offers for what I am calling the generic interests conception of the common good. Finnis, like Taylor, embraces a realist, perfectionist view of the common good. He says, "there is a 'common good' for human beings, inasmuch as life, knowledge, play, aesthetic experience, friendship, religion, and freedom in practical reasonableness are good for any and every person" (2011, 155). Also like Taylor, Finnis argues that the "point or the common good" of the polit-ical community is securing the "ensemble of material and other conditions that tend to favour the realization, by each individual in the community, of his or her personal development" (2011, 154).

Like Rawls, Finnis treats certain goods as fundamental because of the crit-ical role they play in realizing the personal development of the individual. This shared interest in personal development grounds a claim to access these goods and constitutes the focus for social collaboration. In this sense, we might say that Finnis offers a view that is both political and metaphysical. It is political in the Rawlsian sense of offering a set of reasons that have purchase on, or constitute reasons for, reasonable individuals who are pursuing diverse conceptions of their individual good. But it is metaphysical in the sense that personal development is treated as an objective good that is enriched by the constitutive goods of life, knowledge, play, aesthetic experience, friendship, and so on. In this regard, Finnis can be seen as holding that the highest-order standpoint that Rawls regards as a purely political perspective represents a deep moral insight into the human good—that is, into the nature of the first-order life plans that individuals should be encouraged to adopt and pursue.

For my present purposes the point is that, despite this disagreement, these thinkers can be seen as supporting a version of what I am calling the basic or generic interests conception of the common good. In different ways, they each recognize that individuals share in common a set of fundamental interests that relate to their ability to formulate, pursue, and revise a life plan and to engage in relationships of meaning with others and that it is the purpose of a just social order to provide the supports necessary for individuals to enjoy the fair value of this capacity.

4.6.4 An Institutional Utilitarian Formulation

Finally, in different ways, each of the thinkers just mentioned argues against the adequacy of purely consequentialist moral or political theories. Nevertheless, the generic interests conception of the common good can also be formulated within a broadly consequentialist framework. For brevity I mention two strategies for doing this. The first is what Russel Hardin calls institutional utilitarianism (Hardin 1988). This is a form of utilitarianism in that it holds that the goodness of outcomes is the foundational concern of morality and that the good should be understood in broadly welfarist terms. However, unlike traditional act utilitarianism, which brings this foundational concern to bear directly on the evaluation of individual acts, institutional utilitarianism brings this foundational concern to bear on the choice of institutions that are to regulate social interaction.

Hardin justifies this focus on institutions on several grounds. One is the common assumption that individuals are generally better judges of their interests than third parties and that institutions that empower individuals to advance their own welfare will produce a greater net utility than institutions that attempt to allocate advantages and burdens directly to individuals.

A second, and related, ground is that we often lack the information necessary to make meaningful interpersonal comparisons of welfare. [21] This ground can have two interpretations. On the contingent interpretation, such information is available in principle but gathering and processing it in practice would be so expensive and morally intrusive that it is either infeasible or possibly self-defeating. On a more substantive interpretation, such information is unavailable because it simply doesn't exist. This can be because there is no way to construct a single, coherent interpersonal utility that can preserve the many different valuations of the diverse individuals in a society. But even if this skeptical view is mistaken, it is not sufficient to establish that such a utility function is possible. Rather, it must also be the case that there is a single, unique way of constructing such a utility. Otherwise, the problem is that there are too many ways of doing this and there are no value-neutral grounds for preferring one representation over another.

In the absence of social consensus regarding the information that should be used to generate interpersonal welfare comparisons, Hardin argues, we should seek to design institutions that "secure mutual advantage for all even though there can be no interpersonal weighings of advantages" (1988, 76). We do this by erecting institutions that protect certain basic interests of persons, securing the integrity and security of their person, their holdings, their privacy, and securing their ability to speak, associate, and form relationships of meaning and significance.

The argument for basic rights in this approach is Paretian: guaranteeing basic rights makes no one worse off and creates the institutional setting in which individual and collective action can take place through which persons can advance their own interests as they understand them. Rights are essential to addressing collective action problems that would arise without the security they provide. As a result, on this view, "We constrain individuals' choices of strategy in order to produce a better outcome than would have resulted from unconstrained choices" (Hardin 1988, 80).

Institutional utilitarianism supports the generic interest conception of the common good to the extent that it marks out certain interests of individuals as sufficiently fundamental that we are justified in erecting social institutions to safeguard and advance their cultivation and pursuit. Moreover, social institutions are to safeguard these interests not for a select few, but for every person.

---

[21] I discuss the issues raised in this paragraph in more detail in §6.7.3.

4.6.5 An Objective Consequentialist Formulation

A different, although not mutually exclusive, way to formulate the generic interests view of the common good within a broadly utilitarian framework is to deny that the good is a single dimension onto which the diversity of all value can be mapped. If there is a diversity of goods that cannot be commensurated onto a single scale of comparison, then there is no single domain of goodness for decision-makers to maximize. At best, there is a set of dimensions of goodness, each of which is capable of ranking or ordering alternatives for choice, but which cannot be reconciled into a single, all-things-considered utility function.

There is a sense in which Henry Sidgwick was a pluralist of this sort in that he argued that there is no single standpoint from which to integrate or reconcile the claims of individual self-concern and impartial social concern. This is analogous to positing two goods, each of which make normative claims on us, but whose respective demands cannot be reconciled in a single perspective—such as a weighted average.

Sidgwick represents the subjectivist wing of utilitarian theories. In contrast, David Brink (1989) has defended what he refers to as "objective utilitarianism," where the modifier "objective" is intended to provide a contrast with subjective theories that reduce human welfare to mental states such as pleasure or desire satisfaction. Brink claims that it is this subjectivism that makes classical utilitarian theories prey to objections concerning the distribution of welfare because the subjective mental states of each individual are summed together to give a single aggregate utility score to the community. Instead, he proposes a non-reductive, naturalistic account of human welfare whose primary components include the reflective pursuit and realization by agents of reasonable life projects and the development of personal and social relationships of mutual concern and commitment.

Brink argues that his objective account of the good is distribution-sensitive because basic goods such as health, nutrition, and education are either necessary conditions for the existence of value, or they are all-purpose means that enable individuals to pursue a wide range of individual life plans (1989, 272). Brink's theory is still utilitarian, in that it is consequentialist and welfarist—it is just that this view treats welfare as a set of objective goods that cannot be reconciled into a single higher-order good. By defining welfare in terms of the development and exercise of certain basic intellectual and affective capacities, he argues that objective utilitarianism does not permit trade-offs between access to basic goods for increases in social utility.[22]

The point of these remarks is to illustrate that the generic interests conception of the common good can be formulated within a variety of theoretical frameworks and that within these different frameworks those interests help to define the terms on which the basic social institutions of a decent society should be regulated and organized. It is also helpful to survey the justificatory strategies that different approaches use in supporting institutions that safeguard and advance these generic interests, since many of these justificatory strategies can be deployed outside of the narrow frameworks in which they are discussed here.

For instance, the arguments deployed by institutional utilitarians are available to a wide range of non-utilitarian frameworks. This is because other frameworks often recognize the importance of consequences, individual welfare, and collective action, even if they also recognize as fundamental other normative claims that utilitarians reject or view as derivative from specifically utilitarian assumptions.

In the course of the present work, I gravitate toward Rawls's purely political presentation of the highest-order perspective from which individuals

---

[22] See Brink (1992). One reason that this conception of the common good may go unrecognized, or may be greeted with skepticism, is that certain of its formulations are easily confused with the corporate conception. Classical utilitarianism resembles the corporate conception because it identifies the good with a subjective mental state, such as pleasure, and then evaluates states of affairs in terms of the net utility score of the social aggregate. One of the basic objections to classical utilitarianism is that its focus on aggregate utility makes it insensitive to questions of the distribution of welfare between individuals. In principle, if persecuting a minority yields a higher aggregate utility score than a policy of equal treatment, then it would be justifiable. As Rawls puts it, "classical utilitarianism treats the political community as a single entity, thereby focusing moral and political deliberation on how best to maximize the overall well being of this corporate individual" (1971, 22–33). What is important for our present purposes is not the accuracy of Rawls's objection, but the fact that it appears to target what I am calling the corporate conception of the common good.

Other versions of utilitarianism, however, attempt to avoid this pitfall.

This is a generic interests conception of the common good, then, in the sense that it defines the common good in terms of a set of interests that members of the community share and have reason to promote both in their own case, and with respect to every other member of the community as well. On this view, pursuit of the common good involves creating the personal and social conditions that enable agents to develop and exercise these basic capacities, including steps to provide agents with access to the basic material resources and conditions required for the exercise of these capacities.

Brink's objective utilitarianism is an ambitious attempt to provide a thick, non-reductive, naturalistic account of human welfare that can serve as the centerpiece of a consequentialist moral theory. Contractarians who embrace the generic interests conception of the common good reject consequentialism and its derivation of the right from the good. They are also deeply impressed by the pluralism in contemporary society surrounding thick conceptions of the good and are, therefore, dubious of the prospect of achieving societal consensus about such complex issues. Whereas Brink deploys his arguments as part of a larger program of naturalistic moral realism, Rawls sees these constraints as constructs that result from an overlapping consensus.

can see themselves as sharing a set of basic interests. This is because I take this approach to have the broadest appeal in the sense that it presupposes the weakest premises. That is, this purely political perspective allows us to identify interests that others may wish to ground in more metaphysically baroque frameworks, or within larger traditions that Rawls regards as comprehensive conceptions of the good, without having to take a stand on which of those comprehensive theories of the good is correct. I am not opposed to efforts to vindicate such theories; I merely regard them as relying on stronger premises than are needed for the purpose of the argument I am making here.

Finally, I gravitate also to Hardin's institutional utilitarianism since it allows us to consider and respond to collective action problems while recognizing that in a pluralistic society in which there are potentially as many ways of making interpersonal comparisons of welfare as there are distinct conceptions of the good life, we should evaluate the effects of social institutions on terms that respect the highest-order interests of each person in having real freedom to pursue the projects and plans from which they derive personal welfare or well-being.

4.7 The Egalitarian Research Imperative

4.7.1 Stating the Imperative

Traditional proponents of a research imperative equated the common good with the corporate conception. By arguing that "ordinary" sources of avoidable morbidity and mortality do not pose a threat to the common good, Jonas relegated research with human subjects to the realm of the private ends of private individuals. In light of the analysis provided here, we can say that Jonas was correct to argue that there is no social imperative to carry out research grounded in the corporate conception of the common good.

In contrast, the generic interest conception of the common good does ground a social imperative to support a wide range of research, not only in the sphere of individual and public health but with respect to the operation of any social institution that impacts the basic interests of that community's members. Because this imperative is grounded in the fundamental interests of individuals and not in the role-related obligations of any profession, it is binding on, and applies to the conduct of, a much wider range of stakeholders than frameworks in orthodox research ethics. However, because the PC on the pursuit of the common good is much more robust, this research imperative does not empower professionals to make arbitrary judgments against research participants. This is because the research enterprise itself must be consistent with respect for the generic interests of both the stakeholders to the research enterprise and the members of the larger community in whose name research is carried out and who are expected to be the eventual beneficiaries of the advances it creates.

To unpack these various claims, it is useful to begin by formulating what I call the egalitarian research imperative:

The Egalitarian Research Imperative: There is a strong social imperative to enable communities to create, sustain, and engage in research understood as a scheme of social cooperation that respects the status of stakeholders as free and equal and that functions to generate information and interventions needed to enable their basic social systems to equitably, effectively, and efficiently safeguard and advance the basic interests of their constituent members.

Clarifying how this imperative is grounded in the basic interests conception of the common good will enable us to justify its particular relevance to health-related social systems, to explain the sense in which research must be understood as a scheme of social cooperation between free and equal people, and to explain two senses in which this is an egalitarian imperative.

4.7.2   Grounding the Imperative

The egalitarian research imperative is grounded in three claims. The first is that a decent social order strives to preserve and advance the common good, understood as the set of basic interests that individuals require to be able to formulate, pursue, and revise a life plan. These interests can be set back or thwarted by ignorance, poverty, crime, oppression, social exclusion, lack of access to economic opportunity, environmental hazard, contagion, sickness, and disease. To avoid these pitfalls and to realize the fair value of these interests, a decent social order will include a wide range of social institutions designed to safeguard the basic interests of individuals across this diversity of spheres and domains.

Because the basic interests of individuals can be set back by sickness, injury, disease and other threats to individual and public health, a just social order will include social institutions for safeguarding and advancing the basic interests of individuals in the sphere of public and individual physical and mental health. These social institutions include health care systems, such as hospitals, clinics, and similar venues for health care delivery, as well as the various organs of public health and health policy within a community.

The provision of medical and public health services is thus part of the basic structure of a just society because the provision of these services is necessary to preserve or to realize the ability of community members to function as moral and political equals—to have the real opportunity to exercise their moral powers, free from arbitrary social interference, to formulate, pursue, and revise a reasonable life plan. Rawls makes a similar point when he argues that the provision of medical care falls into the category of a primary good—a good that is valuable to individuals because of its ability to support the generic interests needed to pursue any from among a wide range of life plans. As he puts it,

> provision for medical care, as with primary goods generally, is to meet the needs and requirements of citizens as free and equal. Such care falls under the general means necessary to underwrite fair equality of opportunity and our capacity to take advantage of our basic rights and liberties, and thus to be normal and fully cooperating members of society over a complete life. (2001, 174)

Second, the egalitarian research imperative is grounded in the claim that the generic interests of individuals define the space of moral and political equality. Because individuals share the generic interest in having the real freedom to formulate, pursue, and revise a life plan and because these interests are fundamental to the agency and welfare of individuals, these interests define the respect in which community members have equal claim to equal treatment. Every community member has an equal claim on the basic social institutions of their community that function to secure and preserve the fair value of their basic interests.

As a result, there is a moral and a political imperative that social institutions that affect the basic interests of community members function effectively, efficiently, and equitably. The imperative that such systems function effectively is grounded in the importance of the basic interests of individuals to their ability to function as agents and to shape and pursue a life plan of meaning and significance. It is not sufficient that such institutions be designed with the intent or the purpose of securing the fair value of these interests. They must possess the knowledge and the means of intervening in the world to bring about these ends in actual practice.

There is a moral and a social imperative that those institutions function efficiently, in the sense of securing and advancing the basic interests of community members with as little wasted effort and the fewest wasted resources as possible. This imperative derives from the fact that these institutions must meet the needs of all community members within resource constraints. These resource constraints can derive from various sources, including the fact that just limits must be set on the share of social resources dedicated to social systems in different spheres. No community can dedicate all of its social resources to education or to health care. Rather, every community is constrained to secure and advance the basic interests of its members across a range of spheres, including education; protecting and promoting safety, security, and human rights; and ensuring fair equality of opportunity in social and economic spheres and in the realm of health. Reducing wasted time, effort, and human and material resources allows institutions to achieve better outcomes or to achieve the same outcomes for more people with the same bundle of resources.

Finally, there is also a moral and political imperative for the basic social institutions of a community to function equitably—to preserve and advance the generic interests of all community members with equal safety and efficacy. The imperative of equity derives from the equal claim that all community members have on the basic structures of their society. Disparities in the ability of basic social institutions to advance this end for different members of the community in one sphere can translate into disparities in the ability of those community members to take advantage of opportunities in other spheres (Bloom and Canning 2000; Jamison et al. 2013). This includes increasing the burden of avoidable sickness, injury, disease, and premature mortality (Dwyer-Lindgren et al. 2017; Forde et al. 2020). If such disparities are not addressed, they can produce gaps in opportunity for affected community members that persist and compound over time (Jamison et al. 2013; Bloom and Canning 2000; Ridley et al. 2020).

For example, disparities in access to nutrition or basic public or individual health services can prevent individuals from taking full advantage of educational opportunities. Shortfalls in each of these areas can translate into a lack of effective access to social and economic opportunities that would otherwise be available to the individuals in question. Physical environments that exclude persons with disabilities reduce their ability to access opportunities in a range of spheres, including education, health care, participation in social life, and the ability to participate meaningfully in the political process. Even when such exclusions do not result from social animus, they can produce cascades of deprivation that prevent individuals with particular traits from being able to enjoy the fair value of their basic interests in being able to formulate, pursue, and revise a life plan.

In other cases, disparities in the operation of a community's basic social institutions stem from and perpetuate histories of unequal treatment rooted in prejudice, domination, and abuse (Cogburn 2019). Racism, sexism, ableism, and other forms of unfair and oppressive treatment deny the moral equality of individuals on the basis of an arbitrary characteristic and translate into social practices that deny and erode the freedom of individuals in those groups to enjoy the fair value of their most basic interests.

The imperative that the basic social institutions of a community function with equity entails a moral and political responsibility to identify and then to address gaps in the ability of these institutions to secure and advance the basic interests of community members. This imperative is particularly strong in cases where patterns of disparity persist through time and reflect histories of indifference toward, or unjust treatment of, individuals in particular groups, such as groups defined by racial or ethnic characteristics, religious or sexual orientation, gender, or disability status.

Thirdly, the egalitarian research imperative is grounded in the intimate connection between the evidence and information that research produces and the ability of the basic social systems of a community to effectively, efficiently, and equitably safeguard and advance the generic interests of the individuals and groups who depend on them. In particular, how to safeguard and advance the basic interests of persons involves inherently causal questions, and in areas such as individual and public health, the state of current knowledge is not sufficient to support the development of safe and effective interventions (understood broadly to include policies, practices, procedures, drugs, and devices) without carefully controlled empirical testing. As a result, research with human participants is often the only way to generate the knowledge necessary to understand the factors in a particular sphere that influence the basic interests of individuals and to understand the relative merits of different strategies for securing or advancing those interests for the diverse constituents of a community.

The imperative to ensure that a community's basic social institutions can safely, efficiently, and effectively secure and advance the basic interests of its members combined with the dependence of such efforts on carefully designed empirical testing entails a social imperative to use social authority and resources to promote research that generates the information necessary to improve the ability of basic social institutions to fulfill their special moral purpose.

Moreover, because the research enterprise is understood broadly, as a division of social labor among a wide range of parties, this imperative is also understood broadly. It includes investing social resources, founding institutions, and establishing the rules and norms that are necessary to promote scientific research across the full lifecycle of knowledge development and deployment. It also includes the use of social authority to align the incentives of a wide range of actors who produce health-related information with the common good. Intellectual property laws, patent protections, the evidentiary thresholds necessary to secure regulatory approval, and the scope of the indication for which interventions can be marketed and sold are a few examples of policy decisions that shape the incentives of funding agencies, private sector firms, researchers, regulators, and other actors. Because these activities involve the exercise of state authority and because these decisions impact which questions are likely to be investigated in research and whether gaps in the ability of basic social institutions to advance the basic interests of community members are widened or closed, they implicate questions of justice and must be justifiable to community members as advancing the common good.

How the research enterprise is organized is a question of justice because that enterprise calls into action the social authority, institutions, and resources of the state to create a division of social labor that must advance a particular social purpose. This moral purpose is generating information that is necessary to close gaps in the ability of the basic social institutions of a community to secure and advance the basic interests of its members. The point is not that health or health-related research is a key to solving or resolving all social ills—it is not.[23] Rather, the point is that the ability of individuals to be

---

[23] Discussing my human development approach to international research, Shamoo and Resnik characterize my view as holding that researchers have a duty to do more than ensure fair benefits: "They must rectify past injustice and promote social, economic, and political development in the host nation" (2009, 335). I discuss the inadequacies of the fair benefits view in chapter 8 and elaborate the human development approach in chapter 9. Shamoo and Resnik appear to confuse two ideas that are related to the current discussion. The first idea is that the entitlements of community members are shaped by a range of background considerations of justice. In particular, community members have a claim on one another to social institutions that advance their common good, and the organs of research are such institutions. Additionally, inadequacies in the capacity of a community's

able to formulate, pursue, and revise a life plan is affected by the way a variety of social arrangements are designed, implemented, and regulated. The health-related institutions within a community are one element within this larger social division of labor, and their ability to fulfill their special social mission effectively, efficiently, and equitably is closely connected to the terms on which the research enterprise is organized.

Additionally, the moral and social imperative to support research with humans represents the fact that the evidence and information that it produces is an important public good on which a diverse array of stakeholders rely to discharge important moral and social responsibilities. To illustrate this point, it is worth considering the sense in which knowledge is the most important output of research with human participants, the sense in which this knowledge represents an important public good, and how myriad stakeholders rely on this good to discharge important responsibilities.

4.7.3 The Knowledge Research Produces Is a Public Good

Although it is common to speak about drugs, devices, policies, or practices as the units of translation—as the entities that move from the bench to the bedside and that are the fruits of research—this view is fundamentally inadequate (Kimmelman and London 2015). In particular, although the drug, device, or other intervention may be the most tangible product of research, these concrete products alone have no social utility. A drug, for example, is merely a substance that at one concentration may be effectively inert and at

---

basic structures to fulfill their social purpose is often a major source of avoidable morbidity and mortality in a community and such inadequacies can result from a variety of causes, including domestic injustice and unjust dealings with foreign entities. The second idea is that these background considerations have to factor into our evaluation of cross-national research initiatives. Shamoo and Resnik assume that this second idea entails that researchers alone are responsible for rectifying all of the injustices in a community. This erroneous interpretation of my view results from trying to shoehorn questions of justice, at a social level, into the narrow confines of the IRB triangle. The obligation to ensure that the basic structures of a community fulfill their social mission is shared by a wide range of parties. But researchers are not charged with rectifying all past wrongs in a community. Rather, they have a duty to ensure that research with humans addresses the priority health needs of host communities and expands the capacity of their health-related social systems to advance the common good. They share this duty with numerous parties, including local governments. Recognizing that research is part of a larger social system, recognizing that how research functions can affect the operation of key aspects of these social systems, and requiring researchers to take this into account when planning and engaging in research activities is not the same as holding that researchers have the kind of expansive duty that Shamoo and Resnik infer.

other concentrations can be lethal. A device alone is a piece of hardware. In order for these things to produce a net advantage—a benefit that is sufficient to offset any attending adverse effects—they must be used properly. For simplicity, we can limit our discussion to drug development, but the claims here generalize.

The true product of drug development is not a compound or an artifact; it is the knowledge of whether and how a particular chemical compound can be used to provide therapeutic or prophylactic advantage to patients. This knowledge is critical to the ability of actors who consume this information to make decisions that implicate the use of scarce social resources and that affect the basic interests of community members.

The knowledge about whether and how a substance can be used to produce beneficial effects includes the set or "ensemble" of factors that modulate its effects in use (Kimmelman 2012; Kimmelman and London 2015). This set of factors includes how to distinguish the population of patients that the drug can help from those it cannot. This is often referred to as the indication for a drug, and it includes understanding how an intervention's effects might differ in patients with various clinical characteristics and which features of patients might put them at elevated risk of experiencing adverse events. This set of factors also includes the knowledge of the dosage at which a drug must be given to unlock its therapeutic potential and the window outside of which it is either ineffective or harmful. It includes the frequency or schedule for delivering a drug to ensure the proper concentration and the window outside of which the drug is likely to again be ineffective or harmful. It includes any special diagnostic steps that might be needed to monitor recipients and any co-interventions that are required to amplify benefits or to mitigate adverse effects. It also includes an understanding of how that drug interacts with other treatments, including which combinations of drugs to avoid because of their potential for producing adverse events.

This practical knowledge is not the only fruit of clinical translation. The results of research also provide information that supports or undermines the larger theories of disease pathophysiology and intervention mechanism that drove the development of that intervention and that are likely to drive further development activities (Kimmelman and London 2015). In particular, intervention development is often driven by background theories about the pathophysiology of disease, factors that increase or mitigate susceptibility or disease progression, and the ability of interventions of a certain kind to alter mechanisms that are important to the lifecycle of disease.

These theories often drive drug development by highlighting mechanisms to exploit and suggesting pathways through which those mechanisms might be influenced with the fewest adverse events. Repeated failures to develop interventions that leverage these insights for therapeutic benefit cast doubt on the credibility of those underlying theories. Likewise, practical success in exploiting such insights reinforces the utility of particular models and encourages their use in understanding the source and nature of disease and how it might be delayed, reversed, or cured in both future research and in clinical practice.

Although a drug or a device may consist of materials that are scarce or that constitute the intellectual property of a particular person or firm, the practical knowledge necessary to unlock its therapeutic or prophylactic potential and the evidence this provides about broader understandings of sickness, injury, or disease constitute a public good. It is a public good because a wide range of stakeholders rely on this knowledge to discharge socially important obligations or to carry out activities that relate directly to the common good and so are the subject of a just social order. It also has features of a public good in the economic sense (Schaefer et al. 2009, 68). This information is non-rival, meaning that these stakeholders can rely on and make use of it without thereby diminishing its content or value or reducing the share of information that is available to those other stakeholders. It is also difficult to exclude others from using that knowledge once it has been disseminated. On the one hand, a drug or a device cannot produce practical benefits without the knowledge of how to use it. On the other hand, the (un)successful development of a particular drug necessarily provides evidence about the utility of the broader theories of disease and drug mechanism that contributed to the intervention's development.

How the research system is organized thus has a profound effect on the ability of a wide range of stakeholders to discharge their moral responsibilities (London 2005, 2019; London, Kimmelman, and Carlisle 2012; Wenner 2016, 2018). These stakeholders include policy makers, health systems, individual health care providers, patients, and the other scientists who build on this information.

Policy makers depend on reliable medical information to determine which health practices to promote or discourage, which public and individual health goals to prioritize, which mix of strategies to adopt to advance those priorities, and where scarce health resources can best be invested in order to promote the efficacy, efficiency, and equity of health systems.

Health systems cannot make an efficient use of scarce resources without information about how best to prevent, diagnose, and treat the wide range of afflictions likely to be represented in the populations they serve. Because of the variability of disease, uncertainty about its etiology, and the likely effects of different strategies for preventing or otherwise intervening on those conditions, carefully controlled trials in humans are often the only way to generate this information.

Individual providers within health systems are similarly dependent on research findings to discharge their fiduciary duties to patients. Their ability to advance the medical interests of patients, consistent with the way those patients understand those interests within their larger conception of the good and their broader life plan, hinges on the quality of the information they possess about the relative merits of interventions and practices available to them.

Likewise, patients cannot effectively engage with health systems and providers to protect and advance their own interests without reliable medical information. This includes the information they need in order to understand their health status, to understand medical conditions they experience, and to comprehend the relative merits and demerits of the options available for prevention, diagnosis, or treatment.

Finally, the process of drug development is itself a collaborative activity that is extended across time in which medical evidence is produced and consumed by a wide range of actors. For example, the information produced in pre-clinical research can have implications for the use of a drug in clinical practice, but it is most directly relevant to other researchers who are also conducting pre-clinical research or who will conduct early phase studies in humans. Similarly, early-phase studies in humans explore the various parameters of a drug's use that must be understood in order to unlock its therapeutic potential. These studies too can be relevant to clinical practice, but their primary and most direct purpose is to identify elements within the ensemble of knowledge and practices that are necessary to use a drug to produce clinical benefit. Once these various elements have been identified, ensembles of materials, knowledge, and practices can be subjected to confirmatory testing in large late-phase trials. These trials are crucial to establishing the relative therapeutic or prophylactic merits of an intervention, and the information that they produce is the most directly relevant to the widest range of stakeholders. Nevertheless, these studies build on a prior network of research and contribute to the evidence base that supports subsequent investigation.

The ability of these various stakeholders to safely, effectively, and efficiently address the health needs of community members in practice, or to carry out the research that is necessary to effectuate this goal, depends critically on the quality of the evidence that is generated in research and its relevance to the ability of that community's basic social structures to secure and advance the basic interests of that community's members. Poor quality research that generates misleading or biased information detracts from the ability of stakeholders in basic social institutions to effectively and efficiently secure and advance the basic interests of community members. Similarly, disparities in which health needs are the subject of research and investigation can create or exacerbate disparities in the ability of these different stakeholders to meet the needs of community members, or to meet those needs with equal efficacy, safety, or efficiency (Dresser 1992; Weijer and Crouch 1999; London and Kimmelman 2016; Basu and Gujral 2020).

The egalitarian research imperative reflects the status of the information that research produces as a public good and the moral importance of ensuring that this information is of sufficient quality, reliability, and relevance that it can advance the moral mission of research. How the research enterprise is organized—from the questions that are chosen for investigation to the methods that are used to generate answers—is bound up with requirements of justice because these issues determine whether this activity can be justified as advancing the common good of community members. In other words, considerations of justice are raised by decisions that determine whether research contributes to improving or reducing the efficacy and the efficiency of practice and whether it serves to reduce and eliminate, or to create and exacerbate, disparities in the ability of health systems to meet needs of community members that relate directly and indirectly to their ability to formulate, pursue, and revise a reasonable life plan. I return to some concrete examples that illustrate these points in §4.9.

Although I have focused on health in this exposition, health systems are not the only social system that affects the basic interests of individuals. As a result, it is important that a framework for research ethics be of sufficient generality that it can apply to a wide range of research involving human participants (London 2005, 2006a, 2009; Kukla 2007; MacKay 2018). For example, both Kukla (2007) and MacKay (2018) discuss research that falls under the umbrella of social systems outside of the health sector, narrowly conceived. These include the effect of early education on opportunity, access to supplemental nutrition within social safety net programs, and the relative efficacy of different policies to prevent homelessness. As I have framed it here, the same arguments that support the egalitarian research imperative in the sphere of health would apply to any other context in which a social system has a direct impact on the basic interests of community members.

4.7.4 Egalitarian in Two Respects

The research imperative articulated here is egalitarian in two respects, each of which is grounded in the idea that free individuals "exist for their own sake and not for the sake of someone else" (Aristotle 982b25–27). It is egalitarian in the first respect in that the interests that it targets are shared by all community members. All community members depend on a variety of social systems, including health systems, to safeguard and advance their basic interest in being able to formulate, pursue, and revise a reasonable life plan. In order to be responsive to the moral and political status of individuals as free and equal persons, social systems must strive to eliminate gaps in the efficacy and efficiency with which they are capable of responding to the basic interests of the individuals in the community they serve. The normative force of the egalitarian research imperative derives from the importance of the needs that basic social systems address and the unique ability of the research enterprise to produce the information that enables those social systems to equitably, safely, and efficiently fulfill their social purpose.

This research imperative is also egalitarian in a second respect. This same concern for the basic interests of individuals that triggers the NC also provides the content to the PC on the forms of social interaction that are permissible means of advancing this goal. Coercion, domination, exploitation, neglect, abuse, and other forms of harmful or unfair treatment violate the practical constraint on acceptable ways of attempting to advance the common good because they undermine the status of the affected individuals as free and equal. They compromise the moral freedom of individuals to the extent that they secure access to their person or their participation in an activity without regard to the place of that activity in the plans or projects of that individual. They undermine their status as moral equals because they treat the interest of some as sufficient to license showing lesser regard to the basic interests of the affected parties.

It is a particular strength of this view that this practical constraint is not an exogenous value imposed on research from the outside. Rather, it is internal to the conception of research as a social undertaking that requires the sustained and voluntary collaboration and cooperation of many different stakeholders over time. The generic interests of the diverse parties who participate in and make this undertaking possible merit equal respect. There are thus no grounds to justify a division of social labor in which some stakeholders are empowered to show less moral concern for the basic interests of others or to relegate them to a position of subordination or domination. The egalitarian research imperative thus does not justify empowering researchers to conscript unwitting participants into medical research as "soldiers of science" or to "play god" by selecting small samples of individuals whose interests can permissibly be sacrificed to the greater good (McDermott 1967, 39).[24] In chapter 6, I outline a framework for evaluating research risks that reconciles promoting the common good with the requirement to show equal regard for the basic interests of study participants in the process.

In the previous chapter I argued that Wertheimer's principle of permissible exploitation (PPE) revealed fault lines running through the foundations of research ethics. One of these consists in the asymmetric treatment of the interests of various parties. In orthodox research ethics, even when individuals suffer from health problems that threaten their capacity to form, pursue, or revise a reasonable life plan, this is not sufficient to generate a duty on anyone's part to carry out research of any kind. Research, even if it would address such basic needs, is treated as a largely optional, private undertaking. Nevertheless, if those same individuals are involved in research, then their basic interests ground robust deontological protections that place what Wertheimer sees as significant limits on the liberties of both researchers and participants. This creates an inefficiency that PPE attempts to resolve by weakening constraints on exploitative, unfair, or disrespectful treatment. As we saw, PPE could be seen as sanctioning some wrongdoing in the form of exploitative, unfair, or unjust research relationships as a way to remedy the overly permissive attitude in orthodox research ethics to the neglect of important health needs without creating an overly demanding set of moral requirements in the process.

---

[24] In this regard, the view I defend here captures the insight of Jonas that "human experimentation for whatever purpose is always also a responsible, nonexperimental, definitive dealing with the subject himself and not even the noblest purpose abrogates the obligations this involves (1969, 220) and Kukla's claim that "the research enterprise gives investigators no license to compromise citizens' moral entitlements to justice, respect, and welfare protection" (2007, 184).

The egalitarian research imperative rejects the fundamentally asymmetric view of the basic interests of persons shared by both orthodox research ethics and PPE. Rather than empowering a few to dominate their compatriots in order to promote social progress, the egalitarian research imperative enjoins communities to provide various social supports for, and to encourage the development of, a division of social labor in which free and equal individuals can serve the common good by voluntarily cooperating within a social system that is arranged to ensure that their cumulative efforts produce an important public good. The same fundamental concern for the basic interests of persons that grounds the imperative to generate the knowledge needed to bridge gaps between the basic interests of persons and the ability of the basic social institutions in their community to meet those needs grounds a social imperative to ensure that these social systems are designed to attract the voluntary participation of study participants, just as it attracts the voluntary participation of researchers and other stakeholders.

The idea that a just community can discharge its responsibilities to citizens without abrogating the rights of its constituent members is neither radical nor new. In the *Politics*, Aristotle argues that "constitutions that aim at the common advantage are in effect rightly framed in accordance with absolute justice," because a polity is a "partnership of free persons" (1279a17–22). Democracies require representatives and leaders, but candidates for these positions are chosen from volunteers who see public service as part of a rewarding personal life plan. Just states need physicians and teachers, researchers and engineers, lawyers and judges, and a dizzying array of professionals who discharge important responsibilities of basic social institutions. A just state cannot operate without these professionals, but they are selected from the ranks of volunteers who see in such careers opportunities to develop their talents and abilities, earn a living, join a profession, and contribute to the common good.

Promoting a system of research involving human participants requires the thoughtful implementation of concrete social incentives that encourage a diverse set of parties to take up, as part of their individual life plan, advancing an important element or component of this larger division of social labor. It also involves providing a system of concrete social assurances that this division of social labor will not be co-opted for parochial or partisan purposes and that in voluntarily participating in this scheme of social cooperation, no stakeholder will be subject to deception, injustice, or abuse (see chapter 7).

4.8 A Scheme of Cooperation among Free and Equal Persons

4.8.1 To Whom Does the Imperative Apply?

At the most general level, the egalitarian research imperative applies to all of the individuals who comprise a community. The reason for this is that it is individual community members who owe duties of justice to one another. However, as we saw in §4.6, a just social order represents a division of social labor through which free and equal people divide responsibility for securing the basic interests of community members. Individual community members thus bear a responsibility to create and to support a division of social labor that advances the common good. One of the ways that individuals discharge the egalitarian research imperative is by delegating to government the critical responsibility to create and maintain the infrastructure, rules, and resources that comprise a functioning research system.

Even if we view individuals as delegating this responsibility to government, they retain at least three important residual obligations. The first residual obligation is to hold political leaders accountable for fulfilling their moral and political obligation to discharge this duty. The second is to refrain from acting in ways that conflict with, subvert, or undermine the ability of the various parties to this division of labor to discharge the responsibilities they take on within this scheme of social cooperation. The third is to be prepared to support the activities of these stakeholders, especially when this can be done in a way that does not require a significant compromise in one's basic or personal interests.

On this view, the primary responsibility for discharging the substantive requirements of the egalitarian research imperative in practice falls to governments. Governments are responsible for allocating resources and creating the institutions and systems of rules that are necessary to effectuate three goals. The first is to ensure that the research enterprise functions to generate the knowledge needed to bridge gaps between the basic interests of community members and the ability of the basic social institutions in their community to meet those needs. The second is to ensure that the system of norms, rules, and incentives that govern the research enterprise align the personal and parochial interests of stakeholders with the promotion of this end. This includes providing credible public assurance to all stakeholders that no party has the ability to co-opt this division of social labor to exclusively advance their own parochial interests. The third is to provide credible public assurance to all stakeholders that as each seeks to pursue their personal interests in this arena—to seek profit, career advancement, or access to novel medical interventions—no party will be subject to domination, exploitation, abuse, or other forms of unfair or harmful treatment.

Exactly how this social division of labor should be organized is a question of mechanism design. Moreover, it seems reasonable that different communities could adopt different approaches that rely, to greater or lesser degrees, on public and private entities. At one extreme would be an effort to fund, regulate, and carry out research entirely with public funds and within public institutions. At the other extreme would be an effort to create a public system of rules and regulations within which the various activities in the research enterprise are carried out entirely by private enterprise. In the United States and most other economically developed nations there is a mix of public funding and public infrastructure, such as governmental agencies and institutions, that interact with a range of private entities in a regulated market. The point I want to emphasize for present purposes is that, however this system is organized, governments retain a duty to monitor and adjust the system of rules and norms that create the strategic environment in which the various stakeholders to the research enterprise interact, with the goal of ensuring that this system advances the goals described in the previous paragraph.

Although national authorities should be regarded as having the default responsibility for fulfilling the egalitarian research imperative, the just and legitimate division of social labor within states entails that responsibility for carrying out particular strategies necessary to satisfy the egalitarian research imperative sometimes fall to regional, provincial or local health authorities. Similarly, it is possible that the community that is bound by the research imperative may be larger than the individual state. This is most clearly the case when states form larger bodies bound by common laws and policies that regulate the provision of individual or public health or the process of research and development. The European Union may represent such a body to the extent that its member states share common structures for drug development regulation and approval.

Larger collectives of this type can be bound by the egalitarian research imperative, but to the extent that national governments delegate responsibilities to such entities, they would nevertheless retain duties that are analogous to the duties that individuals retain when they delegate responsibility for fulfilling the egalitarian research imperative to states. Additionally, such extra-national agreements often utilize the local institutions of the states that are party to the collaboration and rely on the legal authority and enforcement mechanisms of those states to ensure compliance with agreed upon norms (Freeman 2006). Because extra-national agreements often supervene on the structures, rules, and authority of cooperating nations, national governments should still be seen as the default bearer of the responsibility for discharging the substantive requirements of the egalitarian research imperative. How this default is affected by factors such as prior histories of unjust interaction is dealt with in chapter 9.

In this respect, MacKay is correct to say that governments bear key duties in this area, since they have "duties of justice to provide their residents with access to particular types of goods, and/or to realize particular outcomes" (2017, 3). But it would be a mistake to assume that governments are the only parties who bear duties of justice that relate to the organization and functioning of the research enterprise. In particular, citizens retain the three obligations I described previously and private entities that conduct research have a responsibility to ensure that their activities contribute to the common good on terms that respect the status of other participants in this social undertaking as free and equal.

4.8.2 Prior Moral Claims

I argued in chapter 2 that orthodox research ethics tends to treat research as a private activity in the sense that it is not clearly constrained by its relationship to larger social purposes. I also argued that this view is bolstered by the tendency to conceptualize research as a set of goals and purposes that can be taken up by individuals and that stand in contrast to the goals and purposes of medical practice. As a result, orthodox research ethics tends to locate the moral epicenter of research in the IRB triangle, the discrete relationships between researchers and study participants.

The arguments I have presented here offer a very different account of research and its relationship to the larger purposes of a just social order. In particular, it is worth emphasizing that, on the view I am presenting here, the egalitarian research imperative enunciates a duty to create a certain kind of institutional order. This is an institutional order in which a broad range of stakeholders can collaborate in ways that produce an important public good.

This public good is the knowledge and the means necessary to effectively, efficiently, and equitably bridge gaps in the ability of that community's basic social structures to secure and advance the basic interests of that community's members.

Understanding research as a scheme of social cooperation invites us to consider the social arrangements that are necessary to identify priority knowledge gaps of this kind, understand the source and nature of the problems to which they relate, formulate strategies and interventions for addressing them, evaluate the relative merits of those strategies and interventions and then to make this knowledge and these interventions available on a widespread basis so that they can be incorporated into basic social institutions that are charged with securing and advancing the basic interests of community members. These social arrangements include the training of investigators, mechanisms for funding research, the terms on which interventions can be marketed and sold, the standards of evidence required to establish safety and efficacy, and so on.

This perspective also invites us to consider the wide range of actors who play a role in this division of social labor. Beyond the players within the IRB triangle, the stakeholders whose activities affect the ability of research to advance the common good include policy makers who shape intellectual property laws or in other ways influence funding allocations and priorities. It includes biotech companies, pharmaceutical firms, philanthropic organizations, and public institutions that sponsor research or carry it out. It includes regulators in the various institutions that set or enforce the rules for research oversight, and the bodies that perform research oversight functions including regulatory bodies that determine the standards for intervention approval and market access. It includes administrators in health systems and clinics where research is carried out and medical societies and professional organizations that set standards for medical practice and for professional conduct. It includes journal editors and bodies who create publishing guidelines that determine the standards of quality and for disclosure that research must satisfy in order to warrant publication. It includes patient advocacy groups whose lobbying, advertising, or funding activities influence politicians, study participants, clinicians, or other stakeholders.

The imperative to ensure that this division of social labor produces an important, public good entails that prior moral claims constrain how the infrastructure of the research enterprise can be used. The institutions, rules, and human and material resources that facilitate this scheme of social cooperation are not free for entrepreneurial agents—investigators, sponsors, regulators, consultants, or participants—to utilize solely to advance their private purposes, without regard for the way those purposes align with the common good.

Open societies are free to harness the power of the private sector and the profit motive to secure financing and to drive innovation, but it remains a duty of government to ensure that the rules, incentives, and constraints in this system align the parochial interests of these parties with the common good. Private firms may own the resources that they invest in the research enterprise, and public firms may invest resources that are derived from the investments of shareholders to whom they owe a fiduciary duty. But this is consistent with the claim that such resources cannot be deployed in the research enterprise solely to advance the parochial interests of these parties. Rather, engaging in the research enterprise entails a duty to ensure that human and material resources, and the infrastructure on which they rely, are used in the service of ends that contribute to identifying, investigating, and closing gaps in the ability of a community's basic social structures to secure and advance the basic interests of its respective members.

Private individuals and entities, academic researchers, academic medical centers, medical associations, disease advocacy groups, and pharmaceutical firms can play an important role in this division of social labor, but they do not have unlimited discretion over the way this system is used. This is because the prior claims of community members to social systems that safeguard and advance their basic interests constrain the goals that this system can be used to advance and the means that can be used to advance those goals.

Similarly, individual researchers, investors, and biotech or pharmaceutical firms may be drawn to research as an area in which they can use their intellectual, material, and human capital to secure profit, notoriety, and any number of private goods. All of these private goods and the motives that attach to them represent levers that can be used to incentivize participation in this division of social labor. But it is the responsibility of all of the stakeholders in this enterprise, including policy makers and regulators, to ensure that the strategic environment in which these parties interact aligns these parochial motives with the common good and constrains the extent to which those motives might undermine or subvert this end.

Finally, just as prior moral purposes constrain the ends to which the infrastructure of research can be used, the products of research are not a purely private good. Private firms may have intellectual property in the compounds and devices that represent the most visible fruits of research efforts. But, as I argued in §4.7.3, the knowledge that research produces is a public good on which myriad stakeholders rely to discharge important social and moral responsibilities. The conditions under which firms can market and sell products and the quality of the information needed before a product can be approved for use are centrally relevant to research ethics.

Because orthodox research ethics is so centrally focused on protecting the rights and welfare of study participants, it can be difficult to motivate concerns about the quality and relevance of the information that research is likely to produce if the studies in question do not place study participants at elevated risk. On the view I am articulating here, questions about the quality and relevance of the information generated in research, and about the efficiency with which that information is generated are centrally relevant to research ethics because they raise questions of justice. It is worth concluding with some brief examples that illustrate this point.

4.9 Examples of Neglected Issues

Three brief examples illustrate the way in which the activities of what are traditionally seen as private actors in this context raise questions of justice. These examples are drawn from work I have done with Jonathan Kimmelman and are presented in schematic form for brevity. Nevertheless, they provide an important contrast to the parochialism of orthodox research ethics.

Prior to regulatory approval of a new drug, private firms have a strong incentive to quickly conduct well-designed clinical trials. The reason is that they cannot market and sell their product—and thus reap a return on their investment—without generating evidence that establishes its safety and efficacy for a particular indication. The standards for approval set by regulatory agencies like the US Food and Drug Administration (FDA) thus play a critical role in determining the extent and the quality of the evidence that is available to clinicians, patients, policy makers, and health systems about the efficacy of a drug and its anticipated side effects in patients with a wide range of clinical characteristics. As a result, FDA standards for drug approval determine whether a new drug is tested in a narrow and homogenous population or whether it must be tested in more diverse populations that better reflects the characteristics and demographics of the population in which that drug is likely to be used.

Recently, the United States has seen a concerted push on the part of various stakeholders, including patient advocacy groups and pharmaceutical firms, to lower the evidentiary requirements necessary to secure drug approval in order to speed drugs to market. The moral arguments offered in support of such policies focus on the needs of patients who currently lack access to effective interventions and their interest in being able to accept greater risk in return for earlier access to novel interventions.

Reducing drug development timelines in this way, however, raises questions of justice that are difficult to frame within orthodox research ethics because they fall outside the confines of the IRB triangle (London and Kimmelman 2016). In particular, one of the easiest ways to compress development timelines is to test drugs in increasingly homogenous populations. In the United States this often means populations that are Whiter, younger, and healthier than the populations who are likely to use the intervention in practice. Another way is to rely on surrogate endpoints that allow studies to be completed in a shorter time. For example, a cancer trial might use tumor shrinkage over a period of months as a primary endpoint rather than waiting years to collect data about overall mortality.

Within the narrow confines of orthodox research ethics, any objection to proposals to shorten drug development timelines would likely have to be framed in terms of the rights and interests of study participants. But if the individual protocols for such studies are scientifically sound and pose only reasonable risks to participants, then orthodox research ethics would likely have no grounds for concern with such proposals.

Yet, such proposals raise questions of equity and justice to the extent that they allow interventions onto the market when they are supported only by direct evidence about their effects in populations of patients drawn from groups that are already advantaged within the medical system. Younger, Whiter, healthier patients face fewer risks in accessing these interventions in clinical practice than patients who differ from them. This includes much older and much younger patients, patients with additional common medical problems, patients using other medications, and patients from minority populations who are already historically underserved in health systems.

These groups face higher risks when accessing such interventions because their effects have not been established in groups with co-morbidities, who concomitantly use other medications, or whose bodies process medications differently because they are older or younger than trial participants. Uncertainties about dosing, schedule, and effects in such patients elevate risks to patients, both in terms of their expected efficacy and whether they provoke adverse events that reduce their net therapeutic advantage in these different groups. Speeding drugs to market can thus exacerbate inequities in health systems.

Additionally, these efforts offload the burden of generating the evidence necessary to rectify such inequalities from the stakeholders who profit from their sale to the patients, providers, and health systems that pay for them. This is inefficient in that it takes longer, and thus it takes more instances of harm to patients, to detect differential effects of such drugs in other populations when those effects have to be detected in clinical settings. Clinical settings are noisy in the sense that there are many sources of variation that can impact patient health other than the beneficial or adverse effects of the drug in question. Similarly, offloading the cost of generating this information onto consumers and health systems raises questions of fairness since their budgets already strain to meet the full range of health needs in the community.

The standards of evidence that the FDA requires for drug approval thus raise important issues of justice because they impact the extent to which health systems function effectively, efficiently, and equitably. Proposals to reduce drug development timelines may advance the interests of a narrow set of patients, but they also reduce the bandwidth of information that is available to other stakeholders including health systems and clinicians who care for patients who are already not well served by existing health systems. These proposals raise issues of justice that are largely invisible within orthodox research ethics, in part because they involve stakeholders outside of the IRB triangle. But this is also because they implicate issues relating to the quality of the information produced in research that are difficult to make salient within a cognitive ecosystem that is heavily focused on protecting study participants.

The standards regulatory agencies use for intervention approval are a mechanism for influencing the incentives of powerful actors whose decisions determine the bandwidth of information available to stakeholders, how uncertainty is distributed across the different segments of the population, and how the costs and burdens of addressing residual uncertainty are shared across different social institutions. These issues bear on the ability of social institutions to function effectively, efficiently, and equitably, and they would be difficult to address at the level of IRB review. Broadening the scope of research ethics brings these decisions into the purview of the field. It creates conceptual space in which issues of justice can be articulated and it situates those discussions within an institutional context in which mechanisms are available for shaping the incentives of key actors.

As a second example, once drugs are approved for sale, the incentive for firms to fund additional studies attenuates dramatically. In fact, firms may be reluctant to fund additional studies because adverse events or information about an intervention's clinical merits relative to a competitor's alternative put their profits at risk. When post-marketing studies are conducted, however, they are often carried out in ways that are designed more to advertise a drug and to tout its merits than to generate new medical evidence.

If post-marketing studies generate flawed or biased information without imposing risks on study participants, then orthodox research ethics has a difficult time capturing the ethical issues at stake in those studies (London, Kimmelman, and Carlisle 2012). But this parochialism ignores the extent to which a range of stakeholders rely on the evidence that is generated from research. Companies may use private funds to conduct such studies, but the information they generate is a public good, and co-opting this public good allows firms to increase their profits without advancing the medical interests of patients, the evidentiary interests of other scientists, or the informational needs of policy makers and health systems. These practices thus raise important questions of justice that are also largely invisible within orthodox research ethics.

Finally, even when practices do impact the health and welfare of study participants, the parochialism of orthodox research ethics makes it difficult to frame and address the relevant issues. This happens when scientific and ethical issues arise from practices that happen at the "portfolio-level" (Kimmelman et al. 2017). Within orthodox research ethics the unit of evaluation is the individual study protocol. But groups of similar studies constitute a portfolio of trials, and how such sets of studies are organized and which methods they employ determine the bandwidth of information that is produced, whether that information is most relevant to the needs of subsequent researchers or to practitioners, how uncertainty is distributed over different treatment populations, how burdens are distributed across study participants, and how much profit sponsors are able to generate relative to the value of the information their studies produce (London and Kimmelman 2019).

To use a single example, consider a case in which four interventions (w, x, y, z) appear promising as treatments for a particular disease. For simplicity, let's assume that all are owned by a single firm. Orthodox research ethics effectively regards the decision about how to test these different interventions as a private consideration for this private actor. But the alternative approaches a firm might take can influence the bandwidth of information that is available to stakeholders, its relevance to those stakeholders' informational needs, as well as how many study participants are likely to be harmed in order to generate the same quantity of information.

In particular, a firm might decide to evaluate these interventions by testing each in a separate trial in which participants are randomized to the investigational intervention or to usual care. The result is four different trials, each of which must recruit a particular number of participants in order to detect a particular effect at a predetermined level of statistical significance. Orthodox research ethics would look at each of these protocols and require that they meet particular ethical standards: subjects must provide free and informed consent and risks must be minimized and must be reasonable in light of the evidence studies are likely to produce. If each individual protocol passes muster on these grounds, they will each be approved.

Orthodox research ethics operates on the background assumption that if each protocol is approved, then the set of protocols must be ethically permissible. But this assumption is false. To see this, consider the bandwidth of information produced from these distinct studies compared to a possible alternative approach. In particular, it is possible for firms to design each of these studies so that a finding that x is superior to usual care and y is superior to usual care may not reveal much about the relative merits of x and y. One factor, for example, concerns the extent to which usual care in these two protocols is standardized so that it is effectively the same. If what constitutes usual care differs between the trials, then a firm might be able to sell more than one intervention as an effective treatment for the condition in question without ever generating evidence that supports a reliable comparison of the relative merits of x and y.

In contrast, if the firm were to run a trial in which w, x, y and z are all compared against one another and against a usual-care control arm, then it could generate a wider bandwidth of information while subjecting fewer participants to the risk of harm. The bandwidth of information is wider because such a design allows for a determination not just about whether both x and y are better than usual care, but about the relative merits of x and y. This information is more relevant to stakeholder needs because it eliminates the inefficiency associated with deploying two interventions in clinical practice in those cases where one provides a superior net therapeutic advantage to patients over the other. Additionally, fewer patients might be harmed in such a trial because the overall population needed to generate this evidence can be smaller than the total population in the four pairwise trials described above.

The approach in which all of these interventions are tested within a unified study design shows more respect for the health and welfare of participants, makes a more efficient use of their time and commitment, and better addresses the informational needs of a wide range of stakeholders. But using this approach can conflict with the firm's pecuniary interests. If fielding two interventions allows a firm to maximize profits by better segmenting the market, then this more unified approach jeopardizes profit. In cases where x is owned by one firm and y is owned by another, this more unified approach is in direct conflict with the financial interests of each firm. Each might prefer to split the market rather than take the gamble of losing out altogether.

Orthodox research ethics doesn't address such portfolio-level questions— they fall outside of the IRB triangle and they implicate questions of justice that revolve essentially around questions that are difficult to frame within the paternalistic focus of orthodox research ethics. Nevertheless, these decisions affect how effectively health systems meet patient needs and how efficiently they use scarce resources. As a result, they raise issues of justice and the framework articulated here captures the key respects in which those issues are morally salient.

4.10 Conclusion

Orthodox research ethics has avoided connecting research to larger social purposes, in part, from fear that those social purposes might license the abrogation of individual rights and the denigration of individual welfare. In this chapter I have argued that there is a conception of the common good that grounds a social imperative to carry out research that is designed to close knowledge gaps between the basic interests of community members and the ability of that community's basic social structures to safeguard and advance those interests. However, because this imperative is grounded in a concern for the basic interests of individuals, it requires that research be organized as a scheme of social cooperation that respects the status of its various stakeholders as free and equal persons.

I also showed that although this conception of the common good is capable of grounding such a social imperative, it is not uniquely dependent on a single, substantive conception of the good or on a particular philosophical approach to social or political philosophy. Rather, this conception of the common good can be formulated within frameworks that span important philosophical divides, including communitarian or liberal starting points and contractarian or consequentialist frameworks.

Finally, the egalitarian research imperative has important implications for the range of issues that fall into the scope of research ethics and the range of stakeholders whose conduct is a legitimate target for assessment. As we will see again in subsequent chapters, this framework provides a more unified and consistent foundation for some established requirements in research ethics while drawing coherent connections to a broader range of issues that are more difficult to formulate and address within the narrow confines of orthodox research ethics.

5

Two Dogmas of Research Ethics

5.1 Is There a Dilemma at the Heart of Research with Humans?

The historical reluctance in research ethics to embrace or recognize a social imperative to carry out medical research grows out of the worry that such an imperative too easily overrides and overshadows the rights and interests of individuals. I argued in the previous chapter that this worry is well founded when such a social imperative is cast in terms of the corporate conception of the common good. In contrast, the egalitarian research imperative that I outlined in §4.7 is predicated on the idea that advancing the generic interests conception of the common good through research with human participants is not fundamentally inconsistent with respecting the rights and welfare of study participants. In fact, the view I defend goes further, holding that respect for the status of individuals as free and equal is an integral, enabling component of the research enterprise understood as a voluntary scheme of mutual cooperation aimed at producing an important public good.

Even if we accept that the social imperative to create a system of research that advances the common good is also an imperative to ensure that such a system represents a voluntary scheme of mutual cooperation among free and equal persons, doubt might remain as to whether medical research can operate on those terms. Put another way, even if it is possible to ground some social or political institutions in the generic interest view of the common good, and to organize them in ways that are consistent with its requirements, it does not necessarily follow that the research enterprise is such an institution. In particular, the way that research exposes participants to risks, and the way that research ethics evaluates whether or not risks are reasonable or acceptable, might pose special problems for the egalitarian research imperative.

For the Common Good. Alex John London, Oxford University Press. © Oxford University Press 2022.
DOI: 10.1093/oso/9780197534830.003.0005

As we saw in §2.2, Walsh McDermott thought that the rule of law and freedom from arbitrary interference could not be extended into the realm of research with human participants because of the "moral dilemma of clinical investigation" (1967, 40–41). A moral dilemma is a situation in which every option an agent faces violates or transgresses some important norm or value. Agents who face a moral dilemma have to make tragic choices in the sense that every option available to them results in doing or allowing something that is bad or wrong (Levi 1986). They cannot extricate themselves from such a situation without incurring a moral loss. Even if more recent commentators reject McDermott's claims about the scope of researcher discretion, many share the fundamental perception that "tragic choices [are] involved in designing a system for research on human subjects" (Menikoff and Richards 2006, 19).

In this chapter I show how some of the problematic commitments that I identified in §1.2 and chapter 2 create a conceptual ecosystem in which the proposition that there is a deep and ineliminable conflict at the heart of research with human participants appears to be analytic, a conceptual truth about the nature of research and research risk. In particular, I show that these problematic commitments are often shared by protagonists on opposite sides of prominent debates and that this obscures their role in structuring the problem being discussed and the options for resolving them that are seen as salient or feasible. This critical or deconstructive work is thus necessary to clear the requisite conceptual space for an alternative framework for risk assessment and management within research ethics. In the next chapter I present such a positive framework and demonstrate how research risks can be managed in a manner that is consistent with a principle of equal respect that satisfies the requirements of the egalitarian research imperative.

This chapter examines a series of arguments that purport to show that there is a moral dilemma at the heart of research with human participants. Examining these positions highlights the central role of two largely unquestioned dogmas of research ethics. The first is the claim that the ethical norms that govern this activity derive from role-related obligations of professionals. The second is that clinical research is an inherently utilitarian undertaking. These dogmas are supported by, and lend support to, a functional view of clinical medicine and medical research that effectively identifies these activities with a set of goals and reasons that direct the individual decision-maker to optimize two incompatible metrics: as a clinician the decision-maker is obligated to provide optimal care to the individual patient but as a researcher the decision-maker is obligated to generate the information that will advance the medical interests of future patients. Together, these dogmas structure the conceptual ecosystem in which genuine (but ultimately manageable) tensions within research appear to pose a fundamental dilemma that calls for tragic choices.

I have tried to order these arguments from those that are more general and wider in scope to those that only apply to research with particular features. In §5.2 I examine the most philosophically general argument which holds that the fiduciary duties of clinicians are necessarily incompatible with the utilitarian goals of research. In §5.3 I argue that statements about the logical or conceptual incompatibility of the ends of research and medical practice show only that these are distinct activities and do not establish that they cannot be organized in a way that reconciles respect for individual interests with pursuit of the common good.

The remaining arguments rely on more contingent features of the research enterprise to generate a moral dilemma. Nevertheless, they share a number of assumptions in common, and it is important to highlight the role of those assumptions in these arguments. To do this, in §5.4 I present what I call the *template for the appeal to uncertainty*. The template provides the most general formulation of the claim that uncertainty about the relative therapeutic, prophylactic, or diagnostic merits of a set of interventions for a particular problem offers a way to reconcile respect for the interests of study participants with the generation of socially valuable information. Whether this argument is sound depends on how a number of key claims are spelled out in practice.

Stating this position in its most abstract form and highlighting the role of these key claims that must be further specified is important for two reasons. First, the positive view I elaborate in the next chapter includes a version of this appeal. So, it is important to establish that there are many ways in which this template can be filled out, some of which resist the objections that are discussed in this chapter. Second, it allows us to show how arguments to the effect that the position outlined in the template are unworkable presuppose very particular ways of filling in some of its key features.

In §5.5 we examine one of the earliest and most influential views that fills out the template for the appeal to uncertainty on terms that have come to dominate the literature. In particular, Charles Fried (1974) argues that if studies begin in the relevant state of uncertainty—given the perhaps unfortunate name "equipoise"—and if they are designed to disturb that state of equipoise, then they can reconcile the individual clinician's duty of personal care and the researcher's obligation to generate valuable information. Fried fills out the template in terms that presuppose a particular conception of uncertainty and that locate that uncertainty in the judgment or in the head of the individual clinician-researcher. Within the conceptual ecosystem of orthodox research ethics this way of filling out the template is natural and intuitive. But I show in §5.6 that it is also doomed to failure. This approach produces self-defeating practices that neither generate sound scientific evidence nor safeguard and advance the interests of individuals.

The failure of Fried's view and the fact that it appears natural and intuitive within the conceptual ecosystem of orthodox research ethics encourages the appearance of an intractable dilemma that arises from practical features of particular studies. But this natural and intuitive view, and the conception of equipoise that it entails, is only one from among a much larger universe of possible views. In particular, where Fried embraces a relatively fragile conception of uncertainty that is located in the head of the individual clinician-researcher, Benjamin Freedman articulates an alternative under the heading of "clinical equipoise" that locates the relevant uncertainty in the expert medical community, and that recognizes that uncertainty can arise from the conflicting assessments of experts who are not themselves uncertain about the merits of the interventions in question.

The fact that these views are often confused in the literature illustrates how deeply ingrained the two dogmas of research ethics are within the conceptual ecosystem of orthodox research ethics. Moreover, I show in §5.7 how the force of those dogmas has led even staunch proponents of clinical equipoise to question its moral relevance and to supplement that view with requirements that effectively recapitulate the problems associated with Fried's view. The upshot of these arguments is to show that common and intuitive ways of completing the template for the appeal to uncertainty are unworkable, but that the intuitive force of these views is rooted in the two dogmas of research ethics that I ultimately argue we should reject.

In §5.8 we turn to an argument that is still narrower in scope than those discussed previously but that appears to be more straightforwardly successful. This argument holds that the dilemma at the heart of research follows from the fact that research often requires participants to undergo risky or burdensome procedures that are not offset by the prospect of direct benefit to those same participants. This poses a special problem for any view that appeals to the template outlined in §5.4 (including Freedman's clinical equipoise) since few experts are likely to be uncertain about the fact that study-related procedures impose risks and burdens on participants that are not offset by the prospect of direct benefit to those same individuals.

More generally, however, this argument has been used to show that research participation is antithetical to the rational self-interest of individuals and that this conflict between the rational self-interest of individuals and the value of research to the community produces a coordination problem known as the prisoner's dilemma (Heyd 1996; Wertheimer 2010, 9). As a result, studies that contain such purely research-related procedures are supposed to be antithetical to both the clinician's fiduciary duty to patients and to the participant's own rational self-interest.

In §5.9, however, I argue that any moral standard that treats the risks and burdens of purely research-related study procedures as antithetical to the clinician's fiduciary duties would be so restrictive that it would prohibit a variety of ethically permissible practices in clinical medicine. Since clinical medicine is the domain in which the clinician's fiduciary duties should be most clearly exemplified, the arguments of this section show that research ethics retains a last vestige of unjustified medical paternalism.

I also argue that arguments purporting to show that research participation is a prisoner's dilemma rely on a conception of individual welfare that is excessively narrow and limited to individual health interests. I show that if such arguments were sound, they would not only apply to research participants, but to researchers. Once we recognize that the way health interests factor into a person's life plan can differ across individuals, the claim that research poses a prisoner's dilemma is undermined.

Ultimately, this long chapter concludes with reasons to reject both dogmas of research ethics and the way that they create a conceptual ecosystem in which several types of morally relevant diversity are obscured. The first is diversity in the expert medical community regarding scientific and medical questions. The second is diversity in democratic societies regarding the life plans that individuals adopt and pursue and the way those diverse life plans shape individual attitudes toward various risks and benefits. These forms of diversity are morally relevant, in part, because a requirement of justice in a decent society is to create social space in which individuals have the real freedom to pursue a life plan of their own. It is precisely this diversity in first-order life plans that makes it possible to satisfy the egalitarian research imperative.

In the following chapter I articulate the integrative approach to research risk. Like some of these early views, it holds that credible uncertainty has a special role to play in research ethics: ensuring that research with humans has scientific and social value and reconciling research participation with equal respect for the rights and welfare of study participants. Unlike those views, however, it rejects both dogmas of research ethics. As a result, it does not frame the central problem as reconciling the moral duties of conflicting social roles, and so the solution that it provides is not constrained by assumptions that are built into the traditional way of framing the problem. Readers who are primarily interested in my positive view can turn directly to that chapter.

5.2 Incompatible Ends?

5.2.1 The First Dogma: Moral Norms from Role-Related Obligations

The idea that there is a dilemma at the heart of medical research is bound up with two dogmas of research ethics. The first dogma is that the relevant ethical norms in this domain grow out of, and are grounded in, role-related obligations. Miller and Brody express this idea when they argue that in this domain "the basic goal and nature of the activity determines the ethical standards that ought to apply" to it (2003, 22 and 1998) and that the goals of clinical medicine and the goals of clinical research are "logically incompatible" (Brody and Miller 2003, 332). As a result, they argue, the dilemma at the heart of research ethics is a fundamental conflict between the incompatible demands placed on a single decision-maker by the moral duties of two conflicting social roles—that of the clinician and that of the researcher.

To understand the dilemma at the heart of research ethics, on this view, we need to understand the sense in which clinical medicine and clinical research are logically incompatible. This, in turn, involves seeing these activities as structured by different frameworks of reasons that can diverge in both principle and in practice. Since the social roles in question are roles for a single agent, if the reasons that structure them cannot be mutually satisfied, then research ethics will necessitate tragic choices between a set of basic and irreconcilable values.

5.2.2 Hippocratic Obligations: Patient-
Centered Consequentialism

Within research ethics, the role of the clinician tends to be understood and explicated in very traditional, Hippocratic terms. For example, the *Belmont Report* provides a standard expression of the physician's duty of personal care when it says that "the Hippocratic Oath requires physicians to benefit their patients 'according to their best judgment'" (National Commission for the Protection of Human Subjects of Biomedical and Behavioral Research 1979). The World Medical Association's 1964 *Declaration of Helsinki* holds that, "The Declaration of Geneva of The World Medical Association binds the doctor with the words: 'The health of my patient will be my first consideration'" (1964). The idea that the health of the patient must be the researcher's first concern was made more explicit in subsequent versions of the Declaration. For instance, the version from 2000 says, "In medical research on human subjects, considerations related to the well-being of the human subject should take precedence over the interests of science and society" (2000). The fundamental moral duty of the clinician is thus defined by the therapeutic obligation (Hill 1963; Fried 1974; Peto et al. 1976; Peto and Baigent 1998; Sackett 2000; Miller and Weijer 2006), sometimes called the "principle of therapeutic beneficence." The underlying idea is that "physicians should promote the medical best interests of patients by offering optimal medical care; and the risks of prescribed treatments are justified by the potential therapeutic benefits to patients" (Miller and Brody 2002, 4).

This traditional view of the provider-patient relationship has a relatively clear structure to it. There are two principal parties, the clinician and the patient. The patient relies on the clinician's expert knowledge and skill to advance the patient's medical best interests. In return, the clinician has a fiduciary duty to use his or her best medical judgment to advance the interests of the patient. When deciding whether or not to conduct a procedure or offer a test, the clinician thus has to consider the likely outcomes of that procedure and how they will affect the medical best interests of that patient. Other concerns are either irrelevant or have the status of secondary considerations that can play a role in decision-making only so long as they do not interfere with the morally primary goal of advancing the patient's medical best interests.

The Hippocratic conception of the clinician-patient relationship thus has the structure of a patient-centered consequentialism. It is a form of consequentialism because the right act for the clinician to perform is determined solely by the goodness of the outcomes it is likely to produce. Like other forms of consequentialism, Hippocratic patient-centered consequentialism is grounded in the value of beneficence—the main moral consideration used to evaluate acts is their likely impact on the good of those affected. Like other forms of consequentialism, it also involves an optimizing conception of rationality. The clinician's duty is to choose the optimal act—the one that brings about the best consequences. However, unlike other forms of consequentialism, which tend to evaluate the consequences of acts in terms of their outcomes for all affected parties, impartially considered, Hippocratic ethics is patient-centered. This means that the consequences that matter when evaluating actions are limited to their impact on the individual patient. Similarly, whereas most forms of consequentialism are concerned with the goodness of outcomes in a very broad sense of the good, Hippocratic ethics is focused on the health or medical best interests of patients.

Thinking of the clinician-patient relationship in these terms dovetails nicely with the idea that clinicians have a special, fiduciary relationship with patients. In a fiduciary relationship, the clinician has a special moral duty to put the interests of the patient above all other concerns—including their own private and professional interests. The ground for this duty traditionally hinges on several factors. Clinicians have expert knowledge and skills that patients lack but which patients rely on to advance their medical interests. This creates an asymmetry in knowledge and power between the two parties. By entering relationships with clinicians, patients become dependent on clinicians in a morally special respect—they rely on the expert knowledge and skill of clinicians to safeguard and advance their medical interests without necessarily having the ability to independently assess and monitor the actions of the clinician to make sure that they are aligned with the patient's best interest. Asymmetric knowledge and power create a relationship of dependence fraught with the potential for domination and abuse. Treating the clinician patient relationship as fiduciary in nature helps to facilitate social trust by articulating clear expectations about the relationship between patient interests and competing concerns. The social enforcement of these expectations provides public assurance that breaches of that trust will not be tolerated (Miller and Weijer 2006).

Hippocratic patient-centered consequentialism internalizes the fiduciary nature of the social relationship between clinicians and patients into the morality of medicine itself. It erects the health interests of the patient as the good to be optimized and it places the physician under a duty to use her best medical judgment to always choose the act—the intervention or course of care—that is most likely to bring about the best medical outcome for that individual.

When deliberating about how to manage the potential therapeutic advantages of an intervention given its possible adverse effects, the clinician has a moral duty to choose the course of care in which potential burdens and risks of care for a patient are offset by the prospect for therapeutic advantage for that same patient. As a result, "when physicians of integrity practice medicine, physicians' and patients' interests converge. The patient desires to regain or maintain health to relieve suffering; the physician is dedicated to providing the medical help that the patient needs" (Miller and Brody 2003).

When Miller and Brody say that the ends of clinical medicine and the ends of research are logically incompatible, they are asserting that these activities are structured by different frameworks of reasons that can diverge in both principle and in practice. If the defining goals of clinical medicine involve advancing the health interests of the individual patient, then there are no circumstances in which the reasons that are internal to clinical medicine should ground conduct inconsistent with the medical best interests of patients. The goals of clinical medicine and the interests of patients are aligned, in this view, because the framework of reasons that structure that activity necessarily tracks patient interests.

5.2.3 The Second Dogma: Research as Inherently Utilitarian

In contrast, "clinical research is dedicated primarily to promoting the medical good of future patients by means of scientific knowledge derived from experimentation with current research participants—a frankly utilitarian purpose" (Miller and Brody 2003, 21 see also 2007, 162). The claim that research with human participants is an inherently utilitarian undertaking is a second dogma of research ethics.[1] One reason for its status as a pervasive and often unquestioned assumption is that it appears to be analytic—a

---

[1] Miller and Brody here give voice to a set of ideas that is often expressed in different terms. For example, it was common in earlier discussions to speak more explicitly of the "problem of experimentation" as setting the terms on which it is permissible to take some lives in order to save more lives (Calabresi 1969) or in which the interests of some must be traded off against the interests of others (Fried 1974).

conceptual truth derived from reflection on the point and purpose of the research activity. If the goal of research is to generate the knowledge necessary to advance the medical interests of large numbers of future patients and if the goals of this activity define the norms that govern it, then researchers have a duty to act so as to generate the knowledge that will bring about these advances in future medical care. Without any clear check or constraint on the methods that researchers can use to promote this end, this position is treated as permitting trade-offs between the welfare of study participants and future beneficiaries of research.[2]

Treating the role-related obligations of clinicians and researchers as different forms of consequentialism sharpens the distinction between these activities in a way that makes them appear "logically incompatible." Whereas the ethical duties of the clinician have the form of patient-centered consequentialism, the ethical duties of the researcher have the form of an impartial, utilitarian consequentialism. As forms of consequentialism, both of these moral frameworks share a slightly narrower focus on health-related outcomes. Both also presuppose an optimizing rationality grounded in beneficence, directed at evaluating the rightness of individual acts by assessing the consequences those acts are expected to bring about. They diverge, however, in their accounts of whose interests matter when it comes to evaluating those consequences: the interest of the individual patient alone or the interests of all future patients who stand to benefit from improvements in the standard of care.

Because Hippocratic, patient-centered consequentialism focuses solely on the medical interests of the individual patient, the expert decision-maker is faced with a problem of comparing the relative value of different health states for the same individual. This is a kind of *intrapersonal* comparison of utility: will the burdens, harms, or risks associated with treatment A be outweighed or offset by sufficient benefits to make the provision of A superior to the provision of treatment B, given its burdens, harms, or risks and the offsetting benefits that might result to the patient?

In contrast, utilitarianism requires that the decision-maker go further and compare the value of outcomes across different individuals. These *interpersonal* comparisons traditionally involve summing the value or disvalue that

---

[2] Strictly speaking, from the narrow claim that the production of socially valuable information is a necessary condition of ethically permissible research, if follows only that research that lacks social value is morally impermissible. Nothing follows about the extent of the demands that can be placed on the interests of free and equal persons in pursuit of this goal. I return to this point near the end of the present chapter.

results for different individuals from different courses of action (Sen 1979). As a result, the considerations that determine whether to perform a test or to administer an intervention to one set of people include the likelihood that doing so will generate information necessary to improve the standard of care that is available to a different set of future people. Moreover, if research is a utilitarian enterprise and if performing procedures or providing interventions that expose study participants to serious harms or risks is necessary to bring about a sufficiently significant benefit to a large enough group of future people, there are no grounds internal to the research enterprise itself on which to block or prevent such sacrifices. As a result, in this view, there is no in-principle alignment between the interests of study participants and the framework of reasons that structure the research activity.

5.2.4 Reasonable Risk: Trading Risk to Some for Benefits to Others

That research is an inherently utilitarian undertaking seems to be reflected in the way that reasonable risks are defined in the field:

Definition of reasonable risk: Risks to subjects that are not offset by the prospect of direct benefit to the participant must be reasonable "in relation to the importance of the knowledge that may reasonably be expected to result" from the study (45 CFR 46.111[2]).

A trial can pose an acceptable degree of risk to participants even if those risks are not offset by the prospect of direct medical benefit to participants themselves. Rather, such risks can be justified if they are offset by the prospect that they are necessary to generate sufficiently valuable information. This seems to countenance the permissibility of trading risk of harm to a small group of study participants if it will purchase sufficient social benefit for others.

This conceptual analysis outlines the conceptual ecosystem within which disputes play out over how to reconcile this fundamental tension. It sets the terms in which debates are framed, and the interlocking claims that go into this formulation of the problem constitute assumptions common to otherwise warring camps. For instance, disputes about how to respond to this tension often take place against a shared framing of the problem as a conflict in the vantage point of a single decision-maker. Normally the decision-maker in question is the medical professional who cannot simultaneously satisfy the demands of these competing and incompatible forms of consequentialism.

Even when they disagree about how to respond to this problem, competing sides often assume that the problem arises because the individual decision-maker has a duty to do what in her best judgment will bring about the best outcome. As a result, the idea that the central tension in research is a conflict in the objectives to be advanced by a single, rational optimizer is baked into the problem from the start. Against this backdrop the conflict hinges on the different metrics this individual decision-maker is required to optimize to bring about the best outcome—the medical best interests of the present patient or the medical interests of a large group of future patients.

5.3 No Easy Analytic Answers

5.3.1 Two Senses of Incompleteness

The claim that there is necessarily a moral dilemma at the heart of the research enterprise appears to represent a deep philosophical truth that follows from a conceptual analysis of the role of clinician and the role of researcher. Against the backdrop of the first dogma of research ethics, this focus on social roles makes sense because the moral norms that govern this sphere are taken to derive from role-related obligations. Each of these social roles pursues a logically distinct set of ends which are part of distinct systems of norms and obligations. The moral obligations of the clinician represent a form of patient-centered consequentialism while the obligations of researchers represent a form of impartial utilitarianism. Against the assumption that these frameworks are to be implemented by the same individual decision-maker, it looks like such a person would necessarily face a choice between optimizing two different metrics: fidelity to the interests of the patient before them and fidelity to science and the greater good.

Even if we assume for a moment that this argument is sound, what does it show? The main point I want to make here is that, although it establishes that these are conceptually distinct activities that advance different ends, it does not show that these activities cannot be integrated in practice in a way that respects the rights and welfare of study participants while generating socially valuable information. In part, this is because professional norms are incomplete in two ways: their guidance may not always be adequate in the face of uncertainty and their guidance may not reflect broader considerations that fall outside the narrow confines of issues recognized by professional roles. Finally, conceptual arguments about the nature of professional roles are often insufficient to answer substantive moral questions because professional roles can be defined in myriad ways, each of which incorporates different responsibilities.

To make these arguments, it is helpful to make explicit an idea that tacitly motivates the conceptual analysis offered in the previous section and that has deep roots in Western philosophy. This is the idea that professions, such as medicine, are distinct bodies of craft knowledge, each of which can be defined by the distinct end that it pursues. For ancient Greeks, craft knowledge or *techne* is the paradigm of a body of knowledge, covering a discrete domain, geared to bringing about or producing a discrete set of ends or outcomes. Different forms of craft knowledge are defined by the pursuit of different ends: blacksmiths make implements from metal, carpenters make objects from wood, generals understand strategy and how to use troops and tactics to achieve victory. Similarly, medicine has a long history of being conceived of as a craft whose purpose is to benefit the patient through the production of health.[3]

Whether the guidance provided by such bodies of technical knowledge is authoritative depends on two kinds of incompleteness. The first concerns whether it has sufficient knowledge to reliably produce the well-defined products or outcomes that define them. Even when it is clear what properties an object or outcome is supposed to have, the guidance of such a body of knowledge becomes less authoritative as its ability to reliably produce that product decreases. The second concerns the degree to which one craft relies on some other body of knowledge to determine what properties its products ought to have in order to serve the larger purposes and ends of the user.

Although different bodies of technical knowledge are distinct and can therefore make competing demands on the same individual, they can also be mutually supportive in actual practice. The reason, as Aristotle was well aware, is that no narrow branch of professional knowledge has as its subject overall individual flourishing. Rather, each has as its defining end the production of some relatively narrow good—health, wealth, victory, and so on. But the question of how to make a good life out of those goods is not a

---

[3] In the opening of the *Republic*, Plato has a protracted discussion of medicine as a craft distinct from the craft of money-making. For its continued relevance to today, see London 2000a and 2020.

technical question. It falls into the domain of ethics and what Aristotle calls *phronesis* or practical wisdom, which, at the social level, is the domain of political philosophy. As a result, the all-things-considered judgments that we make about the limits on professional powers and prerogatives and the constraints on their conduct must be informed by a larger conception of the way that the goals and activities of various professions fit into a social order that reflects the fundamental value of individuals and their interests in making momentous decisions for themselves and in forging and pursuing a good life.

5.3.2 The Incompleteness of Medicine

Medicine is incomplete in both of these respects. First, it is often not clear how to safeguard or advance the health of a patient. For example, we may not understand the pathophysiology of a novel disease and there may not be direct evidence about the effects of various interventions on that disease. At best we may have a range of hypotheses about the mechanisms through which the disease attacks the body and about which possible interventions might represent the best way to bring about a clinical benefit in patients with this disease.

In situations in which it is not clear how to advance a patient's medical best interests, the guidance of individual experts becomes less authoritative. The reason is that the warrant for the claim that some act or course of care is obligatory is grounded, ultimately, in the prospect that it will actually benefit the patient. As it becomes uncertain whether patients are better off receiving one form of treatment for a particular medical condition rather than another (for example, intervention A or B), then randomizing that patient to receive A or B has the advantage of generating reliable medical evidence without knowingly compromising the health and welfare of study participants. We will consider this argument in more detail in a moment (§5.4).

Second, medicine is also incomplete in the second sense outlined previously. Even if we assume that the clinician's moral duties are appropriately modeled as a kind of patient-centered consequentialism, it is simply false that choosing an act that is less than optimal from this standpoint is the kind of wrong that creates a moral dilemma in this space. The reason is that the dilemma in question concerns the rights and interests of study participants and it is perfectly reasonable and ethically permissible for patients or study participants to make choices that are not strictly optimal from the standpoint of the individual Hippocratic clinician. Moreover, the case for this claim is most compelling in precisely those circumstances in which the moral case for conducting research is the most compelling.

Consider the following example (London 2020). At the inception of the SARS-CoV-2 outbreak there was considerable uncertainty about the pathophysiology of this novel disease and about the best methods for preventing its spread and for treating infected patients. Experts relying on hypotheses about disease pathophysiology and about intervention mechanism constructed a list of at least a dozen interventions they regarded as likely to produce a therapeutic effect in patients. It included prednisone, dexamethasone, baricitinib, methylprednisolone, enoxaparin, colchicine, remdesivir, favipiravir, ivermectin, tocilizumab, lopinavir/ritonavir, azithromycin chloroquine/hydroxychloroquine, and convalescent plasma (Herper and Riglin 2020).

Imagine that for each of these n interventions there was a passionate group of clinicians who, looking at the largely indirect evidence that was available, was convinced that their favored intervention was likely to produce the best outcomes for patients. If we assume also that the morality internal to the role of caregiver requires that each recommend for their patients what each believes is likely to maximize the patient's health interests, then it would be impermissible for such researchers to recommend anything but their favored intervention to patients. This means that it would violate their Hippocratic duty to recommend participation in a clinical trial and it is difficult to see how they could refer a patient for a second opinion if they know that their colleagues prefer different treatments as likely to be best.

Paradoxically, however, it would be permissible for each patient to seek a second, or a third, or an nth opinion. Imagine, then, that some patients visit each of these n groups of experts who each favor a different intervention as likely to be medically best for this patient. It is permissible for each of these patients to decide which clinician they want to care for them, even though doing so results in a choice that $n-1$ experts regard as suboptimal. In other words, if a patient agrees to be treated by a clinician who recommends one of these interventions, then all of the others might regard this as a bad choice. But it is not wrong to permit patients in this situation from making such choice.

So here we have a case in which different clinicians recommend different treatments to a patient as likely to be best. If it is permissible for each to make such a recommendation, then it is not wrong for each to act in a way that n-1 experts regard as likely to bring about less than the best outcome. Similarly, the patient chooses an option that n-1 clinicians regard as violating their Hippocratic duty to do what is in the best interests of the patient, but this choice is not morally wrong.

As we will see in this and in the next chapter, if it is permissible for patients to choose at random which experts should provide their care, then it should also be permissible for those same individuals to choose the option of participating in a well-designed trial in which they would be randomized to one of these n interventions. For now, my point is simply that the abstract argument from the previous section fails to capture the two important respects in which medicine is incomplete. As a body of knowledge about how to produce health, it is incomplete in the sense that there will arise cases in which there is uncertainty or conflicting expert judgment about how to best advance the medical interests of patients. In those cases, research provides a way to generate this knowledge and, as I will argue in more detail in the next chapter, this can be done without compromising the rights or welfare of study participants. These activities may be conceptually distinct, but not only may their ends not be incompatible, but in order to fulfill its mission of translating therapeutic intent into actual benefits for patients, medicine may require the thoughtful conduct of well-designed research (London 2020).

Similarly, medicine is incomplete in the sense that the goal that it produces is not the highest good there is. Health is an important good, but its value relative to other ends is a question that falls outside of the technical bounds of medicine. Even if clinicians are bound by Hippocratic duties to always act in what they regard as the patient's best interests, patients are morally permitted to act in ways that subordinate their narrow medical interests to the pursuit of other goals and commitments. In the example just discussed, this takes the form of deciding to allow themselves to be randomized to 1 of n alternative treatments for their medical condition rather than deciding at random to receive care from one or another expert clinicians. In this case, participating in research advances an important social good without necessarily requiring a sacrifice of self-interest on the part of the participant. We will revisit this point several times in the remainder of this chapter.

5.3.3 The Incompleteness of Research

It is worth noting that research, as a technical body of knowledge, is also incomplete in this second sense. If we think of research as something like the craft whose domain is the scientific and statistical methods needed to generate reliable knowledge about the safety and efficacy of various kinds of interventions, then this craft is incomplete to the extent that it relies on other disciplines—such as health policy informed by a proper concern for the freedom and equality of community members—to articulate what knowledge gaps ought to be addressed and to articulate the constraints on permissible methods of addressing those gaps.

When it comes to determining what the constraints are on permissible research studies, the kind of conceptual analysis described in §5.2.1 is not sufficient to answer this question. It is helpful to see that this point can be put in two different ways. In both cases, even if we assume that the purpose of research is to generate knowledge that will advance the interests of future patients, it does not follow that such research is inconsistent with respect for the rights and welfare of study participants.

The first way to make this point is that if we follow the second dogma of research ethics and we grant that research is an inherently utilitarian undertaking, it does not follow that it is wrong, all things considered, not to conduct studies that are regarded as optimal from this narrow viewpoint. Studies that optimize social value may be morally wrong, all things considered, if they do so by abrogating the rights and interests of study participants. Many of the studies described by Beecher fall into this category (§2.2.3). Likewise, studies that fall short of optimality when narrowly considered may be ethically preferable to studies that are optimal in the narrow sense, if they generate sufficient social value to improve the capacity of social institutions to meet the needs of community members without violating or diminishing the rights or welfare of study participants in the process.

In fact, if it is a conceptual truth that research is in some sense an inherently utilitarian activity, then we might also say that it is axiomatic in research ethics as a field that this utilitarianism must be constrained. Asserting the conceptual incompatibility of the norms of research and any other set of norms simply amounts to saying that when research operates under such constraints it may not be optimally utilitarian. But so what. The question is whether, from the standpoint of a just society, it can produce the information necessary to improve the capacity of basic social structures to meet, secure, and advance the basic interests of its various members on terms that respect the status of individuals as free and equal. No purely conceptual argument about the proper ends of this activity can establish that this cannot be done in actual practice.

5.3.4 If External Constraints Are Unnecessary the Second Dogma Is False

Alternatively, research can be defined in various ways and some have argued that the norms for limiting the demands that research can place on study participants can themselves be derived from features internal to the research enterprise. For example, it has been argued that, unlike physicians, who have a fiduciary duty to their patients, researchers have only the weaker obligation not to exploit study participants (Miller and Brody 2002, 2003). If this duty of non-exploitation is internal to research, then research isn't a fundamentally utilitarian undertaking after all and the second dogma of research ethics is false.

Research isn't a fundamentally utilitarian activity, on this assumption, because utilitarianism recognizes only a single duty—to perform the act that brings about the greatest good (see §3.4.3). But if researchers are forbidden from bringing about some real benefit if it involves exploiting study participants, then research would not be utilitarian. Among its goals and ends there would be a set of considerations of sufficient moral import that they sometimes outweigh the production of information necessary to improve the medical care of large numbers of future people. Views that contain considerations of sufficient weight to outweigh the production of greater good are not consequentialist and so cannot be utilitarian.[4]

Now the question arises as to why we ought to adopt this particular definition of research. After all, we can think of at least three conceptions of the research enterprise. Call the first "research," which is defined as a body of knowledge with the purely utilitarian end of maximizing the knowledge necessary to advance the standard of care for future patients. Call the second

---

[4] Such views are not consequentialist because consequentialism is the view according to which the goodness of outcomes is the only factor that determines the rightness or wrongness of an act (Kagan 1998). Views that accept that the goodness of outcomes matter, but hold that there are additional constraints on which actions are right or wrong, are forms of moderate deontology because they recognize constraints of sufficient strength that they sometimes outweigh the production of good outcomes.

"research*," which is defined as the production of such knowledge within the constraints imposed on that activity by a duty of personal care. Call the third "research**," which is defined as the production of such knowledge within the constraints imposed on that activity by the duty of non-exploitation.

By now it should be clear that for any package of constraints [x, y, z,] we can define a conception of "research***" that pursues those constraints by definition. In the face of competing definitions of competing practices, it is a substantive ethical and political question whether we ought to permit the conduct of research, since the demands that it can place on participants are not constrained by anything other than the prospect of helping future people. Perhaps, instead, we ought to forbid the practice of research and only allow the conduct of research*, since that produces socially valuable information and forbids the violation of a fiduciary duty to participants. Or perhaps we should forbid the practice of both research and research* and allow only the practice of research** or research***.

The point is that conceptual analysis can help us differentiate research from research* or research**, and so on, but it cannot settle the substantive moral question concerning which of these practices we ought to promote and how we ought to design the institutions that promote them. Substantive moral questions of this type cannot be derived from analytic claims, since such claims merely tell us how to define our words and concepts. Even if research and medicine are distinct bodies of technical knowledge, how their respective ends should be pursued in a just society and how their pursuit should be reconciled with ends of other activities and the needs of community members are substantive questions of ethics and policy that fall outside of the parochial expertise of either set of professionals.

The upshot of the argument so far is that the conceptual argument for the logical incompatibility of medicine and research cannot ground any substantive claims about how to tackle the challenge of integrating the potentially competing demands of these different disciplines within a just social order. At best, this argument shows that these undertakings are distinct, guided by different ends and responsive to different reasons. The norms that are internal to these activities and that are grounded in an understanding of the ends they pursue are technical norms about how to effectively apply these bodies of knowledge to bring about ends of a particular sort. All distinct bodies of technical knowledge are governed by distinctive norms of this type. But this does not pose an all-things-considered moral dilemma at a level of ethics or policy since the narrow, technical norms of such disciplines do not extend into the larger ethical and political domain of how to integrate various activities within a just social order. Rather, what the scope of these productive disciplines should be, when to call on the one rather than the other, and how to reconcile their pursuit in a just society are substantive ethical and political questions that requires a broader set of values and concerns than the narrow technical norms internal to these disciplines.

5.4 Reconciliation through Uncertainty: The Template

The argument of the previous section rebuts the claim that from the fact that clinical medicine and research are conceptually distinct we can show that there is an inherent moral dilemma at the heart of research ethics. Even if the arguments made earlier are correct, however, there may be more practical grounds for concern about our ability to reconcile substantive requirements pertaining to the welfare of individuals with the features studies require to generate scientifically sound and socially valuable knowledge.

To motivate these worries we need to return to one of the arguments I outlined in §5.3.2. I used that argument to show that the goals of research are not necessarily inconsistent with the interests of study participants. I will first present this argument in schematic form as a kind of template in the sense that a number of its key propositions must be specified in more detail in order for the content of the argument to be clear in operational detail.

Understanding what I refer to as the *template for the appeal to uncertainty* is important for two reasons. First, I show how the two dogmas of research ethics make one way of filling out this template seem natural and intuitive (§5.5). The problem is that the resulting view is unworkable and doomed to failure. Because this view is often seen as the only way to complete this argument, the fact that this common and intuitive way of completing the template is unworkable reinforces the perception that there is a fundamental dilemma at the heart of research ethics.

Second, it is important to understand that the intuitive and natural way of completing this template is unworkable because of flaws that derive from the two dogmas of research ethics and not from flaws inherent in the template itself. Establishing this point is essential, in part, because in chapter 6 I provide a way of operationalizing the template that avoids those problems and redeems the ambition of reconciling the pursuit of social value with respect for the welfare of individuals. Since these are both ways of completing the same general template, it is important to recognize how these views differ so that we can avoid confusion.

To lay out the template for the appeal to uncertainty, it is helpful to begin by giving more precise definitions to two requirements that appear to be in conflict. I will define the first, the Social Value Requirement, in a way that reflects the content of the egalitarian research imperative:

Social Value Requirement: Research with human participants is only justified if it is reasonably expected to generate the knowledge necessary to develop interventions, policies, practices, or other advances that will enable a community's basic social structures (such as its health-related institutions) to more effectively, efficiently, or equitably safeguard and advance the basic interests of its constituent members.

The social value requirement states a necessary condition for ethically acceptable research with humans. It is seen as in conflict with the following requirement:

Concern for Welfare: It is impermissible to knowingly expose a person to interventions, practices, or procedures that are known or credibly believed to be worse than another available option.

One of the most enduring and important ideas about how to reconcile concern for welfare with the social value requirement appeals to the existence of credible uncertainty. The template for this argument, in its most general form, can be stated as follows:

Template for the Appeal to Uncertainty: When there is credible uncertainty about the relative merits of the set of interventions available for addressing an important health problem, it does not violate concern for the welfare of study participants to allow them to be allocated to an intervention from that set by a method (such as randomization) that facilitates the production of reliable medical evidence.

The idea is that when it is clear that such a state of uncertainty obtains, a trial designed to resolve that uncertainty—to bridge that knowledge gap—can generate socially valuable knowledge without requiring the denigration or abrogation of participant welfare.

Consider first the claim that studies designed to address such uncertainty are likely to have significant social value. If there is uncertainty about which of several treatment options is best for patients with a given condition, then research that provides the evidence necessary to vindicate the clinical merits of one alternative over the rest would have a strong chance of altering clinical practice in a way that renders care more effective and efficient. In fact, uncertainty about the merits of the interventions being tested seems to be a necessary condition for sound science since research is a tool for learning, and if the answers to the questions posed are already known, then there is nothing to learn.

Uncertainty about the relative merits of interventions being tested also seems to be a necessary condition for socially valuable research since resolving uncertainty of this kind enables various stakeholders to better discharge important moral or social responsibilities. Clinicians can prescribe optimal care to patients. Patients have greater assurance about the likely effects of various courses of care. Health systems can make a more efficient use of scarce resources by implementing the best therapeutic, prophylactic, or diagnostic options and eliminating less effective care or practices. Policymakers will know which courses of care to promote, and perhaps also which lines of research to foster and support and which to abandon or demote.

Now consider the proposition from the standpoint of participant welfare. If the relative clinical merits of a set of interventions are uncertain, then there are no credible grounds for treating one intervention as superior to the rest. In this case, being allocated to one intervention, rather than the others, does not involve knowingly providing that person with a level of care that is known to be worse than another available option. In this case, allowing a patient to be randomized to the alternatives in this set does not violate or contravene the clinician's duty of personal care. Problem solved!

Unfortunately, matters are not so simple. What I've outlined previously is the template for the argument that scholars who appeal to uncertainty want to make. Part of the problem, however, is that the template is ambiguous about a nexus of specific claims or views that are tightly connected. To give this nexus of views specific content is to fill out the details of a framework of moral assessment within which the appeal to uncertainty has substantial moral content. As those views are given more precise content, the credibility of the argument that results can be evaluated more precisely.

The following four questions capture the nexus of issues that must be specified in order for a framework involving this kind of appeal to uncertainty to have determinant content:

1. **Normative Basis:** What is the normative basis for focusing on uncertainty?
2. **Whose Uncertainty:** Whose uncertainty matters when contemplating these issues?
3. **Model of Uncertainty:** How is "uncertainty" to be understood and modeled?
4. **Epistemic Threshold:** What is the window that determines when the relevant uncertainty obtains and when it has been removed or disturbed?

Against the background of the two dogmas of research ethics, what appears to be the most intuitive and natural way of specifying these views results in a position that cannot support or redeem the ambitions of the template I have laid out. Rather than rejecting the claim that uncertainty plays an important role in bridging concern for individual welfare and social value, as some have, I argue that we should reject the background views that make those unworkable assumptions seem so natural and intuitive. In order for uncertainty to play a critical role integrating ethical and scientific aspects of research, we must dispense with the two dogmas of research ethics.

5.5 The View of Equipoise That Refuses to Die

5.5.1 The Normative Basis for Appealing to Uncertainty

Proponents of the principle of equipoise, like Charles Fried (1974), Benjamin Freedman (1987, 1990), Paul Miller and Charles Weijer (2006a, 2006b) and proponents of the uncertainty principle (Hill 1963; Peto et al. 1976; Peto and Baigent 1998; Sackett 2000), ground the normative basis for focusing on uncertainty in its ability to render research participation consistent with the clinician's duty of personal care, or the fiduciary obligation to provide optimal care to each individual patient. On this view, uncertainty provides the key for turning one dogma of research ethics against the other: the best way to limit the inherent utilitarianism of the research enterprise is to circumscribe the obligations of one professional role within another. The demands that can be exacted from patients are limited to those that are consistent with the clinician's duty of personal care.

5.5.2 Whose Uncertainty Matters

Thinking of uncertainty as a bridge between the goals of science and the moral duties of the individual clinician or researcher entails a particular view of the second question that fills out the template for the appeal to uncertainty, regarding whose uncertainty matters. If the moral obligations of researchers are derived from the physician's duty of personal care, then it follows that the duty of personal care binds the individual physician in the clinical context. Each physician is charged with benefiting their individual patients according to their best judgment. As a result, this requires that the *individual clinician or researcher* must be uncertain about the relative net therapeutic merits of the available interventions in order to recommend that a patient enter into a clinical trial. As a result, Fried (1974) and others (Peto 1976; Chard and Lilford 1998) argue that the uncertainty must reside in the mind of the individual clinician or researcher. After all, individual clinicians or researchers have a special moral obligation to the individuals in their care and they must enroll participants in studies or perform study procedures on individual participants.

The individualistic nature of the provider-patient relationship and the duties of clinicians seems to require that the relevant uncertainty must be located in the mind of individual clinicians. As one proponent of the uncertainty principle puts it:

> An ethical physician must do what is best for his or her patients. She cannot participate in a controlled trial if she is certain that one arm is superior to the others and that some of her patients will receive an inferior treatment by participating in the trial. It does not matter whether her certainty is based on formal scientific studies, on personal experience, on anecdote, on tacit understanding, or rules of thumb. Whether her certainty is in accord with or diverges from the view of the medical community is irrelevant. Uncertainty is a moral prerequisite for a controlled study. If we know what we should do, we should do it, not study it. (Enkin 2000, 758)

Here, the focus on uncertainty in the mind of the individual clinician is combined with a relatively fragile epistemic threshold according to which uncertainty is the absence of even anecdotal reason to expect that at least one of the interventions under consideration is superior to the rest.

5.5.3 Modeling Uncertainty

With regard to the third question about how to understand uncertainty, the focus on the judgments of the individual clinician or researcher who must discharge a duty of personal care to each individual before her suggests that uncertainty should be understood as a subjective state of the individual decision-maker. The traditional, Hippocratic understanding of the duty of personal care models it as a duty to choose optimal care for each individual. As a form of patient-centered consequentialism, the right act is the one that is best for the individual in question. In a situation in which the effects of interventions are known with certainty, then the clinician's obligation is to choose the option that will produce the largest net benefit to the individual. When the effects of interventions are not known with certainty—when they are subject to some element of chance or when the information that we have about them is scant or unreliable—then standard theories of individual rationality hold that the best option is the one that has the highest expected value. Expected value is the product of two factors: the magnitude of the expected net benefit to the individual and the probability of that benefit being realized or obtaining in practice.

In order for the clinician's duty of personal care to permit participation in a study where an individual will be provided one intervention, chosen by a random process, from a set of several options, the clinician must believe that none of those options is likely to be better than the rest. Against the background of the traditional, Hippocratic conception of the therapeutic obligation, this state obtains when there is no difference in the expected value of the interventions in the set of treatment options. In this case, each of these interventions is an equal bet in prospect, meaning that each has the same expected value for the participant. This also seems like a fairly natural and straightforward way to interpret the concept of equipoise—the expected value of each intervention is such that the judgment of the expert is "equally poised" between them.

5.5.4 The Threshold of Uncertainty

At what point has uncertainty been disturbed such that providing a patient with a particular option or set of options from the available set would violate the clinician's duty of personal care? On the view we have been entertaining so far, uncertainty is disturbed as soon as the clinician regards one intervention as having a higher expected value than the rest. Once one intervention has a more favorable expected value than the other options, the clinician's duty of personal care is no longer indeterminate. Rather, their duty is to provide the option that they regard has the highest expected net benefit for the patient in question.

5.6 Doomed to Failure

5.6.1 The Fragility of Individual Uncertainty

One of the most damning objections to this very natural and intuitive way of understanding equipoise is that it is incapable of supporting or redeeming the project of reconciling concern for the welfare of study participants and the production of valuable scientific information. The source of this failure lies in its conception of individual uncertainty, which is so fragile and evanescent that it rarely obtains. As Marquis (1983) and others (Gifford 1986; Hellman 2002) argue, only in relatively rare circumstances will a physician believe that it is equally probable that two or more therapeutic options offer a particular patient the same degree of benefit. There will almost always be some bit of information or some aspect of one intervention that tips the balance of the clinician or researcher's subjective assessment in favor of one intervention over others. Because such a fragile state of uncertainty will rarely exist, clinical trials between therapeutic alternatives cannot ethically be initiated.

Alternatively, even if such a fragile state of uncertainty did obtain at the start of a trial, critics argue, it would vanish as soon as evidence from the trial emerges (Hellman 2002). As a result, equipoise will not persist long enough to bring a clinical trial to its desired conclusion. As soon as the trial generates its first data points the physician is obligated to update her beliefs about which intervention is most likely to best advance the patient's health interests. If one option appears to fare better than another, the hypothesis that one option is inferior to the other would be more probable than its complement. As

Marquis argues, this means that the clinician's therapeutic obligation is no longer neutral between available options since, "A physician should not recommend for a patient therapy such that, given present medical knowledge, the hypothesis that the particular therapy is inferior to some other therapy is more probable than the opposite hypothesis" (1983, 42). Once this fragile state of uncertainty is disturbed, the trial can no longer be justified.

Since the point of the appeal to uncertainty is to reconcile the production of socially valuable knowledge with respect for the welfare of study participants, the considerations laid out in this section are sufficient to show that the particular conception of equipoise we are discussing here is an abject failure. In the rest of this section I show that this view is subject to additional shortcomings. Before moving on to the additional problems with this view, however, it is important to understand exactly what the objections in this section show.

Because the conception of equipoise that refuses to die is often treated as synonymous with equipoise in general, some critics take the argument in this section to show more than it does. In particular, they take it to show that there is a moral dilemma in research in which we can either respect the individual welfare interests of study participants or we can generate the information necessary to promote scientific progress. We can't do both (Marquis 1983; Gifford 1986; Hellman 2002; Miller and Brody 2003). But this is a mistake.

The arguments in this section drive a stake into the heart of a very particular way of filling out the content of the template for the appeal to uncertainty. In particular, we have shown only that these objections apply to a very specific view, namely, the conception of equipoise in which the uncertainty in question resides in the head of the individual clinician or researcher and is represented as a subjective judgment that the interventions in question have equivalent expected therapeutic value. From the fact that this conception of equipoise prohibits the vast majority, if not the entirety of socially valuable clinical research, it does not follow that the template for the appeal to uncertainty is unworkable. That is because there are other ways that the template can be filled out. In particular, Freedman rejects the view of equipoise that locates the relevant uncertainty in the mind of the individual researcher, in part, to avoid these very objections. In the following chapter I argue for an alternative that is sufficient to reconcile respect for the welfare of participants with advancing the common good.

The point of these remarks is to highlight the significant influence of the various background claims and presuppositions that structure the conceptual ecosystem in which this view of equipoise most naturally arises. If we accept all of those presuppositions, then not only does there appear to be a dilemma at the heart of clinical research, but it appears to be stark and bleak. On the one hand, if we endorse the idea that the best way to make sense of respect for the welfare interests of study participants is to appeal to the individual clinician's duty of personal care, and we retain the traditional, Hippocratic conception of that duty, then we have to bite the bullet and hold that most clinical research is unethical. Alternatively, if we step back from all of this, and examine our intuition that a good deal of sound clinical research is not morally objectionable, then we seem to have to bite a different bullet and infer the utilitarianism of clinical research has to take priority over concern for individual participant welfare. This is why it is critical to distinguish the template for the appeal to uncertainty, and the range of alternatives for completing its practical content, from this particular attempt to specify its content.

5.6.2 Permitting Senseless Studies

The previous section recapitulated some prominent arguments in the literature on equipoise. Those arguments show that the view of equipoise that refuses to die is overly restrictive in that it would prohibit scientifically and socially valuable research from ever starting and that, even if such research can be initiated, this framework would prevent it from generating sufficiently reliable information to alter clinical practice and advance the standard of care.

One potential weakness of that argument is that proponents of the conception of equipoise that refuses to die might bite the bullet and simply hold that it is not permissible to violate the clinician's duty of personal care as they conceive it. The important insight in this response is that the arguments in the previous section rely on an independent judgment that clinical research is sufficiently valuable and important that a view which would prohibit all research must be morally flawed. Without independent support for the value of research, the previous argument might be seen as begging the question—as asserting that research is morally acceptable when the argument in question gives us credible reasons to believe that it is not. As a result, it is important to consider other weaknesses in the view of equipoise in question that do not rely on any claims about the moral value of activities that such a view prohibits.

The next argument points out something that is not well understood in the larger literature: the view of equipoise that locates uncertainty in the mind of the individual clinician and treats it as a fragile state of equivalence in prospect is too permissive—the studies that most clearly satisfy its requirements can lack significant social value.

On the view of equipoise in question, research is permissible when the expert clinician or researcher does not have a preference between any members of a set of interventions. This condition occurs when the expert judges that the members of that set have equal expected value. If a clinician believes that interventions A and B have equal expected value, then, on this view, it is permissible to allow study participants to be randomized to receive either of these interventions. The objections of the previous section target the state of affairs in which we need new information to clarify the relative merits of a set of interventions in order to close a knowledge gap. I say they target this case because closing an information gap is a paradigm case of a study with social value—generating reliable information in that case has a high likelihood of altering clinical practice and providing patients and other stakeholders with the information they need to make momentous decisions. The point of the objections of the previous section is that the conception of equipoise that refuses to die is incapable of generating information of this kind.

But consider the case in which an agent's belief that the interventions in the relevant set are of equivalent clinical value rests on considerable prior evidence. In this case, subjecting these interventions to further testing would not have significant social value and so would not be a wise use of scarce resources since we are asserting, by hypothesis, that there is no evidence gap that needs to be filled to improve the care of future patients. Nevertheless, it would be the case that such a study is morally permissible on the view of equipoise under consideration since the individual clinician or researcher has no grounds on which to prefer one intervention over the others. Although there is no social value in initiating such a study, the conception of equipoise in question regards the study as morally permissible because it begins in a state of equipoise—the individual researcher regards the relevant interventions as an equal bet in prospect.

Moreover, this study represents one of the rare cases in which this view of equipoise can support a trial that runs to completion. In other words, if the interventions in question really are of equivalent value, then it would be possible to run the study to completion as long as interim evidence accurately reflects their equivalent practical utility. But the fact that such studies could be run to completion cannot be used to rebut the present objection since the probability that such a study runs to completion is in inverse proportion to the social value of the study. The less likely it is that we will learn anything new, the more likely it is that such a study will remain permissible on this (faulty!) conception of equipoise.

The argument in this section does not rest on any question begging assumptions about the relative importance of generating socially valuable information compared to the importance of respect for participant welfare. Instead, it shows that the conception of uncertainty that motivates this common and intuitive view of equipoise does a poor job of tracking the social value requirement, since the clearest cases in which this type of equipoise is likely to obtain are the least likely to generate information that will close important information gaps.

5.6.3 Conflicting Judgments and
Self-Defeating Requirements

There is an additional argument against the conception of equipoise as a fragile state of uncertainty in the mind of the individual clinician that does not rest on what the proponents of that view may be motivated to regard as potentially objectionable premises about how to trade off one value against another. In particular, this conception of equipoise is self-defeating in the sense that it sets back the legitimate interests of a range of stakeholders without advancing any countervailing interests. Part of the problem relates to the reason why Freedman rejected this view of equipoise, namely, it is incapable of addressing a common kind of medical uncertainty precisely because that uncertainty is not to be found in the head of any particular expert.

One of the reasons that Freedman rejected the view that equipoise is a state of uncertainty in the mind of the individual clinician is that he had a clear sense that this focus is too narrow. In particular, there is often reasonable diversity in judgment among well-qualified and informed medical experts. Any conception of uncertainty that focuses solely on the judgment of a single medical expert will fail to capture an important form of uncertainty that clinical research should play a key role in addressing. This is uncertainty in the form of conflicting expert judgments or conflicting medical assessments.

To illustrate this point, let us more carefully consider what states might count as examples of medical uncertainty. The view of equipoise that frames uncertainty as a feature of the decision process of an individual decision-maker can recognize two states of affairs that count as exemplifying medical uncertainty.

I call the first state of affairs *clinical agnosticism*. This state obtains when the individual decision-maker does not have a considered expert judgment about the relative merits of a set of medical interventions for patients with a specific medical condition. For instance, we can imagine a condition for which there are no interventions that have been established as effective treatments and there is a novel intervention that has been shown to be safe in healthy adults. Now consider a proposal to test the efficacy of this novel intervention in a trial in which all participants receive usual medical care and randomization is used to determine which patients receive a placebo and which receive the novel, investigational intervention. In this case, the set of relevant interventions includes A, the investigational drug, and B, the placebo. An expert clinician is agnostic about the relevant merits of A and B if that expert considers the evidence so sparse or unreliable that it doesn't favor one option over the others.

Clinical agnosticism is different from what I will call *clinical equivalence*. This is because the agnostic clinician is unable to form a preference of any kind between the interventions in question. In other words, the expert is unwilling to say that A is preferable to B, that B is preferable to A, or that A and B are of equivalent value. In contrast, clinical equivalence is the state in which the expert believes that the evidence is sufficient to warrant a judgment about the relative merits of the interventions in question and, on the basis of that information, concludes that they are of equivalent expected value.

Clinical equivalence may itself come in different forms or flavors. For example, if the evidence about the relative merits of A and B is relatively sparse, then the assessments of the likely expected value of each intervention might involve probability distributions that are very wide and encompass a broad range of possibilities. In contrast, as evidence accumulates about the merits of A and B, that uncertainty might narrow, indicating a greater confidence on the part of the expert about what to expect from the provision of these interventions.

For our present purposes, the main point is that neither clinical agnosticism nor clinical equivalence can capture another state of affairs that seems to represent a paradigm case of medical uncertainty. I call this state *clinical conflict*. The state of clinical conflict obtains when one group of well-informed and expert clinicians have a strict preference for one option over the others (for example, these clinicians regard A as a superior treatment option to B) but there are other, equally well-informed experts who regard B as the superior treatment option to A. This is a case of clinical conflict because every expert clinician has a definitive expert judgment that one intervention is superior to the others, but the judgments of these well-informed medical experts do not agree. In the example I've just given, no individual expert is in a state of clinical agnosticism or clinical equivalence with respect to A and B. Nevertheless, the community is in a state of clinical conflict because some judge A to be superior to B while others judge B to be superior to A.

Freedman rejects the idea that equipoise is a state of uncertainty in the mind of the individual clinician precisely because he recognizes that what I am calling clinical conflict is a form of medical uncertainty in which there is "a split in the clinical community, with some clinicians favoring A and others favoring B" (1987, 144). This is why he is at pains to say that his favored position, what he calls *clinical equipoise,* is "consistent with a decided treatment preference on the part of the investigators. They simply recognize that their less favored treatment is preferred by colleagues whom they consider to be responsible and competent" (1987, 144).

Freedman makes this move because he recognizes that there is significant social value in conducting research that has the prospect of reducing conflict among expert clinicians. If it is the case that one group of clinicians is correct, and that, for example, the clinical merits of A dominate the merits of B, then demonstrating this fact will reduce inefficiencies in current practice since, without the study, some experts would provide B to patients. Not only are some patients receiving inferior medical care, but scarce resources are being spent on the provision of inferior care. Reducing or eliminating such inefficiency will directly benefit patients and help health systems steward shared resources to more effective uses.

The problem, however, is that the view of equipoise that we have been entertaining here—the one that Freedman rejects and that refuses to die—cannot permit research that is designed to address a state of conflict among well-informed medical experts. The reason for this is simple: no expert is uncertain in the sense of uncertainty that defines that view. In a case of clinical conflict, every expert has a definitive expert judgment in favor of one option and no clinician is in a state of clinical agnosticism or clinical equivalence. Those who favor A over B thus see themselves as having a duty of personal care to their patients to provide them with A and to prevent them from being randomized to B. Similarly, those who favor B over A see themselves as having a duty of personal care to their patients to provide them directly with B and to prevent them from being randomized to A. Because no clinician is uncertain, if the view of equipoise that refuses to die is correct, a trial that would establish the relative merits of A and B cannot be run.

This result, however, is absurd. Patients who happen to live in one place, or who happen to have a particular insurance provider, or who happen to be assigned to a particular clinician, will receive intervention A. Other patients, who happen to live in a different place, or who happen to have a different insurance provider, or who happen to be assigned to a different clinician, will continue to receive intervention B. Each clinician believes she is doing what is best for her individual patient, and each disagrees with the treatment recommendations of other equally well-informed medical experts. Prohibiting patients from being randomized to A or B results in a situation where arbitrary differences in location, insurance coverage, or other circumstances result in some patients receiving A and some receiving B, but under conditions in which the relevant merits of these interventions cannot be compared. The prohibition on randomization thus deprives a wide range of stakeholders of information that is relevant to decisions that affect people's health and welfare without advancing any countervailing interest.

Now consider the situation in which we allow patients to be randomized to A or B. In this case, some patients receive intervention A and some receive intervention B—just as in the status quo. Only now, randomization creates the conditions under which the effects of each intervention are statistically independent of a wide range of factors that might influence and confound the observed outcomes. As a result, the random allocation creates the conditions under which we can discern the relative clinical merits of A and B. We can learn, that is, whether one of these interventions is superior to the other.

Prohibiting this trial makes no one better off. It doesn't advance the interests of any person. Nor does it protect patients from receiving substandard care since prohibiting the trial permits both A and B to be provided by clinicians who favor them. All it does is deprive clinicians, patients, and other stakeholders of the information they need to better advance the health needs of people with this medical condition. Similarly, permitting this trial does not make anyone worse off. Each participant receives a level of care that would be recommended for them by an expert clinician. But when participants are matched with treatments by a random process, we can expeditiously learn about the relative merits of these interventions and improve medical practice.

Prohibiting a patient from being offered the option of being randomized to A or B in the presence of effective study oversight is self-defeating. It removes an option that does not adversely affect any interest of any stakeholder, but which does represent an avenue through which participants can contribute to the resolution of a clinically meaningful question. Blocking research as an avenue through which patients can contribute to the common good, in the sense defended here, is an unjustifiable restriction on individual liberty. Because it also prevents the generation of a social good without any offsetting benefit to participants, it stymies a socially beneficial undertaking without warrant. The myriad stakeholders who rely on the information such studies are intended to generate are deprived of that information, setting back the interests of the various stakeholders who depend on them, without an offsetting benefit.

The argument outlined here represents a powerful objection to the view of equipoise that requires uncertainty in the mind of the individual researcher. It identifies an area of uncertainty—clinical conflict—which that view is incapable of accommodating. Nothing in these arguments presupposes controversial claims about how to trade off risks to participants against the likely gains in socially valuable information. Rather, the kind of case outlined here represents a situation in which the interests of participants and the requirements of sound science are not in conflict. The fact that the conception of equipoise that refuses to die prohibits research in this case reveals the extent to which it is misguided, and its normative foundations fail to track the ethically relevant issues.

5.6.4 Confusion in the Field: The Uncertainty Principle, Equipoise, and Clinical Equipoise

Too often, the view that treats the relevant uncertainty as a fragile subjective state of the individual clinician is treated as synonymous with *the* equipoise requirement, or as capturing the essentials of all variants of the equipoise principle. For example, Ashcroft describes clinical equipoise as

> equipoise in the mind of the intending physician regarding treatment options. In many ways, this remains the best formulation. For clinical equipoise is a necessary condition on entering a patient into a trial, and if any clinician is not in clinical equipoise regarding a patient of a trial, then this

(or any other of his patients) should not be entered by him or her into the trial. The ethical duty of the physician here is clear enough. (1999, 320)

Equating this position with clinical equipoise is a mistake. Nevertheless, it is a mistake whose seeds were sewn at the birth of the concept of clinical equipoise. When Freedman opens his seminal paper "Equipoise and the Ethics of Clinical Research," he writes:

> In the simplest model, testing a new treatment B on a defined population P for which the current accepted treatment is A, it is necessary that the clinical investigator be in a state of genuine uncertainty regarding the comparative merits of treatments A and B for population P. If a physician knows that these treatments are not equivalent, ethics requires that the superior treatment be recommended. (1987, 141)

In this general introductory statement, Freedman is following Charles Fried's formulation in which the uncertainty that is required to justify the trial is situated in the mind of the individual clinical investigator. This gives readers the false impression that Freedman is expressing his own, considered view in this passage. The problem is that Freedman does not endorse this view. He calls it "theoretical equipoise," which he rejects.

According to the view of clinical equipoise that Freedman actually endorses, the requisite uncertainty is located in the larger expert medical community. Equipoise obtains when "there is no consensus within the expert clinical community about the comparative merits of the alternatives to be tested" (1987, 144). Moreover, Freedman explicitly states that clinical equipoise can exist in situations in which no individual clinician is uncertain. This happens when there is "a split in the clinical community, with some clinicians favoring A and others favoring B." In this case, he argues, clinical equipoise is "consistent with a decided treatment preference on the part of the investigators. They simply recognize that their less favored treatment is preferred by colleagues whom they consider to be responsible and competent" (1987, 144). Finally, Freedman adopts a more robust epistemic threshold, according to which the relevant uncertainty persists until evidence for the superiority of one intervention emerges that would be sufficient to forge a consensus in the relevant expert clinical community (Freedman 1987, 1990). This threshold requires that the evidence supporting a claim to superiority on behalf of one intervention from among the set under consideration must be sufficiently compelling that it will influence the practice behavior, not just of one physician, but of the community of physicians.

What Ashcroft identifies as "clinical equipoise," therefore, is actually what Freedman identified as "theoretical equipoise" and what Fried had referred to simply as "equipoise." Adding to the confusion, within literature from the United Kingdom this latter position (what Freedman calls "theoretical equipoise") is commonly referred to under the name of "the uncertainty principle" (Hill 1963; Peto et al. 1976; Peto and Baigent 1998; Sackett 2000). In contrast, what Freedman actually describes as "clinical equipoise," Ashcroft calls "collective or professional equipoise," a term that is also more common among writers from the United Kingdom (e.g., Chard and Lilford 1998).

As a result, when the concepts of equipoise or clinical equipoise are invoked in all but the most scrupulous literature, they are often glossed in the terms I outlined in §5.5—as a requirement that the individual researcher believe that the interventions in question are an equal bet in prospect. Even when scholars distinguish the concept of clinical equipoise from other variants of equipoise, the former view is frequently mislabeled. Given the proliferation of different nomenclatures, this has created a fair amount of both confusion and frustration.

As a result, the view I've outlined is like a character from a horror film. It can be shot, stabbed, and burned, but just when you divert your attention it rises again to stalk the pages of journals and lecture halls, reigning terror in its wake. In part, this happens when scholars who believe they have vanquished this view under one label—they have repudiated it under the label of "theoretical equipoise," for example—go on to invoke the content of theoretical equipoise in some more restricted domain (§5.7). In other cases, rampant confusion over what constitutes equipoise in general, or clinical equipoise in particular, promotes the tendency to (mistakenly) explicate any proposal made under this moniker by reverting to the terms of the view it is intended to displace. This process is undoubtedly fueled, in part, by the fact that the term "equipoise" seems to connote something like views that are "equally poised" on a scale or an edge of some sort.[5] This imagery, in a conceptual

[5] Eyal and Lipsitch (2017) is a recent example in which equipoise is rejected under the assumption that it requires individual uncertainty and an equal balance of probabilities.

ecosystem structured by the two dogmas of research ethics explicated previously, creates a set of entailments that seem entirely natural and straightforward. As a result, this conception of equipoise is the philosophical equivalent of the alien that has laid its egg in the stomach of its unwitting victim so that the monster can dramatically burst forth from the victim's chest, only the victim here is clinical equipoise and the view that bursts forth is the view of equipoise it was meant to supplant and replace.

For the moment, the point I want to drive home is that the view of equipoise that refuses to die—what Freedman calls "theoretical equipoise" and what Charles Fried simply called equipoise—cannot provide a workable foundation for scientifically and socially valuable research. This failure reinforces the perception that there is a fundamental conflict—a moral dilemma—at the heart of research ethics. As I showed in the previous section, Freedman had already recognized some of the weaknesses in this view and they drove his attempt to defend an alternative view that might avoid these shortcomings.

Freedman's core innovation was to move the uncertainty that is relevant to establishing the boundaries of morally permissible research out of the head of the individual clinician. I think that this move was largely correct, and I extend and build on it in the next chapter. However, because Freedman continued to ground his view in the role-related obligations of physicians, his view also suffers from significant problems.

Before turning to those arguments, it is important to consider a recent challenge to Freedman's conception of equipoise that has been articulated, perhaps surprisingly, by two of its most ardent defenders. Miller and Weijer (2006b) argue that clinical equipoise is insufficient as a moral safeguard on research because "clinical equipoise does not adequately specify the doctor-researcher's duty of care to the patient-subject" (2006b, 546). Examining their claims will underscore the extent to which a focus on the moral responsibilities of individual clinicians has such a powerful hold on the moral debate in this area. It also allows us to investigate the merits of an alternative formation of Fried's equipoise in which the relevant uncertainty is located in the mind of the individual clinician, but the fragile threshold for disturbing equipoise is replaced by a more robust, social threshold.

5.7 The Duty of Care Revisited

5.7.1 Does Clinical Equipoise Address the Wrong Issue?

Miller and Weijer frame the fundamental problem of research ethics in terms that recapitulate the first dogma of research ethics. On the one hand, randomized clinical trials (RCTs) are designed to produce the public good of generalizable medical evidence. On the other hand, physician-researchers owe patients a "duty of care" that requires that they exercise their discretionary powers to advance patient interests "to the greatest extent possible" (2006b, 545). They thus hold that the "central dilemma of the randomized clinical trial" arises "because offering patients enrolment in RCTs imperils the doctor's duty to act in their interests" (542). The core question to be resolved, then, is "when may physicians, consistent with their duty of care to patients, offer them enrolment in an RCT?" (542).[6]

Miller and Weijer are proponents of clinical equipoise, but they part ways with Freedman when they argue that "clinical equipoise does not adequately specify the doctor-researcher's duty of care to the patient-subject" (2006b, 546). Their argument for this claim involves several steps. First, they note, correctly, that questions about the social value of a trial and the reasonableness of the risks that it involves must be addressed at the point when a study protocol is being formulated and prior to the enrollment of study participants. In other words, before participants can be approached with the possibility of participating in a study, an IRB must find that the study is ethically permissible.

Second, Miller and Weijer argue that Freedman's clinical equipoise is the appropriate standard for approving a study protocol. In other words, IRBs can ask whether there is honest and informed disagreement among experts in the relevant medical community about the interventions to be tested in a study and, if this is the case, they can permit a trial to move forward. Miller and Weijer refer to this as fulfilling the state's obligation in protecting the "agent-neutral interests of patient-subjects" (2006, 543). Although they do not define the term "agent-neutral interests" the idea appears to be that these are interests that agents can be presumed to have insofar as they are patients with a particular medical condition who meet the conditions listed

---

[6] There is a minor typographical error in this passage that I have corrected in my quotation.

in the protocol's inclusion criteria and who lack the various characteristics listed as exclusion criteria. When IRBs find that clinical equipoise exists— that there is honest disagreement about the merits of the interventions in a trial for patients who meet the stated inclusion criteria and lack character- istics in the exclusion criteria—then the IRB ensures that participants "will not be asked to accept substandard treatment to participate in clinical re- search" (544).

Thirdly, they argue that because IRB approval is limited to the protection of these agent-neutral interests, such approval "does not entail the moral or legal acceptability of enrolling particular patient-subjects in research, nor does it entail the acceptability of their continued participation in the study, as these acts engage the agent-relative interests of patient-subjects" (2006, 545). Once again, the term "agent-relative" interests is not defined, but from the context it appears that it refers to specific or unique interests that pertain to individual subjects. Thus, for example, if the specific medical history of a patient suggests that receiving a particular intervention A would be "unduly harmful" (2006, 546) then it would be impermissible to enroll such a person in a study in which they might be randomized to A, even if that patient has the medical condition that A is intended to address.

As a result, Miller and Weijer argue that clinical equipoise captures a duty that the state owes to individuals who agree to participate in research to en- sure that their agent-neutral interests will be protected in the course of such participation. However, as they understand it, "clinical equipoise does not contemplate the particular circumstances of individual patient-subjects. Therefore, it is not, and indeed cannot be, considered to be an adequate spec- ification of the duty of care of doctor-researchers, because they are bound to protect the agent-relative welfare interests of the patient-subjects" (2006, 546). In effect, they argue that clinical equipoise is a solution to the wrong problem: the fundamental dilemma at the heart of research is about how to reconcile research participation with the clinician's duty of personal care—a subject, they argue, Freedman's clinical equipoise simply doesn't address.

5.7.2 The Clinical Judgment Principle

As a result, Miller and Weijer claim that although clinical equipoise is a nec- essary condition for ethically initiating a trial, no person can be enrolled into a trial solely on the basis of clinical equipoise. Rather, to reconcile study participation with the physician's duty of personal care, it must also be the case that the individual physician-researcher regards study participation as consistent with that duty. And, like Fried and others, Miller and Weijer argue that the duty of care requires the exercise of discretionary powers for the sole purpose of advancing the individual patient's medical best interests.

Miller and Weijer take themselves to be showing that clinical equipoise and Fried's equipoise are not mutually exclusive. The former governs the review of study protocols by IRBs and the latter states the conditions under which individuals can be recruited into a study. How then do they propose to avoid the problems that led Freedman to reject Fried's view in the first place—the problems we canvassed in §5.5–5.6?

Miller and Weijer argue that it is a mistake to assume that the clinician's duty is based on a fragile epistemic threshold in which a mere hunch that one intervention is superior to the rest is sufficient to trigger the physician's duty of personal care and require the provision of that intervention and no other. Instead, they argue that individual researchers are subject to what they call the "clinical judgment principle," which holds that if an RCT has been approved by an IRB, "the physician may offer patients enrolment in a trial unless (1) they believe that it would be medically irresponsible to do so and (2) this belief is supported by evidence that ought to be convincing to colleagues" (2006, 546).

How is this clinical judgment principle supposed to avoid the problems that plague Fried's equipoise? Presumably, the idea is that this principle has a more robust epistemic threshold. Recall that on the more fragile view, a clinician would be obligated to provide A over B if she had a mere hunch that A was superior to B. On the present view, presumably the clinician could permit a patient to be randomized to A or B, even if she had a hunch that A was better, as long as that hunch is not supported by evidence that "ought to be convincing to colleagues." Presumably, if there is evidence that ought to be convincing to colleagues that A is superior to B, then it would be impermissible to allow that patient to be randomized to A. In fact, it may be medically irresponsible to allow randomization in that case. In effect, Miller and Weijer want to hold that clinicians who favor one intervention over another (e.g., A over B) can still allow their patients to participate in a study in which they will be randomized to A or B as long as doing so does not represent a medically irresponsible action, where "medically irresponsible" is a higher threshold than the standard of providing what the individual clinician actually believes is optimal care.

5.7.3 A Dilemma for the Clinical Judgment Principle

Miller and Weijer's proposal reflects the profound influence of the idea that the central issue to be resolved in research with human participants is to reconcile the duties of the individual clinician with respect for the welfare of the individual patient. Appealing to a more robust epistemic threshold is supposed to allow them to have the cake of locating uncertainty in the mind of the individual clinician even after having eaten the cake of avoiding the problems that plague the conception of equipoise that refuses to die.

But their view seems to face a difficult dilemma. Recall that Miller and Weijer find clinical equipoise deficient because it does not adequately address the duty of care of physician-researchers who must exercise their judgment and discretion in order to advance the agent-relative welfare interests of their patients to the best of their ability. But what is the relationship of the clinical judgment principle to the expert's duty of personal care? Either the clinical judgment principle is weaker than the clinician's morally and legally recognized professional duty to her individual patient or it is not. If it is weaker, then Miller and Weijer's own view can be rejected for not addressing what they regard as the central problem to be resolved, namely, reconciling research participation with the clinician's actual duty of personal care. If it is not weaker, then it is unclear how their position on this question differs from Fried's and therefore avoids the deep problems that his view faces (§5.6).

Although this dilemma can be easily stated, it cannot be easily addressed. We can amplify these concerns by revisiting the extent to which locating the focus of moral uncertainty back in the head of the medical expert recapitulates one of the very problems that clinical equipoise was developed to resolve—failing to recognize disagreement among experts as a kind of uncertainty that clinical trials ought to address (§5.6.3).

5.7.4 Conflicts over What Is Medically Irresponsible

A second major problem with this approach helps to flesh out the concern raised in the previous section. In particular, because the clinical judgment principle locates the relevant uncertainty in the head of the individual clinician, it cannot cope with situations in which expert disagreement runs so deep and is so polarized that the various sides question whether the care recommended by the others is ethically responsible.

Imagine a case in which some clinicians not only favor one intervention (e.g., A over B) but regard the other as medically irresponsible. Imagine further that other clinicians favor a different intervention (B over A) and regard the other as medically irresponsible. Now imagine further that each individual physician bases their judgment, not on a mere hunch, but on medical evidence that each regard as of sufficient credibility that it ought to be convincing to their colleagues. On the view articulated by Miller and Weijer, a protocol that would randomize individuals to these interventions could be approved by an IRB because such a body would correctly judge that clinical equipoise obtains—there is honest disagreement in the expert medical community about the relative merits of these interventions.

However, on Miller and Weijer's view, no clinician could permit her patients to enroll in such a study because doing so would violate the clinical judgment principle. That is, proponents of A would argue that it is medically irresponsible to allow their patients to be randomized to B and proponents of B would argue the same about being randomized to A. By reintroducing uncertainty in the mind of the individual clinician, Miller and Weijer's view recapitulates the same problems that we saw in §5.6—it prohibits socially valuable research without making anyone better off in the process.

5.7.5 Epistemic Humility

Miller and Weijer might argue that these last two objections misunderstand the force of the "ought" in the second condition of their principle of clinical judgment. In this view, if at least a reasonable minority of expert clinicians regard the evidence in support of A as sufficiently compelling that it ought to convince their colleagues, and a different group of at least a reasonable minority of experts believes the same about B, then both groups *ought* to update their beliefs and adopt the view that both treatments are above the threshold of medically responsible care. In other words, responsible medical professionals should show a modicum of epistemic humility in the face of such disagreements. Although this is a promising response, it suffers from several problems.

First, and most importantly, urging epistemic humility does not vindicate the importance of embracing uncertainty in the mind of the individual physician; it makes it irrelevant. This is because once we have established that clinical equipoise exists, we have established that there is sufficient evidence to support A and sufficient evidence to support B that reasonable experts "ought" to regard randomization to each of these interventions as being consistent with competent or morally acceptable medical care. But, in this case, all of the real moral and epistemological work is being done by clinical equipoise and by an auxiliary claim that when clinical equipoise exists, reasonable clinicians ought to, in some sense, recognize the validity of the expert judgments of their honest and informed colleagues.

Second, this auxiliary claim is itself a substantive position that may seem plausible, but as a descriptive claim it need not be true and as a normative claim it requires substantive defense. In other words, it is not clear that it is irrational or unethical for different individual experts who are fully aware of all of the relevant medical evidence to draw conflicting treatment recommendations from that same set of evidence. The reasons for this claim take us beyond the scope of the current argument, and I will return to this issue briefly in the next chapter. But all that matters for our present purposes is that if clinical equipoise obtains and that is sufficient for the auxiliary claim, then Miller and Weijer's position adds nothing that was not already present in Freedman's view. On the other hand, if clinical equipoise is not sufficient for the auxiliary claim and if experts do not adhere to it in a particular case—if they regard the opposing view as medically irresponsible—then Miller and Weijer's view faces the objection we explored in §5.6; it would prohibit the conduct of a study that has significant social value without advancing anyone's interests in doing so.

5.7.6 Clinical Equipoise and the Particularities of Individual Patients

A second response might be to say that the analysis I have provided so far misconstrues the role of clinical equipoise and fails to take seriously the respect in which Miller and Weijer regard it as inadequate. In particular, Miller and Weijer argue that clinical equipoise only addresses the agent-neutral interests of participants; it does not and cannot address the agent-relative interests of study participants. So, this reply runs, clinical equipoise must be augmented by the judgment of a clinician who has a duty of care toward the *individual* patient in question.

The problem with this reply is that it misconstrues the role that clinical equipoise can and ought to play in research ethics—clinical equipoise need not be limited to the agent-neutral interests of participants. Miller and Weijer correctly note that a trial protocol must be written at a certain level of generality, prior to an encounter with any particular patient, and that the question of whether or not a study would begin in and be designed to disturb clinical equipoise plays an important role in evaluating such protocols. They are also correct to note that inclusion and exclusion criteria are defined at the time the protocol is written and that it is important that these capture a realistic population of patients. Nevertheless, we can concede that they are also correct that if some patients could present with such a unique history—with characteristics that were not anticipated in the protocol's exclusion criteria—then the risks of study participation for that individual could be unreasonable. All of this is correct, as far as it goes.

But it is a mistake to think that just because IRBs must use clinical equipoise to determine whether or not to approve a particular protocol prior to the enrollment of individuals, that is the only place that clinical equipoise can be applied. To apply clinical equipoise at the level of individual patients, we need only ask whether, for each individual from whom consent is sought, experts who favor one intervention for patients with this condition would also regard that intervention as superior to the other alternatives *for this particular patient*. In other words, would those experts who favor treatment A over B for patients with this condition also prefer A over B for *this particular* patient? Similarly, would experts who favor B over A prefer B over A for *this particular* patient? If so, then it is permissible to randomize that patient to either A or B. Notice that it would be morally permissible even if each of these experts regards the evidence in favor of their preferred option as so strong that providing anything else violates Miller and Weijer's principle of clinical judgment.

Miller and Weijer appear to assume that questions about the unique medical history of particular individuals would have to be answered by a single individual and that that individual is the individual researcher. But this assumption is unnecessary. For example, imagine that after receiving IRB approval, a study begins to recruit participants. Each participant is evaluated by an expert who favors intervention A over B to determine whether in fact A would be an appropriate intervention for this person. This expert would determine whether, given the unique medical history of the person before them, there is any reason to think that A would pose unreasonable risks to this person (i.e., whether being given A is inconsistent with this person's agent-relative interests). Each participant is also evaluated by a second expert who favors intervention B (and so on if there are additional interventions). If one or more of these experts finds that a particular person should not receive the intervention that they tend to favor for patients of this type, then such a person could be excluded from the study, or could be prevented from being randomized to that intervention if there are others (e.g., B and C) that are regarded as not unduly risky for this individual by the experts who regard each of those interventions as best for patients of this type. A design of exactly this type (only each expert is replaced by a computer model of the considerations that they regard as relevant to their clinical assessments) is described in Kadane (1996).

In such cases, no expert is asked to alter her beliefs in light of the conflicting judgments of other experts. Each is asked to make a medical judgment that best advances the interests of the patient before them. Nevertheless, no single individual expert need be uncertain about the relative merits of the interventions in question and, in fact, each can regard the views of the others as representing irresponsible medical care. This demonstrates how, contrary to the claim of Miller and Weijer, clinical equipoise can be used to regulate both the approval of the study protocol and the inclusion of individual participants and that clinical equipoise is sufficient to safeguard the agent-relative interests of individual patients.

In summary, then, Miller and Weijer's view is least objectionable when it is interpreted in a way that simply uses the existence of clinical equipoise to determine what individual clinicians ought to believe. To the extent that their view deviates from the requirements of clinical equipoise it recapitulates some of the problems that plague Fried's view. Ultimately, the analysis presented here shows that their argument for departing from Freedman's position rests on an unreasonably narrow understanding of how conflicting professional judgments can be used to evaluate both study protocols and the inclusion of individual study participants. The framework that I defend in the following chapter illustrates how a principle similar to clinical equipoise can address the concerns that motivate Miller and Weijer's departure from clinical equipoise without recapitulating the errors of Fried's view.

The arguments of this and the previous several sections provide strong reasons to reject any view in which uncertainty in the mind of the individual clinician is treated as a necessary condition for ethically acceptable research. Because this view is often treated as the only way to fill out the content of the template for the appeal to uncertainty, it is often assumed that the failure of this position demonstrates that there is a moral dilemma at the heart of medical research. In truth, it shows only that this is a misguided way to fill out the details of the template.

In this section I argued that Freedman was aware of some of the limitations of treating the relevant uncertainty as located in the mind of the individual clinician. His claim that the relevant uncertainty should instead be treated as a function of beliefs of different experts in the medical community is important, and the view that I develop in the next chapter incorporates this insight. As we will see, however, the view I defend goes farther and rejects the commitment that Freedman shares with these other positions, namely, that the normative ground for the appeal to uncertainty is to reconcile role-related obligations of medical professionals with the demands of clinical research.

5.8 Purely Research-Related Risks

5.8.1 No Uncertainty about Purely Research-Related Risks

Even if it is possible to fill in the content of the template outlined in §5.4 in a way that avoids the problems discussed so far, it might be argued that this establishes that research can be organized to avoid a moral dilemma only if we limit ourselves to the interventions to which participants will be allocated. The next objection holds that there is, nevertheless, a dilemma at the heart of all research in which study participants are exposed to risks that derive from procedures or interventions that are necessary to advance the scientific aims of research and which are not offset by the prospect of individual benefit to participants. In other words, sometimes medical research requires tests or procedures that are performed solely to advance the purposes of research. They are necessary because they play a role in generating the data a study requires to assess the chosen endpoints or because they contribute to some other purely research-related desiderata, such as controlling bias. The worry, therefore, is that research that exposes participants to risks that are not offset by the prospect of direct medical benefit to those same participants poses a moral dilemma because it requires those participants to sacrifice their own welfare for the greater good.

This argument can be formulated in two ways. In §5.8.2 I present the version that focuses on the moral obligations of clinicians and researchers. In §5.8.4 I present a more general version that focuses on what it is rational for potential study participants to choose. The latter version of this argument is of special interest since it is widely seen as grounding the claim that research participation represents an instance of the prisoner's dilemma.

The goal of this section and the next is to demonstrate that these arguments presuppose a conception of individual interests that is unjustifiably narrow. This view of individual best interests produces a conception of the clinician-researcher's duty of care or fiduciary duty that is so restrictive that it would rule out as inappropriate activities that are widely regarded as ethically permissible in the very area from which it is supposedly derived, namely, clinical medicine. As a result, I demonstrate in §5.9.1 this conception of the researcher's moral obligation to study participants is unjustifiably paternalistic. A parallel argument in §5.9.3 holds for the conception of individual interest presupposed in the claim that research participation constitutes a version of the prisoner's dilemma.

Together these arguments reveal the extent to which the first dogma of research ethics contributes to a conceptual ecosystem in which the appearance that research participation requires tragic choices is almost inescapable. Because Freedman's conception of clinical equipoise accepts this dogma of research ethics—it frames the point of the appeal to uncertainty as reconciling the clinician's duty of personal care with the demands of sound science—the problems discussed in this and the following section reveal important shortcomings in Freedman's conception of clinical equipoise. Together, these arguments illustrate the importance of finding an alternative normative ground for the appeal to uncertainty and reconsidering the first dogma of research ethics.

5.8.2 The Clinician-Centered Formulation

The *clinician-centered formulation of the argument from purely research-related risks* begins with the claim that a great deal of medical research involves practices, procedures, or interventions that are "not clinically indicated" (Wertheimer 2010, 9). These are interventions that would not be performed on a person in the context of direct medical care. Rather, they are provided because of the contribution they make to some important aspect of a research study. For example, in order to measure concentrations of a drug in a participant's blood, a study protocol may require study-related blood samples at regular intervals. In order to measure the effect of a drug on a tumor, the protocol may require multiple biopsies at pre-specified intervals. In more extreme cases, in order to ensure that study participants cannot tell whether they received the active intervention in a trial or the control intervention, some study participants may be exposed to sham procedures. In the most benign cases, these procedures may involve mostly theater— surgeons reading a script, making superficial incisions in a participant's skin, and pretending to insert an arthroscope into the participant's knee, for example. But in other cases, the sham procedure can involve drilling a hole in a participant's skull and inserting a cannula which will deliver the investigational drug to those in the active arm and a placebo substance to those randomized to the control group (London 2006b, see also London and Kadane 2002, 2003).

The second claim is that the provision of such procedures cannot be justified by any view that requires research participation to be consistent with the individual clinician's duty of personal care. In particular, if that duty is understood along traditional, Hippocratic lines, then the clinician cannot recommend any course of care that is less optimal than some other possible course of care. But purely research-related procedures are provided solely to advance the scientific goals of a trial and not to advance the interests of the individual participant. As a result, clinicians who act on their fiduciary duty to put the interests of their patients above all other concerns, and who act on their duty to provide optimal courses of care to each patient, will not be able to support participation in any trial that exposes participants to such purely research-related risks.

To put matters in terms that link it more directly to the template outlined in §5.4, the risks and burdens of purely study-related procedures cannot be justified by the presence of uncertainty *no matter where it is located*. The risks and burdens of study-related procedures are usually not subject to the relevant kind of uncertainty—clinicians are not likely to be agnostic about whether such procedures align with and advance the interests of study participants. Rather, the opposite is likely to be the case—their risks and burdens are known and not reasonably seen as being offset by the prospect of direct benefit to the patient. Similarly, no clinician is likely to hold that the option of being exposed to such procedures in the course of a clinical trial has the same expected value for a patient's health interests as the option of foregoing study participation and receiving medical care directly. If everyone agrees that a given intervention or procedure carries risks and burdens that are not offset by the prospect of individual benefit, then there is also no clinical conflict about their relative therapeutic, diagnostic, or prophylactic merits.

Even if uncertainty can bridge the divide between the clinician's duty of personal care and the demands of scientific research when it comes to the provision of alternative medical treatments or investigational interventions that are being tested as candidates for treatment, the objection currently under consideration holds that it can't play this role for purely study-related procedures. If a study protocol requires a set of blood draws or biopsies that would not be required in the context of normal medical care, then it is unlikely that even a reasonable minority of expert clinicians would regard those procedures as potentially beneficial to the individual trial participant. But if such uncertainty does not obtain, then we cannot appeal to the existence of uncertainty to reconcile study participation with the fiduciary duties of caregivers. Therefore these procedures appear to pose a dilemma for research ethics.

5.8.3 Compromising the Duty of Personal Care

The objection from study-related risks relies on a contingent feature of research, since different studies involve purely study-related procedures or interventions to varying degrees. In principle as well as in practice it is possible to design valid studies in which the relative merits of a set of interventions are explored without exposing participants to purely study-related procedures or interventions. This would be the case, for example, if the merits of these interventions are compared only on the basis of endpoints and measures that are routinely used in the course of delivering those interventions in clinical practice. Nevertheless, most studies with human participants do expose participants to purely study-related procedures that carry some risk or degree of burden. When this is the case, such research would be regarded as ethically impermissible on any view that requires its conduct to be consistent with the clinician's duty of personal care, understood as optimizing the medical interests of individual patients.

Even advocates for clinical equipoise seem to accept the conclusion of the argument in §5.8.2. In particular, the proponents of what is called "component analysis" restrict the scope of the equipoise requirement to interventions that are provided with "therapeutic warrant" (Weijer 1999, 2000; Weijer and Miller 2004). This includes interventions whose diagnostic, prophylactic, or therapeutic merits are in question and under scrutiny in a particular study. As such, all purely research-related aspects of a study must be assessed on terms that reflect the weighing of different interests, as reflected in the definition of reasonable risk outlined in §5.2.4.

But adopting two standards for assessing research risks, as component analysis does, is a tacit admission that it is not possible to reconcile all aspects of clinical research with the clinician's duty of personal care. Since exposing individuals to procedures that, as Wertheimer puts it, are "not clinically indicated" cannot be reconciled with the clinician's duty of personal care, then critics can insist that component analysis shows that it is not possible for research to proceed on terms that are consistent with the clinician's duty of personal care. If what we "ought" to do is reasonably limited to what we "can" do (if "ought" implies "can"), then the proponents of component analysis must admit that it is permissible to carry out research on terms that diverge from the clinician's duty of personal care.

I have explicitly formulated the argument of this section as applying to the project of reconciling research participation with the role-related obligations of caregivers. This is an important objection and, as I argue in §5.9–5.10, it reveals a genuine problem for views that accept the first dogma of research ethics. Before turning to that discussion, however, it is important to present an alternative formulation of this argument that seems to have even broader scope and even more important implications. In particular, if it is true that research in which individuals are exposed to purely research-related risks cannot be reconciled with the clinician's duty of personal care, and if the clinician is seen as the fiduciary of the interests of the individual patient, then it seems to follow that participation in any such research is against the interests of individual participants and so not a rational choice for those individuals.

5.8.4 The Participant-Centered Formulation

In the previous three sections I explicated what I called the clinician-centered formulation of the argument from purely research-related risks. In this section I introduce a related version of this argument that I refer to as the *participant-centered formulation of the argument from purely research-related risks*. What makes this formulation appear to be distinctive is that it seems to bypass an appeal to the role-related obligations of health professionals altogether, holding instead that research participation is fundamentally inconsistent with the individual participant's concern for her own welfare. In other words, for any individual who is primarily concerned with her own medical best interests, clinical research appears not to be a rational choice.

Something like this argument seems to motivate the assertion of Menikoff and Richards that "tragic choices [are] involved in designing a system for research on human subjects" (2006, 19). Tragic choices are required because:

> Doing research involves *intentionally* exposing persons to risks, and *not for the primary purpose of treating them or making them better*, but rather to answer a research question. And, given the sorts of things that are commonly done in research studies, being a research subject in many cases will indeed be a bad choice for someone who is mainly concerned about his or her own best interests. (18)

If a person is "mainly concerned about her own best interests," then she will avoid participating in research because such participation so frequently involves being exposed to interventions, practices, or procedures that expose participants to burdens and risks without the offsetting prospect of direct, personal benefit.

5.8.5 Is Research Participation a Prisoner's Dilemma?

The idea that research participation is antithetical to the best interests of participants entails that if those individuals are choosing rationally, they will do all that they can to avoid research participation. At a social level, this creates a kind of paradox: although we all want to benefit from advances in the standard of care brought about by the conduct of well-designed research with human participants, none of us wants to be such a participant. The postulated moral conflict at the heart of medical research thus manifests at the social level in the form of a serious social dilemma.

The claim that medical research poses a social dilemma has been made by several scholars. David Heyd (1996) argues that research participation poses a social dilemma that is "reminiscent of the Prisoner's Dilemma" (193) because each potential participant would prefer to receive care directly from their clinician than to participate in a randomized clinical trial. If each person pursues what is in their individual interest, it forecloses advances in medical understanding. But, in order to agree to participate in a randomized clinical trial, an individual would have to choose an option that is not as good as the available alternative from the standpoint of her narrow self-interest.

Alan Wertheimer makes a similar argument:

> Hence, we face a form of prisoners' dilemma. Suppose that the best available information suggests that it is 60% likely that intervention X is superior to intervention Y. Although it is in the *ex ante* interest of each individual not to participate in research and to simply receive X, it is in the interest of many others (including future persons) that a sufficient number participate in research to determine whether X is superior to Y with a greater level of certainty. Moreover, even if it were 50/50 as to whether X is superior to Y, it would be a bad choice to enter such a trial if one has to undergo procedures that were not clinically indicated or one were otherwise inconvenienced by participation. (2010, 9)

Wertheimer's claim that research with human subjects has the basic structure of a prisoner's dilemma draws on two sets of considerations that we have examined so far. The first (discussed in §5.6) is the idea that equipoise, conceived of as uncertainty in the mind of the individual expert, is fragile and evanescent—it will rarely obtain and even when it does it will not persist until the conclusion of a trial. The second is the idea that clinical research often involves tests or procedures that are not aimed at the medical best interests of participants. In both cases, Wertheimer argues that it is against the interest of potential participants to participate in research.

Wertheimer's formulation of the claim that research ethics requires tragic choices reveals the close connection between the clinician-centered and the participant-centered formulations of the argument from purely research-related risks. In particular, both arguments rely on a particular conception of the relationship between rational choice, welfare, and the health interests of the individual. In the participant-centered formulation, rational choice is equated with choosing the option that best advances the interests of the agent, where those are equated with that person's narrow health interests. The same view is presupposed in the clinician-centered formulation to the extent that it relies on the traditional, Hippocratic conception of the caregiver's duty of personal care. On that view, the duty of personal care requires clinicians to choose the option available to her that best optimizes the individual's medical best interests.

Purely study-related procedures and interventions appear to create a dilemma for research ethics because they are inconsistent with the medical best interests of participants. After all, these procedures or interventions are used, not because of the prospect that they will help the individual participant, but because of the way they contribute to a scientifically sound or socially valuable study design. A clinician who is obligated to choose only interventions or procedures that advance the narrow medical best interests of the patient before her cannot choose to expose individuals to such interventions. Similarly, if we assume that rational choice requires individuals to choose options that are in their own medical best interests, then no individual would rationally choose to participate in a study in which she is exposed to burdens and risks that are not offset by the prospect of direct, individual benefit.[7]

In the following section I deal with each of these arguments in turn. In §5.9.1 I argue that the clinician-centered argument from purely research-related risks is unjustifiably paternalistic and that we have independent grounds to reject this conception of the relationship between the duty of personal care, health, and patient welfare. I then argue in §5.9.2 that we have equally strong grounds to reject the more general position that individual rationality somehow requires individuals to choose only acts that optimize their narrow medical best interests.

---

[7] Although the *clinician-centered* and the *participant-centered* formulations of the argument from purely research-related risks are closely connected, the nature of that connection might differ, depending on how one approaches a larger set of questions. For instance, what we might call the *strongly role-related argument* holds that clinicians are obligated to advance the narrow medical interests of individuals for whom they are responsible because of the special role-related duties of caregivers. For example, one might argue caregivers have a special obligation to focus on patient health interests because of the centrality of health to their social role.

The *weakly role-related argument* holds only that caregivers are obligated to advance the best interests of individuals as those individuals understand them. Here, the clinician's focus on the narrow, medical best interests of individuals does not derive from anything internal to their professional role. Instead, it derives from (a) the deeper claim that in order for individuals to make rational choices they must choose the option that best advances their interests and from (b) the further claim that in matters of health, this necessarily involves choosing the act that optimizes their narrow health interests. If individuals understand their best interests as extensionally equivalent to whatever is in their narrow health-related interests, caregivers would inherit this focus on the patient's narrow medical interests.

As I proceed here, my critique of the clinician-centered argument dispenses with the strongly role-related version of this position (§5.9.1) and my critique of the claim that research participation is not in the narrow self-interest of participants dispenses with the weakly role-related argument (§5.9.2 and 5.9.3).

5.9 Well-Being and the Life Plan of Persons

5.9.1 Arbitrarily Restricting Individual Liberty

In §5.8.2 we saw that the clinician-centered argument from purely research-related risks is predicated on a fairly traditional, Hippocratic understanding of the clinician's duty of personal care. As a form of patient-centered consequentialism, it holds that "Physicians should promote the medical best interests of patients by offering optimal medical care; and the risks of prescribed treatments are justified by the potential therapeutic benefits to patients" (Miller and Brody 2002, 4). I now argue that we have independent grounds for rejecting this interpretation of the physician's duty of personal care. Rejecting this understanding of the duty of personal care removes one formulation of the argument which holds that there is a dilemma at the heart of research ethics.

Ironically, the grounds for rejecting the traditional, Hippocratic interpretation of the duty of personal care stem from applying it to the realm from which it is supposed to be derived, namely, clinical medicine. In fact, it is surprising that the Hippocratic conception of the duty of personal care persists in research ethics since the rejection of this view was one of the main drivers of contemporary medical ethics.

For the duties of Hippocratic patient-centered consequentialism to be aligned with patient interests it must be the case that health and health-related interests are the highest and most authoritative of the patient's interests (Goldman 1980). Although this is often the case, it is not always—and so not necessarily—the case. Patients sometimes have interests that take priority over their strict medical interests or that so color and shape those interests that it is difficult to disentangle their strict, medical interests from the larger set of interests that define their particular life plan. As a result, the larger contours of a person's distinctive life plan can lead them to make decisions that are at odds with what the Hippocratic clinician believes to be in their medical best interests.

To illustrate this point I want to focus, for the purposes of the present argument, on particular aspects of clinical medicine that bear structural similarities to purely research-related interventions or procedures. In particular, there are a range of practices in which patients undergo risks and burdens in clinical medicine solely for the purpose of assisting other people. Some examples involve relatively minor burdens and risks, such as blood donation.

Others involve more significant burdens, such as bone marrow donation. Still others involve even more significant burdens and medical risks, as when clinicians use their medical knowledge and skill to remove an organ or a portion of an orgen, such as a kidney or a lobe of the liver, from one person and transplant it into another.

If saving the lives of people in medical distress is an important project in a person's life plan, then the narrow medical or health risks of blood donation, organ donation, and other such procedures must be evaluated in light of the contribution that these activities make to the welfare of that same agent. Because some of these very acts are performed in both medical and research contexts, we can make the following direct argument. If the risks and burdens associated with drawing a person's blood violate the clinician's duty of personal care when performed in the context of a clinical trial, then those same risks and burdens must violate the duty of care when performed in the context of donations to be used by others in need. By modus tollens, because it is not impermissible for patients to donate blood for the purpose of advancing the interests of other people in the clinical context, it is not impermissible for study participants to donate blood in a clinical trial for the purpose of generating valuable information that is required to advance the interests of other people.

This argument demonstrates that the Hippocratic interpretation of the duty of personal care is more restrictive than the way that very same duty is interpreted in clinical medicine. Moreover, this is the same duty in both contexts. So, if the interpretation of that duty that is used in the clinician-centered argument is correct, then it would also rule out bone marrow donation, living organ donation, medical quarantine, and routine vaccination since all of these medical procedures impose some burdens or risks on one person for the purpose of generating a benefit that accrues to others. Since these activities are not regarded as inconsistent with the clinician's duty of care, then the we must reject the formulation of the clinician's fiduciary duties that animates the clinician-centered argument.

I have focused on cases that have a structural similarity to clinical research, because the Hippocratic conception of the duty of personal care requires medical procedures to advance the narrow medical interests of patients. Procedures such as vasectomy and tubal ligation are often not performed to rectify a medical pathology—to heal or alleviate pain or suffering or to restore what Daniels (1985) calls typical species functionality. Rather, those procedures are performed in order to assist individuals in carrying out life plans in which they wish to engage in sexual activities without having to worry about procreating in the process. Those procedures would be regarded as ethically impermissible under the Hippocratic conception of the duty of personal care because they expose patients to medical risks and burdens to achieve goals or purposes that derive, not from addressing physical ills or medical pathologies, but from the goals of the individual's larger life plan.

Similarly, cosmetic procedures expose patients to risks that are not necessarily in the strict medical best interests of patients. Reshaping the contours of a fully functional nose, cheek, chin, breast, belly, and so on, are optional undertakings, often driven entirely by aesthetics. Many may question the wisdom of undergoing such procedures, and others may hold that because they are ethically optional undertakings there is no duty to use scarce resources to pay for them. But these are not the issues in question. On the argument we are considering here, offering such procedures to patients would be unethical because doing so violates the physician's duty of personal care—such procedures are intended, not to restore functioning or to treat disease, but to achieve aesthetic ideals.

The moral permissibility of medical procedures performed on patients for the benefit of others, or to advance goals other than a patient's strict medical interests follows from the rejection of medical paternalism. This was, in part, a rejection of the idea that the medical profession's specialized knowledge of health and disease was sufficient to understand the way that health or its absence influences patient welfare (Goldman 1980, 156–230). If health and the avoidance or amelioration of disease are sovereign values, the highest goal for any rational patient, then clinicians would have special insight into patient welfare in virtue of their special medical knowledge. But if health and the avoidance or amelioration of disease cannot necessarily be presupposed to be a person's highest goal or sovereign value, then which medical care best advances—or is most likely to frustrate—the interests of patients must be determined for each patient in light of that person's larger life plan.

The rejection of medical paternalism involved the recognition that the value of a state of affairs or of an outcome for a patient is not solely a function of that person's narrow medical interests; it depends on how those states or outcomes are situated relative to a patient's larger life plans (Goldman 1980). The very idea that a patient could have the right to refuse unwanted medical care—to withdraw a ventilator even when it is certain to fulfill its proper medical function of sustaining and extending that person's life—requires recognition that health states that one person may regard as valuable and worth experiencing might be regarded by others as undignified and worth avoiding.

The reasonable diversity of life plans entails that although some individuals would not want to take any degree of personal risk or bear any burden to advance the health interests of others, other people view this as a calling and an avenue through which to express important values such as love, compassion, charity, solidarity, or reciprocity. Although some people would forego the prospect of extending their life if the means of doing so were painful, protracted, invasive, or risky, others often decide differently. Similarly, there are differences of judgment about the wisdom and value of reshaping one's body for motives other than the restoration of prior form or typical functioning and whether the attending risks are reasonable in light of the expected benefits, if any. This reasonable diversity in judgment about the risks and burdens of common medical practices stems from the reasonable diversity of life plans. This point is a concrete illustration of the respect in which the narrow technical perspective of medicine is incomplete (§5.3). How risks or burdens to a person's narrow medical interests impact that individual's welfare or wellbeing depends on their relationship to the projects and plans in that individual's larger life plan (see also §5.9.2 and §5.11). This information derives, not from the technical expertise of medicine, but from the reflective self-understanding of the individual whose interest medicine is expected to serve.

The rejection of medical paternalism was not a rejection of the idea that physicians and other health professionals have a fiduciary duty to individual patients. That duty is morally sound and important. Rather, the rejection of medical paternalism was a rejection of the idea that the traditional Hippocratic interpretation of the clinician's duty of personal care is a morally appropriate model of the relationship between patient health and patient welfare. That view has been repudiated in clinical medicine—the very domain in which it is supposed to be sovereign—because treating health as a proxy for individual well-being misconstrues the nature of human welfare. Equating welfare with a person's health elides the texture and complexity of the diverse life plans individuals in a free society can reasonably embrace. But it also gives too much authority to the social role of the clinician. In both cases, it arbitrarily restricts the autonomy of patients.

In the grip of the first dogma of research ethics, the field has retained the traditional, Hippocratic conception of the duty of personal care even after that view was repudiated in the context of clinical medicine. The upshot of the argument of the current section is that the claim that the Hippocratic conception of the duty of personal care accurately reflects the content of the clinician's fiduciary duty to the individual patient is false.

If the clinician's fiduciary duty is interpreted, instead, as a duty to advance an individual's medical best interests as those interests emerge within that person's life plan, then this duty is not necessarily inconsistent with the performance of purely study-related procedures—even if those procedures carry affirmative risks and burdens. Rather, the permissibility of these procedures will depend on the extent to which the individual in question regards them as necessary and proportional burdens undertaken in the course of advancing an important project or plan. This point provides a kernel of insight on which we will draw in our response to the deeper and more philosophical problem about the relationship between rational choice, individual interests, and health, to which we now turn.

5.9.2 Personal Risks Are Not Irrational

It is important that when Menikoff and Richards assert that research participation is often a bad choice they scrupulously state that it is a "bad choice for someone who is mainly concerned about his or her own best interests" (2006, 18). This addition might seem trivial, since it might seem to be trivially true that every individual is mainly concerned about his or her own interests. But, in the sense in which this statement is trivially true, it is not necessarily inconsistent with an individual's best interests to participate in research in which they are exposed to burdens and risks that are not offset by the prospect of direct medical benefit. The reason is simple: if a project is sufficiently important to an agent that advancing it is a personal priority, then undertaking risks that are necessary to further that project is consistent with advancing their best interests.

On the other hand, if we understand concern for one's interests in such a way that it excludes accepting affirmative risks to one's health or welfare in the course of activities that primarily benefit others, then this claim is not only *not trivial*, it is so strong that many life choices would also pose a moral dilemma—including the decision of a young student to pursue a career as a physician or a medical researcher! We can elaborate the points in these last two paragraphs one at a time.

For the sake of the argument, let's assume that there is a tight motivational and rational connection between what an agent has a reason to do, what an agent is motivated to do, and what is in an agent's best interests. In particular, let us grant that if x is in an agent's interest, then that agent has a reason to support or engage in x and, conversely, that if x is not in an agent's interest then that agent has a reason to discourage or avoid x. Given these assumptions, it is critical to clarify what it means for something to be in an agent's interests.

Consider first the idea that an agent has an interest in x—that x is in the interest of an agent—if x is a constituent of that agent's life plan or if x is an instrumental means of advancing a project or element of such a life plan. This way of conceiving an agent's interests dovetails nicely with our previous claims about a close connection between x being in an agent's interest, that agent having a reason to do x, and being motivated to do x. In fact, this connection seems almost trivially true since it basically says that agents have a reason and a motivation to support or pursue whatever is a constituent of, or an instrumental means of effectuating, their particular life plan.

On this view, a wide array of things can feature into the life plan of an agent: careers, hobbies, ambitions, social connections or affinities, personal relationships and affections. In each of these cases, what constitutes advancing the agent's interest need not directly involve or appeal to any aspect of that person's health, physical status, or psychological state. Pursuing a career as an engineer, for example, can involve long hours dedicated to understanding the principles that organize some domain of the physical world and developing the knowledge and the means to use that knowledge to build structures, synthesize materials, or design and construct some other form of physical system. Success in the pursuit of such a career involves achieving the excellences that are associated with understanding the relevant systems, creativity in design, implementation or construction, efficient and safe use of resources, and so on. In such cases, an individual's life plan can revolve around an activity—such as designing and constructing a large and complex structure—to such a degree, and can involve exposure to such a range of associated risks, that pursuing that person's goals and ambitions can come into conflict with that individual's narrow health interests.

Civil engineers often work on construction sites in which there are positive risks of injury or death. Chemical engineers handle chemicals that can cause blindness, injury, or death. Similarly, physicians and medical researchers risk contracting illness from their patients, whether through direct exposure or from accidents such as needle sticks.

Part of the refutation of medical paternalism involved precisely this insight—that, in many areas of life, the life plans of individuals elevate the pursuit of other goals or ends over the maximization of individual health. The point of this insight is not to deny that health is an individual interest; it is simply to dethrone the idea that health is an agent's sovereign interest, trumping all others. Once we recognize that a person's life plan can elevate accomplishing some goal or set of goals above advancing their narrow health interests, then we can no longer assume that expertise in medicine provides sufficient insight into a person's interests to warrant empowering clinicians to subvert the freedom and choice of individuals in order to advance those individual's narrow health interests.

On this view, although it is almost trivially true to say individuals have reason to act in their own interest, and to avoid acting in ways that are not in their interest, the fact that participation in a study might expose a person to risks that are not offset by the prospect of direct medical benefit is not sufficient to establish that study participation is against that person's interests. If it were, it would establish that being an engineer or a clinician or a researcher is also against a person's interests. But such claims are false because a person's interests are not defined by their direct physical or mental status, but by the larger contours of their individual life plan. To know whether accepting such personal risks is consistent with or conflicts with a person's interests we have to know how those risks relate to the projects and goals that define their individual life plan.

If helping others plays an important role in one's life plan, and if donating blood is a means of helping other people in need, then when such a person donates blood, they are advancing their interests (the goal of helping others after a natural disaster, for example) despite the fact that the blood draw exposes them to both risks and burdens. Likewise, if finding a cure for a disease is one of a person's goals, and if extra blood draws are necessary to run a scientifically sound study, then undergoing those blood draws as a participant in a study can be in a participant's interests.

For many people, activities in which they take on risks and burdens to themselves in order to help others is a normal feature of everyday life. For example, people in many faith communities are called to engage in community service activities. Volunteers repair homes, provide care to the sick, and perform other tasks that are attended by personal risks and burdens. Similarly, many people identify deeply with their professions, including medical researchers. But medical researchers are often in contact with needles, blood, and pathogens that they can and sometimes do contract. These hazards are often not discussed in public discourse and so researchers and participants are treated as though their respective pursuits are structurally very different—researchers advance their own interests and those of the larger community by conducting activities in which participants are exposed to risks that are inconsistent with their medical best interests.

The point I am making here is that if we focus on the medical best interests of these individuals, both being a researcher and being a study participant can involve risks that are inconsistent with that individual's narrow medical best interests. In both cases, respect for individual welfare requires that those risks be minimized, and gratuitous risks should be eliminated altogether. The key point, however, is simply that the existence of risks to a person's strict medical best interests is not necessarily inconsistent with a person voluntarily accepting those risks in order to advance the plan that imbues their life with personal meaning and social significance.

When Heyd (1996), Menikoff and Richards (2006), or Wertheimer (2010) assert that it is not in an individual's interests to participate in a study that poses some affirmative risks or that requires enduring some burdens or inconveniences, they are asserting a claim that entails that it is also not in an individual's interest to take on the career of a medical researcher. Such a result, however, is absurd.[8] Many people are drawn to a career as a researcher precisely because they see it as a way to use a diverse mix of scientific, mathematical, and social abilities to advance a worthwhile individual and social

---

[8] This narrow position seems more palatable when it is paired with what looks like an innocuous ancillary assumption. This assumption is that being a researcher is not in a person's individual interests until it is attached to a significant salary or elevated to a particular social status. On this view, being a researcher on its own is not in an individual's strict interests, but being a researcher as a way of securing significant wealth or social status renders it consistent with that individual's strict personal interests.

But this ancillary assumption is far from innocuous. In particular, when individuals value wealth or social status then attaching those things to an undertaking represents a way to encourage people to value that undertaking. But this move saves the narrow conception of individual interest by appealing to the broader conception of what it is to be in an individual's interest to which this narrow theory is supposed to be an alternative. In particular, it isn't clear why doing x for the money is supposed to be easier to grasp as a rationale for engaging in x than doing x as an outlet for one's various talents and abilities, or because it contributes to a cause to which one is committed. Making money does not make a direct contribution to one's narrow health interests. Instead, it is either valuable as an end that one embraces for itself, or as a means to advancing the other ends that one embraces, including advancing one's health interests. But developing one's talents and abilities and pursuing one's larger life projects might make an affirmative contribution to one's physical and mental health. Even if it doesn't, developing one's talents and abilities is either an end in itself or a means of advancing other ends that one embraces. As a result, doing x because it advances a life project or represents the expression of one's talents and abilities seems no worse, and possibly better, as an explanation for why x is in one's interests than doing x for the money.

project. Many scientists identify so closely with the ends that they pursue that they have been willing to put their life on the line, whether as a subject in their own study (Altman 1972; Neuringer 1981) or as a researcher in dangerous contexts in which they could contract life-threatening disease or be subject to violence (Green 2014). These behaviors are not only permitted, they are often valorized.

In a community in which different individuals pursue a diversity of life plans, it is likely that many people are willing to accept affirmative risks to their own health if those risks will contribute to the knowledge needed to understand and ultimately alleviate suffering or disability associated with sickness, injury, or disease. In such cases, personal risks may be unwanted and not assumed lightly or without adequate safeguard, but insofar as they cannot be avoided and are tied to activities that are constitutive of or instrumental to a person's life plan, they are not necessarily inconsistent with that individual's best interests. Researchers and study participants differ in many morally relevant respects. In particular, participants are likely to face particular risks with greater certainty because they are part of an explicit and formalized research protocol. Nevertheless, researchers and participants can be symmetrically situated in their acceptance of risks to their narrow, medical interests, in order to advance meritorious social ends.

5.9.3 Study Participation Is Not a Prisoner's Dilemma

The argument in the previous section allows us to demonstrate precisely why research participation does not give rise to a prisoner's dilemma. To make this case, it is helpful to carefully lay out the structure of this particular social dilemma. Doing so reveals an interesting fact—that contrary to the assertions of those who make this claim, research participation is not in fact this type of strategic dilemma. Even so, once we distinguish the impact of participation on an individual's health interests from its impact on their overall interests, we can demonstrate that study participation can be a rational move to make in this kind of strategic situation.

Figure 5.1 contains a simple diagram that illustrates the structure of a prisoner's dilemma.[9] In this example, each individual has to make a choice

---

[9] Although this example focuses on two individuals, this is merely for convenience. Two-person prisoner's dilemmas can be scaled up to n-person prisoner's dilemmas without altering the results.

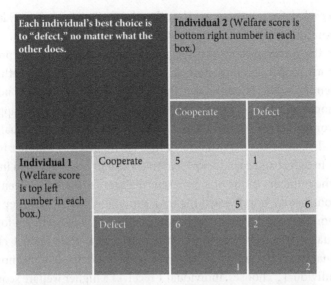

Figure 5.1 Simple representation of a two-person Prisoner's Dilemma. Individual 1's welfare score in each outcome is indicated by the top left number in each box. Individual 2's welfare score in each outcome is indicated by the bottom right number in each box.

between participating in some collaboration or defecting. The boxes represent outcomes that result from the respective choices of each player and the numbers inside each box represent the "payoffs," "utilities," or "welfare score" for each party in that state of affairs. For convenience I have chosen integers to represent welfare scores, but, once again, the structure of the dilemma does not depend on our being able to assign specific numbers to individual welfares. The same dilemma emerges as long as the relative orderings of outcomes depicted in the table are preserved.

In the example from which this problem derives its name, two prisoners are being interrogated by the police. If they both cooperate, and keep silent, they go to jail for only one year. In the matrix in Figure 5.1, this is the cooperate/cooperate square in which each player receives 5 welfare units. But if one player keeps silent and the other defects, blaming his partner for their nefarious activities, then the defecting partner goes free (a score of 6 units) and the silent party goes to jail for the maximum sentence (a score of only 1

The number of parties involved is thus less important than the structure of the problem they face— that is the central issue.

unit). If each defects and exposes the other they go to jail for slightly less than the maximum sentence (2 units each).

From the standpoint of the players in this game, the outcomes produced when both cooperate are preferable to those produced when both defect. The dilemma arises from the fact that in this situation, there is no third-party "social agent" who gets to choose which outcome actually happens. In other words, there is no dictator who can force these two individuals to co-operate. Instead, each party has to choose for themselves whether to coop-erate or to defect and each is expected to choose in his or her own interests, where the numbers in the box represent the agent's interests. Given the as-sumption that each individual makes a rational choice when they choose the option that best advances their own interests, it is not rational for either individual to choose to cooperate. No matter what Individual 1 chooses, Individual 2 receives a higher welfare score from defecting and no matter what Individual 2 chooses, individual 1 receives a higher welfare score from defecting. This result does not depend on complicated solution concepts from game theory such as the Nash equilibrium. It hinges simply on the fact that, for each individual, defecting produces more individual welfare than cooperating regardless of what the other person chooses. In the formal language of game theory, the choice to defect "dominates" the choice to participate.

Prisoner's dilemmas can arise in a wide range of contexts. As such it is best not to think about the motivating story of the two prisoners and to focus instead on the relationships between the payouts in the matrix. Any social interaction in which the interests of the parties are accurately modeled by welfare payouts with these relationships will face this thorny problem. When commentators assert that research participation is a prisoner's dilemma they mean, not that the parties are prisoners of some kind, but that the choices they face have consequences whose values are accurately modeled by the numbers in Figure 5.1.

Despite its allure, the claim that research participation is a prisoner's di-lemma is false. When someone refuses to participate in a study they continue to experience or undergo whatever course of care or state of affairs is the status quo. As a result, the coordination game facing potential participants in medical research is represented in Figure 5.2. For simplicity, the status quo for each party is represented as "0," as neither a gain nor a loss. As a result, the party who defects does not stand to gain something by defecting, at least when measured relative to the status quo. She may gain something relative to

	Participate	Don't participate
Participate	x+y x+y	x 0

Don't Participate	0
	
	    x
		0
		
		      0

Figure 5.2 The coordination game reflecting the strategic decision of parties who must decide whether or not to participate in medical research. Here, x represents the direct positive or negative impact on the health of the agent from participating in the study and y represents the agent's personal valuation of the information that the study is designed to produce.

the other player, however, depending on what is involved in participating in research.

In light of our discussion in the previous section we can represent the effects of participation with two variables. The direct impact (positive or negative) on the health of the agent expected from participation is represented by x. The valuation of participation, as represented by the agent's valuation of the information the study is expected to produce, is represented by y. In Figure 5.2, y is only present in the cell in which both players participate. This is intended to mark the idea—reflected in the original claim that research participation has the form of a prisoner's dilemma—that the social benefits of research require cooperation of other willing participants. In that respect, y only materializes if a sufficient number of individuals are willing to participate that the study can be run to completion with sufficient power. To maintain the simplicity of the representation, therefore, it is best to think of the parties in this example as small groups.

The nature of the strategic situation represented in Figure 5.2 depends on the values that x and y take, but none of these values produces a prisoner's dilemma. The situations associated with the different values of x and y is represented in Figure 5.3. If x offers sufficient prospect of direct personal benefit to participants (x > 0) then there is no dilemma and no coordination problem; everyone prefers to participate rather than not to participate. If study participation involves affirmative risks and burdens (such that x < 0), and no agent values the information the study is likely to produce to such a degree that it would compensate for those personal risks or burdens (x + y < 0) then there also is no dilemma; nobody participates because nobody thinks the study is worth the risk.

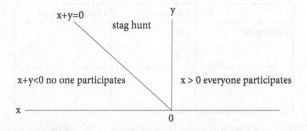

Figure 5.3 The strategic structure of the game represented in Figure 2 depending on the values of x (direct health benefits or burdens to individual participants from study participation) and y (the value to the agent of the information a study is likely to produce) relative to the status quo (represented as 0).

If the study involves affirmative risks to participants (x < 0) but the prospective participants value the information that the study is likely to produce enough that they are willing to accept those risks (x + y > 0), then the game has the form of what is called a stag hunt (Skyrms 2004). In a stag hunt, each individual prefers to cooperate only on the condition that others cooperate as well. Unlike the prisoner's dilemma, defecting is not the dominant course of conduct in a stag hunt. In that regard, the stag hunt is a coordination problem and not a social dilemma. If the agent is convinced that there are other agents who also value generating the evidence the study is designed to produce, and so will participate on condition that others participate as well, then joint cooperation is a rational choice. Put in slightly different terms, under the circumstances just described, participating in research in which the participant will be exposed to some burdens or risks that are not offset by the prospect of direct medical benefit remains an equilibrium of the game and therefore a rational choice for a rational agent.

In a pluralistic community, different agents may have different attitudes toward the same study. Some agents may regard the associated risks as unreasonable in light of the way participation fits into their larger life plan. In contrast, other agents may view study participation as contributing to a worthwhile project or reflecting important aspects of their personal life plan. In such cases, the society is faced with a coordination problem—if enough people embrace a life plan that is advanced by generating information that will help to understand, treat or prevent a debilitating disease and are willing to participate in research, then society need only provide assurance to such individuals that if they participate then enough like-minded people will follow to generate socially valuable information.

The upshot of the argument in this section is that accepting affirmative risks to one's narrow health interests is a routine part of pursuing a distinctive life plan and that, as a result, accepting purely study-related risks when they are necessary to promote an activity that a participant values and wants to promote is not inconsistent with that agent choosing in a way that advances her best interests. From this I showed that research participation is not a prisoner's dilemma.

The arguments of the last two sections show that the participant-centered formulation of the argument from purely research-related risks does not reveal a dilemma at the heart of all research that involves purely research-related interventions or procedures. As a result, any conception of the researcher's duty of personal care or fiduciary duty to the individual that focuses narrowly on that individual's health interests is unduly restrictive and unjustifiably paternalistic.

5.10 Against the First Dogma of Research Ethics

5.10.1 Hippocratic Duty Has Clear Content but Is Unjustifiably Restrictive

Together, the arguments in this chapter provide powerful reasons to reject any view that seeks to constrain research activities by requiring that they be consistent with the individual clinician's duty of personal care. We can express the cumulative force of these arguments in the form of a dilemma. Call this the *dilemma of determinate duties*.

One horn of the dilemma holds that if the caregiver's duty of personal care is interpreted in traditional, Hippocratic terms, as a form of patient-centered consequentialism, then it has independent content that places clear constraints on the practice of research. The problem is that this clarity of content is purchased at an unacceptable price: the limits that it imposes on research are unjustifiably restrictive. This standard would deny individuals who identify with the goals of a socially valuable activity (whether as study participants or researchers) the ability to accept any degree of personal risks or burden in the furtherance of that activity. Not only is such a standard repudiated in clinical medicine—the very context from which it supposedly derives—but its implementation on a social scale would unreasonably restrict the array of life plans individuals in a free society are capable of pursuing and deprive communities of the social benefits generated from the willingness of individuals to adopt life plans that include activities that promote the common good.

If it is consistent with the clinician's fiduciary duty to permit blood donation, bone marrow donation, living organ donation, or cosmetic surgery, then it should be consistent with this same duty to permit study participants to accept those burdens or risks for the purpose of facilitating socially meritorious research. This suggests that when study participants identify with the goals of a clinical trial, study-related blood draws, tumor biopsies, and other procedures can be consistent with the duties and norms of caring medical practice.

5.10.2 Duty of Care That Respects Autonomy Lacks Independent Content

The second horn of the dilemma holds that if we interpret the duty of personal care in a way that is more aligned with how it is understood in medical practice, then we strip from that duty the independent content necessary to set determinant constraints on research risk. In part, this stems from the fact that limits on research risks have to be set prior to the point at which individual study participants are approached with the offer to participate. But if the judgment of the reasonableness of risks requires knowledge of a person's larger life plan, then IRBs would lack the information they need to apply this standard in the evaluation of study protocols.

The problem also stems from the fact that the limits we impose on individual decision-making in clinical practice may be overly permissive. In particular, caring medical practice includes respect for the wishes of competent patients to refuse life-sustaining medical care, hastening the patient's death. It is not clear how this would translate into an analogous standard for limiting risk in research. Would it be permissible for study participants to knowingly hasten their own death in pursuit of research-related objectives? One worry is, thus, that this standard would not provide any substantive constraint on what could be offered to study participants. Instead, it would rely solely on the procedural constraint of whether participants are willing to consent to whatever the study protocol demands, no matter the magnitude of the risks that might entail.[10]

Once it is recognized that reasonable people, with different life plans, can value various health states in different ways, and can have divergent preferences about the means of promoting those health states, then medicine cannot be treated as a form of productive knowledge that has a complete, self-contained understanding of individual patient interests. Rather, medicine is incomplete in the sense that it must look to the larger values and interests of the individual person to fill out the picture of how various health states, and the means to achieve them, fit into an individual's conception of the good life (§5.3.1–2). Making this move brings the content of the clinician's duty of personal care into better alignment with the way that duty is understood in clinical medicine. But it does this at the cost of stripping that duty of its operational content when it comes to regulating research.

The refutation of medical paternalism was not just a repudiation of arbitrary power that had been vested in the hands of physicians; it was a recognition that such power was arbitrary precisely because it did not track the larger interests of individuals as free persons who exist for themselves and not for the purposes of others. Although health is an important good, the place of that good in an individual's larger life plan is ultimately determined by the shape and contours of that larger conception of flourishing and what constitutes a good life. Medicine is an incomplete guide to welfare since the place of health in a person's larger life plan cannot be determined solely by the technical principles of medicine. Rather, that information has to be provided from outside medicine, from the practical judgment of the autonomous individual.

These problems illustrate a point I made in §5.3. Professions are relatively narrow bodies of knowledge that range over distinct domains. But how those domains impact the interests of individuals, and what justice demands of them in a free society, are issues that fall outside the narrow confines of professional obligations. Recognizing this point and repudiating the first dogma of research ethics are essential to understanding how to regulate research risks in a way that is consistent with the requirements of the egalitarian research imperative.

---

[10] For a defense of this position see Rajczi (2004). For a critique see Rid and Wendler (2010).

5.11 Against the Second Dogma of Research Ethics

5.11.1 Utilitarian Assumptions Are Not Necessary

The appearance of a deep conflict at the heart of research with humans is encouraged by the perception that purely research-related risks are necessarily antithetical to a person's interest and, therefore, that the only way to justify their presence in research is by ensuring that they are offset by the expected benefits to future beneficiaries of research. The idea that risks to some must necessarily be traded off against benefits to others is part of the second dogma of research ethics.

The second dogma of research ethics rests on an unnecessarily strong assumption about what is required in order to ensure that research has social value. In particular, even if a frankly utilitarian approach to research risks would be sufficient to promote socially valuable research, it does not follow that it is necessary to achieve this end. But it is the latter, stronger claim that is needed to show that the research enterprise poses a deep conflict with the rights and interests of study participants.

In this chapter I have argued that the perception that research participation is necessarily inconsistent with concern for individual welfare is mistaken. As we attenuate this perception of conflict, we also attenuate the idea that the only way to advance medical science is to be willing to sacrifice individual interests for the benefit of future persons. After all, if scientifically sound and socially valuable information can be generated without requiring compromise in any relevant value—if it does not require breaching participant rights or sacrificing participant welfare—then pursuing the requirement of social value would not be inconsistent with *any* ethical perspective. Even the strictest absolutism about rights and values could support the vision of research participation articulated in the egalitarian research imperative.

I have argued here that when agents adopt socially meritorious ends—ends that involve aiding or assisting others—and those ends cannot be advanced without the agent being exposed to personal risks and burdens, such exposure is not necessarily antithetical to the overall interests of those individuals. This is not to say that it is acceptable for such risks to be gratuitous—it is not. Nor is it to say that such risks should be lightly undertaken. It is to say that when a person donates bone marrow to save the life of another, the pain, inconvenience, and risks of complications that are part of the donation process should be reduced and properly managed, but that they are not antithetical to the welfare of the person making the donation.

To bring what might seem like a counterintuitive claim into sharper relief, it is helpful to contrast two scenarios and the moral principles that might be used to assess the reasonableness of risks in each.

5.11.2 The Principle of Proportionality

Sam is a firefighter who takes great pride in having the strength, stamina, courage, experience, and knowledge necessary to fight fires. Fighting fires, saving property, and rescuing people from hazardous situations are a source of pride for Sam and an outlet through which Sam both experiences certain personal goods and makes a social contribution. Sam's position is paid for by the Township. The Township values Sam as one of its members. It also bears various kinds of responsibility in the case that Sam is injured, becomes disabled, or is killed in the line of duty. Some of these responsibilities are financial. But others relate to the way the Township values people—whether the Township values its workers and its members as free and equal persons or whether it treats them as disposable tools.

In some contexts, Sam appears to be willing to accept greater personal risks than the Township thinks reasonable. The Township therefore wants to limit the risks to which Sam is exposed when acting as an employee of the Township. It relies on the principle of proportionality as a guide to limiting those risks.

Principle of Proportionality: A condition for the acceptability of risks within an activity is that those risks must not be disproportionate in comparison to the goods they are necessary to generate.

Both the Township and Sam agree that this principle allows for different levels of risk depending on the nature of the activity Sam is undertaking. For example, the maximum permissible risk in the course of saving property is lower than the maximum permissible risk in the course of trying to save a person. Even in the latter case, however, there is a limit to what constitutes an acceptable risk to Sam.

5.11.3 The Principle of Utility

In contrast, Pat is an artist whose life plan revolves around exploring personal expression through various visual media. Pat happens to be physically fit and, because of a shortage of firefighters in Municipality, Pat is conscripted into service as a firefighter. Although Pat, like Sam, is physically capable of performing the relevant tasks, Pat, unlike Sam, has no interest in serving as a firefighter. Every moment is an exercise in drudgery and boredom interrupted by moments of sheer terror for Pat.

Municipality invokes the principle of utility to justify selecting Pat to serve as a firefighter.

Principle of Utility: It is permissible to perform an act that decreases the welfare of one person as long as doing so produces a sufficiently large increase in the welfare of others.

In particular, Pat's life plan is set back by service as a firefighter, because Pat values the excellences and experiences of making and appreciating art and every moment spent as a firefighter is a moment taken away from the activities in which Pat finds fulfillment. Nevertheless, Pat's ability to fill this role better than the other candidates is regarded as generating sufficient benefits to others to justify this reduction in Pat's welfare.

Although the principle of utility might entail both the social value requirement and the principle of proportionality, the social value requirement and the principle of proportionality do not necessarily entail the principle of utility. The reason is that the injunction to ensure that the risks a person undertakes in the course of a voluntary pursuit are reasonable in light of the goods they are seeking to produce does not entail the permission to sacrifice the welfare of any agent to promote the good of others.

As we saw in chapter 2, both proponents and critics of the idea that there is an imperative to carry out research conceived of study participation on the model of Pat—as someone whose interests are abrogated or sacrificed for the benefit of others. Implicitly, however, researchers have been treated on the model of Sam—someone who accepts personal risks in the course of an occupation with the noble goal of advancing medical knowledge in order to be a benefactor to humanity. On that model, as we noted previously, the risks that professionals such as clinicians and researchers incur to their health in the course of pursuing their personal and professional objectives are largely ignored. The two dogmas of research ethics perpetuate this asymmetric framing by hard-coding the idea that research necessarily involves trade-offs of the kind to which Pat is subjected.

The egalitarian research imperative that I defend here is an imperative to create a system of knowledge production that gives a symmetric treatment of researchers and study participants on the model of Sam. The goal is to create a social system in which both researchers and participants can participate freely as an avenue through which they have the opportunity to generate an important public good. We have more closely approximated this ideal in the case of researchers and other medical health professionals. In chapter 7 I argue that part of the benefit of a system of prospective review of research before bodies of diverse representation is that it brings us closer to achieving this ideal for research participants as well. Reconceiving research ethics on the model defended in this book would move us much closer to this goal. The point is not to say that researchers and study participants are somehow exposed to the same level or kind of risks—for this is surely not true. Rather, the point is to create a system of voluntary participation in which no person is conscripted like Pat, forced to sacrifice their welfare for the greater good, and in which every participant can be treated on the model of Sam.

In a society in which people pursue diverse life plans, different individuals will be drawn to study participation for different reasons. Whether they are likely to contribute to such research will depend on our ability to provide credible public assurance that the endeavor in which they participate has significant social value, that their participation contributes to the production of an important public good, and that no other party to this cooperative scheme has the ability to co-opt it for their personal, parochial ends (see §5.9.3 and chapters 4 and 7). Although we have seen several arguments that seek to establish that research cannot be organized on such terms, none of those arguments is compelling.

6

The Integrative Approach to Assessing and Managing Risk

6.1 Reconciling Social Value and Equal Concern

The previous chapter presented an indirect defense of the egalitarian research imperative. It was indirect in the sense that it highlighted and then criticized a network of views, some tacit and some explicit, against the background of which it appears almost true by definition that research with human participants poses a fundamental and inescapable moral dilemma. Undermining this network of assumptions clears conceptual room for an approach to risk assessment and management that creates the conditions under which free and equal people, pursuing diverse life plans in a free society, can see research participation as a viable avenue for advancing the common good.

The goal of the present chapter is to demonstrate, in concrete and operationally meaningful terms, how it is possible to reconcile the imperative to support research that advances the common good with the imperative to respect the status of the stakeholders in that undertaking as free and equal persons. What I refer to as the *integrative approach* articulates the conditions necessary to reconcile or integrate these goals.

The integrative approach is grounded in the same concern for the basic or generic interests of individuals that defines the generic interests conception of the common good (§4.5) and that motivates the egalitarian research imperative (§4.7). It is in virtue of this common focus and shared normative foundation that the requirements of the integrative approach are not extrinsic side constraints on research. Instead, they are integral and enabling components of a system of social cooperation in which free and equal persons can advance the common good with credible public assurance that their status as free and equal will not be compromised in the process.[1]

---

[1] The role of prospective review of research before bodies of diverse representation in providing this credible public assurance is the subject of chapter 7.

For the Common Good. Alex John London, Oxford University Press. © Oxford University Press 2022.
DOI: 10.1093/oso/9780197534830.003.0006

In §6.2 I show that pursuit of the egalitarian research imperative that I outlined in chapter 4 entails what I call the principle of equal concern. In §6.3 I present a high-level overview of the three operational criteria that the integrative approach uses to give concrete content to the principle of equal concern. In §6.4 I show how the integrative approach uses insights similar to those in Benjamin Freedman's clinical equipoise to articulate operationally meaningful practical tests for one of these operational criteria. This demonstrates how the integrative approach gives content to what I called the template for the appeal to uncertainty from §5.4 and how it reconciles the social value requirement with concern for participant welfare. In §6.5 I extend this argument to what is arguably the most difficult case to justify for approaches of this kind, namely, research designs that use response-adaptive randomization (a design in which the probability that patients are allocated to various interventions is dynamically adjusted throughout the course of the trial in light of outcomes that are observed in the study's various arms). In §6.6 I show how the integrative approach allows socially valuable research to continue to the point where it is most likely to alter the practice of stakeholders without violating a series of compelling ethical requirements.

The argument presented in these first five sections demonstrates that the integrative approach can reconcile the social value requirement with a set of intuitive and important ethical values. In §6.6 I clarify some of the criteria that should be used to evaluate competing frameworks for assessing and managing risk in the research context, and in §6.7 I highlight some ways in which the integrative approach differs from competing frameworks that also appeal to uncertainty. I conclude with some brief remarks about the distinct advantages of this approach over alternatives that reject the appeal to uncertainty and instead frame the problem of risk in research as an exercise in risk-benefit analysis.

6.2 Two Requirements of the Egalitarian Research Imperative

6.2.1 Social Value and the Public Purpose of Research

We saw in the last chapter that frameworks for risk assessment and management in orthodox research ethics are typically grounded in the moral obligations of medical professionals. This grounding contributes to the idea that the fundamental problem related to risk in research ethics is to reconcile the individual clinician's duty of personal care with the researcher's utilitarian duty to improve the lives of future persons. This framing is understandable for historical reasons, given that research scandals that helped to shape the field often involved clinicians using prerogatives they enjoyed in light of their role as caregiver to conduct research that was antithetical to that role (§2.4). However, this framing creates the appearance of an irreconcilable conflict between the individual decision-maker's pursuit of the epistemic goals of research and a very plausible moral principle that we called the principle of concern for welfare (§5.4):

Concern for Welfare: It is impermissible to knowingly expose a person to interventions, practices, or procedures, that are known or credibly believed to be worse than another available option.

The integrative approach rejects both dogmas of research ethics discussed in the last chapter: it is not grounded in the narrow moral obligations of particular professional roles and it does not presuppose that research is an inherently utilitarian activity. It also rejects the presumption that it is sufficient to think of research in functional terms, as a set of goals and ends that structure the discrete interactions of a set of basically private parties.

Instead, the integrative approach recognizes that research is a scheme of social cooperation that serves a public purpose grounded in considerations of justice. One such consideration of justice concerns the claims that community members have on the goals and ends that are advanced by the research enterprise.

Following the egalitarian research imperative, the public purpose of research is to generate the knowledge necessary to bridge gaps in the capacity of the basic social institutions of a community—such as its system of public health and clinical medicine—to safeguard and advance the basic interests of that community's members. Research programs that satisfy this condition have a strong, prima facie claim to social value. We captured this idea in a formulation of the social value requirement that reflects the content of the egalitarian research imperative:

Social Value Requirement: Research with human participants is only justified if it is reasonably expected to generate the knowledge necessary to develop interventions, policies, practices, or other advances that will enable that community's basic social structures (such as its health-related institutions) to more effectively, efficiently, or equitably safeguard and advance the basic interests of its constituent members.

When research takes place in a community, and it is designed to generate information that is needed to expand the capacity of that community's basic social institutions to safeguard and advance the basic interests of that community's constituent members, then it has a strong claim to represent a just division of social labor and a just use of scarce human and material resources.

6.2.2 The Principle of Equal Concern

Unlike orthodox research ethics, the integrative approach recognizes that research is a scheme of social cooperation involving the collaboration of many different parties, often extended over long periods of time. In order to be consistent with principles of justice, this must be a voluntary scheme of social cooperation in which participants have credible social assurance that in taking on the purpose of advancing the common good they will not be subject to arbitrary treatment, including antipathy or abuse, exploitation, domination, or other forms of unfair treatment.

Following the egalitarian research imperative, in producing socially valuable information this scheme of social cooperation must respect the status of stakeholders—including study participants—as free and equal. This commitment is captured in the following principle:

Principle of Equal Concern: As a necessary condition for ethical permissibility, research with humans must be designed and carried out so as not to undermine the standing of any research participant as the moral and political equal of their compatriots, by either knowingly compromising participant basic interests or by showing less care and concern for their basic interests than the interests of those the research is intended to serve.

The integrative approach to risk assessment and management seeks to reconcile these two requirements by providing a framework that ensures that studies respect the status of participants as free and equal and have a strong, prima facie claim to generating social value. This is a prima facie claim because factors that affect the social value of a study range beyond the set of conditions that determine whether the study is designed on terms that respect the status of participants as free and equal. In order for this prima facie claim to be fully substantiated, additional information may be required about the relationship between the study; the needs of the target community; the ability of that community to use study results to expand the capacity of its health systems without additional assistance; whether necessary assistance is available, if required; and whether there are other ways of addressing those needs that are more effective, efficient, or equitable. Such additional questions are addressed in chapter 9.

The integrative approach thus articulates the conditions necessary for discharging the egalitarian research imperative. In particular, that imperative requires that communities foster research, conceived of as a voluntary scheme of social cooperation that advances the common good. Undertakings that are designed and conducted on terms that satisfy the principle of equal concern create a foundation for voluntary participation in this scheme of social cooperation by providing credible public assurance that in volunteering to advance the common good participants are not sanctioning practices that would make them subject to arbitrary treatment, subjugation, domination, or abuse.

6.2.3 Justice and the Common Good

We can also frame the problem the integrative approach is designed to solve in terms of the conditions we articulated in §4.2.2 on appeals to the common good. Because sickness, injury, and disease threaten the physical, intellectual, affective, or social capacities needed to formulate, pursue, and revise a life plan, they threaten to compromise abilities that are fundamental to the status of individuals as the moral and political equals of their compatriots. This threat to the basic interests of individuals is sufficient to satisfy the triggering condition (TC) for the normative claim (NC). This is a circumstance in which it is permissible to ask individuals to risk, sacrifice, alter, or limit ends or goals that are part of their individual life plan—their personal interests—in the service of an effort to secure the basic interests of others. On the basic or generic interests conception of the common good this means that there are strong moral and political reasons to use social resources and social authority to create cooperative arrangements that promote opportunities for individuals to take up, as part of their personal life plan or as a personal project, activities that advance the basic interests of others.

However, because every community member has an equal claim on the basic institutions of their society to use the best practices available to safeguard and to advance their basic interests, efforts to advance the common good must be consistent with the practical constraint (PC) that the means used must not themselves conflict with or subvert the common good. The principle of equal concern represents the condition necessary to ensure that social efforts to advance the common good do not violate this practical constraint.

The approach to risk that I'm outlining here is "integrative" in the sense that it strives to address social problems by using social resources and social authority to create opportunities for some community members to exercise their shared basic capacities for agency and welfare by taking on personal projects that have as their goal securing these same basic capacities for others (§4.5). At the end of the last chapter we saw that careers in medicine, including careers in medical research, are easily conceived of on these terms (§5.11). They provide a substantive outlet through which individuals can develop and pursue a range of personal talents and abilities while also advancing the common good.

Adhering to the principle of equal concern allows society to treat research participation as an avenue through which its members might advance the common good without compromising their standing or status. To say that being a researcher and being a study participant should each be seen as an outlet for advancing the common good is not to say that the latter offers participants the same kind of outlet through which they can develop and cultivate their talents and abilities as the former. I suspect that this is rarely the case, in fact.[2] The point is not about whether research participation offers the same kinds of opportunities for personal growth as other socially valuable undertakings. The point is to highlight the social value of each of these undertakings, the fact that each imposes risks on those who undertake them, that these risks and burdens must be freely undertaken by fully enfranchised members of a society of free and equal persons, and that conceiving of research participation on these terms entails reasonable limits on the risks and burdens to which participants can be exposed.

---

[2] For the claim that research participation does not offer the same goods as work, see Jonas (1969), Różyńska (2018), and Malmqvist (2019). See also Anderson and Weijer (2002), Dickert and Grady (1999), Lynch (2014), and Lemmens and Elliott (1999).

To make these ideas operational in practice, we need to understand what it takes to respect the principle of equal concern in more concrete terms. Three criteria give operational content to this requirement in practice.

6.3   Criteria for Operationalizing Equal Concern

6.3.1   No Unnecessary Risk

To facilitate concrete risk evaluations, the integrative approach defines three operational criteria to specify the terms on which important research can be advanced without compromising the status of research participants as the moral and political equals of their compatriots. Each of these criteria are to be applied to every study or set of studies under review.

The first operational criterion for ensuring equal concern prohibits arbitrary and unnecessary risks and burdens:

No Unnecessary Risk: To be consistent with the principle of equal concern, the risks to both the basic and the personal interests of participants should be reduced to those that are necessary to produce the knowledge needed to address a gap in the ability of a social system—such as a health system—to safeguard and advance the basic interests of the people they serve.

From this criterion it follows that it is never acceptable to expose research participants to risks that are gratuitous or more significant than is necessary. This requirement is not restricted to basic interests since even though the personal interests of research participants may not be widely shared, they may nevertheless be of profound importance to the particular individual. Where impositions on the personal interests of study participants are foreseeable, such impositions should be reduced so as to ensure that their presence reflects the necessity of their contribution to valuable science and not simply social disregard for their first-order life plan by researchers.

Demonstrating that those risks or burdens are necessary to facilitate the legitimate epistemic goals of scientific inquiry provides credible assurance that decisions that stakeholders make regarding the imposition of risks and burdens track the legitimate social purpose of research. In other words, it ensures that the risks and burdens to which participants are exposed cannot be eliminated without compromising the quality or the integrity of the evidence a study is designed to generate. Satisfying this condition is necessary to ensure that the risks and burdens of research are not arbitrary impositions that reflect antipathy or indifference to individuals or their particular interests (Pettit 1997, vii).

6.3.2 Special Concern for Basic Interests

The second operational criterion for preserving equality is to be applied after the first. It reflects the special normative status of the basic interests of individuals:

Special Concern for Basic Interests: If the basic interests of research participants are threatened or impaired (for example, by sickness, injury, or disease), participants must be provided a level of care and protection for their basic interests that does not fall below what at least a reasonable minority of experts in the relevant fields (e.g., the medical or public health community) would regard as the most beneficial method of response.[3]

This requirement applies to cases in which the basic interests of individuals are threatened. This is a morally important circumstance for two reasons. First, these interests play a critical role in securing the standing of individuals as free and equal persons (§4.5). They are the rudimentary building blocks that individuals need in order to be free to formulate, pursue and revise a distinctive life plan. When the basic interests of study participants are threatened, so is the fair value of their highest-order interest in having real freedom to formulate, pursue and revise a life plan of their own. Second, a just social order is committed to securing and upholding the freedom and equality of persons. The principle of special concern for basic interests provides credible social assurance to study participants that research functions as a division of social labor in which their status as free and equal persons will be respected. As they participate in activities designed to create the means of securing the basic interests of others, study participants can be secure in the knowledge

---

[3] This formulation follows the practice of presupposing that the deliberations in question take place against the backdrop of a particular set of basic institutions. In chapter 9 I argue explicitly for the claim that this principle should be understood as holding relative to the level of care and protection that can be attained and sustained in the basic social institutions of the host community.

that their basic interests will not be treated with lesser regard or subject to antipathy, indifference or neglect.

If an intervention is not regarded as the best way to safeguard or advance the basic interests of a person by even a reasonable minority of experts (in other words, nobody champions that approach as among the best ways to treat, prevent, or diagnose the health problem in question) then I will refer to it as "substandard." The operational test for determining which practices, procedures, or interventions meet this standard is explicated in §6.4.

The focus here on not falling below the standard of what at least a reasonable minority of experts would recommend is meant to capture the idea that even when there is significant uncertainty or widespread disagreement about what constitutes the best or optimal response to a particular problem, it is often possible to identify interventions that would not be regarded as among those likely to be best by even a reasonable minority of the relevant expert community. When the basic interests of individuals are at stake, allocating study participants to interventions that are not regarded as among those likely to be best by even a reasonable minority of the relevant expert community violates the principle of equal concern. In such a case, although different experts might disagree about how best to meet a person's basic interests, they all agree that there are better alternatives to the intervention in question.

When the basic interests of a participant are not at stake, this requirement does not apply. This represents a major difference between the integrative approach and frameworks that first distinguish interventions that are offered with therapeutic intent from those that are employed for purely research-related purposes and then subject interventions in these two different categories to different standards of appraisal. I will return to this point in more detail in §6.7.2. For now, it is sufficient to say that the reason to focus on the interests that are at stake, rather than the rationale for providing an intervention, is that it is the interests of participants that are morally relevant. The distinction between therapeutic and purely research-related study procedures attempts to track this distinction, but indirectly.

This indirect route is problematic because interventions can be delivered with therapeutic intent even when the condition that is being treated does not implicate the basic interests of the recipient. For example, there may be circumstances where researchers want to investigate new prophylactic or therapeutic measures for minor medical conditions, such as minor scrapes and cuts or male-pattern baldness. It may be permissible in such cases to test new interventions against a baseline of no treatment, even if established effective interventions already exist for these conditions (as long as it can be established that such a study still has meaningful social value). This would not violate the special concern for basic interests as long as the conditions under study do not threaten the basic interests of study participants.

Views that hold that interventions administered with therapeutic warrant must be tested against the best available alternative would prohibit studies that allow participants to be randomized to no treatment in such cases. In order to avoid this implication, some have argued that in such minor cases no treatment is often a legitimate therapeutic option. This observation is correct, but it only reinforces the point I am making here. The reason no treatment is a legitimate therapeutic alternative in such cases is explained by the fact that minor, transient, or cosmetic problems do not threaten the basic interests of individuals and, as such, we can legitimately ask study participants to voluntarily forego such interventions if doing so is necessary to conduct a study with the requisite social value (§6.7.2).

A just division of social labor can permit community members to ask one another to risk, sacrifice, alter, or limit ends or goals that are part of their individual life plan—their personal interests—in an effort to secure for others the basic interests that are necessary components of the freedom to formulate, pursue and revise such an individual life plan. This means that it is morally permissible for researchers to ask participants if they are willing to undergo painful but transient procedures, to endure unpleasant but temporary experiences, to bear inconveniences, or to take risks that are unlikely to compromise their basic interests but that different individuals may perceive as more or less significant depending on the way those risks relate to the constituents of their personal life plan. When the basic interests of study participants are not at risk, this permission applies to all study procedures, regardless of the warrant for their use.

When the basic interests of participants are at risk, then there is a strong moral imperative to ensure that participants receive a level of care for their basic interests that does not fall below what would be recommended by at least a reasonable minority of experts. Study participants cannot be offered a course of care for their basic interests that falls below what would be recommended by at least a reasonable minority of experts, and they cannot be subjected to study-related procedures that would compromise their basic interests. It is permissible to ask them to accept risks to their personal interests, from alterations in the course of their care or from purely research-related procedures, so long as the risks and burdens have been reduced as much as possible, are necessary for the conduct of socially valuable science, and are consistent with the provision of care for the participant's basic interests that is not substandard.

The criterion of special concern for the basic interests of participants addresses the question of what it is permissible for researchers to offer to study participants. When research implicates the basic interests of participants, not only must unnecessary risks be reduced, but also researchers cannot offer participation in a study that would provide them with substandard care. They can, however, offer participation in studies in which it is necessary to expose participants to risks and burdens to their personal interests. In all cases this must be done in the context of a process of informed consent in which participants (or their proxies) are given a clear and accessible explanation of the rationale for such risks as well as their expected duration and magnitude. It is then up to individuals to evaluate these offers and to decide for themselves whether those particular burdens and risks are reasonable in light of the goals of the study and their personal values and commitments.[4]

6.3.3 Social Consistency

If the risks associated with research could be limited to the personal interests of participants, then the two operational criteria discussed so far would be sufficient to assess and manage research risks. The problem is that almost every activity poses some degree of risk to a person's basic interests. For example, in the vast majority of cases, a blood draw will expose most people to only brief discomfort and an unsightly blemish. Nevertheless, there is a small but non-zero probability that a blood draw could cause a fatal or debilitating infection. More invasive procedures, such as biopsies or spinal taps, may pose a higher risk of debilitating, permanent, or fatal adverse events, even though the absolute risk of these events may be quite low when they are performed by trained personnel under controlled conditions.

As a result, the integrative approach requires an additional principle for regulating the extent to which stakeholders in the research enterprise can be exposed to risks to their basic interests without violating the principle of equal concern.

---

[4] The wording here is not meant to imply that waivers of informed consent are never permissible. The purpose of these remarks is simply to illustrate the division of moral labor between the risk assessments that structure the way a study is designed and the subsequent requirement to seek the consent of study participants.

The integrative approach uses a third operational criterion to ensure that residual risks to the basic interests of study participants are consistent with the principle of equal concern.

Social Consistency: In all cases, the cumulative incremental risks to the basic interests of study participants that are not offset by the prospect of direct benefit to the participant must not be greater than the risks to the basic interests of individuals permitted in the context of other socially sanctioned activities that are similar in structure to the research enterprise.

The third operational criterion recognizes that respect for the moral equality of individuals cannot require that they be prohibited from voluntarily assuming risks to their basic interests. First, such a standard simply could not be achieved; even routine activities involve some incremental risk to a person's basic interests. Second, enforcing such a standard would not only rule out participating in medical research, but, as we saw in the previous chapter (§5.9–11), it would rule out pursuing a career as a researcher (and many other important social activities and professional roles), since that work can itself involve small but non-zero risks to the researcher's basic interests. The challenge, therefore, is to establish when incremental risks to the basic interests of individuals violate the underlying commitment to moral equality, recognizing that there can be reasonable diversity across a range of different social activities in the extent to which risks to the basic interests of persons can be seen as reasonable.

The third operational criterion addresses this context sensitivity by requiring stakeholders to identify social activities that are structurally similar to the research enterprise and to ensure that incremental risks to the basic interests of participants do not exceed the incremental risks to the basic interests of individuals associated with those structurally similar social activities. The central challenge then lies in delineating criteria for structural similarity that can be used to locate relevant comparison classes of activities and then in determining how to make these comparisons in practice.

The requirement of structural similarity is meant to capture the idea that it is not appropriate to use just any social activity to determine what kind of incremental risks to the basic interests of participants are morally permissible. For example, some people may enjoy auto racing, ski jumping, or hanggliding at least partly because of the thrill that comes from their associated risks. More generally, there may be activities in which individuals willingly engage such that eliminating all risk of physical harm would detract from the underlying value of that activity. In research, however, if it were possible to eliminate all risk of harm it should make participation in this activity more, rather than less, attractive.

This feature of clinical research should therefore be used as a criterion of structural similarity. That is, appropriate comparison classes of activities should be ones whose primary social purpose is to benefit others, where the associated risks are viewed as necessary evils such that reducing or eliminating those risks would render that activity more attractive to participants.

Additionally, when individuals perceive themselves as having control over salient features of an activity, they are often willing to accept greater risks to themselves than in similar activities where they lack such control. This may help to explain why people are willing to tolerate greater risks from driving than from airline flight or other forms of public transportation. Such asymmetries matter in the research context because research participants put their interests in the hands of identifiable parties who possess knowledge and expertise that participants lack, and who pursue a diverse set of interests, some of which may overlap or dovetail with those of participants and some of which may not. This militates in favor of comparing the risks to the basic interests of research participants that cannot be eliminated, to risks to the basic interests of community members that are associated with social activities that involve this kind of principle-agent relationship.

Finally, it is imperative to avoid using activities as comparators in which oversight mechanisms or safety regulations are poorly enforced or are widely recognized to be inadequate. For instance, coal mining has become a safer occupation then it was several decades ago because of tougher safety regulations. However, at the time that I wrote one of the papers on which this chapter is based, there were several high-profile accidents at mines that had been repeatedly cited for safety violations. As a result, the risks that coal miners face in actual practice were clearly higher than what was judged to be socially acceptable, as evidenced by the fact that actual conditions on the ground often fell short of the requirements of existing health and safety regulations. Appropriate comparator activities should not only be the subject of active public oversight, but should have a record of complying with the requirements outlined in such oversight, so that the risk profile associated with the activity can be seen, at least prima facie, as representing a level of risk that is deemed socially acceptable after due reflection.

To be clear, the goal in applying the third operational criterion is to find reasonable criteria of similarity that can be used to identify appropriate comparison classes of activities and then to examine the risk profiles associated with activities that satisfy some or all of these criteria. This process itself may require careful adjustments in the criteria of similarity as well as discerning judgments about whether the activities that meet these criteria ought to be endorsed as appropriate comparators for clinical research. This is therefore an inherently normative or evaluative process. The objective is not to avoid making such normative judgments. It is, rather, to find a reasonable set of criteria that can be used to facilitate this process so that data that exist about the risks associated with socially important activities in one sphere can be used to assess the incremental risks to the basic interests of research participants that come from purely research-related elements of a particular study.

One place to look for appropriate comparison classes of activities might be to public service professions, such as volunteer fire departments or paramedic services. The volunteer nature of these activities combined with their orientation to serving the public interest represent important structural similarities to the research enterprise. Similarly, these occupations are often subject to varying degrees of public oversight. However, because there is no principal-agent relationship in these activities it may not be appropriate to permit in clinical research activities that have a risk profile that is similar to the most dangerous activities that individuals in these roles sometimes undertake.

The idea I am proposing is to use these comparison classes of activities to construct practical tests for this third operational criterion. Such practical tests demarcate an acceptable upper bound on the incremental risks to the basic interests of participants in clinical research. Ideally, most studies would impose risks that fall well short of this upper bound. Where such risks cannot be eliminated and are necessary to produce socially valuable information, the proposal is to ensure that they are not greater than the incremental risks to basic interests that members of helping professions, such as fire fighters or paramedics, face on a routine basis. If a phase I clinical trial involving healthy participants failed to meet such a test, for example, then it would have to be redesigned, delayed until further pre-clinical research could be completed, or the data would have to be generated in some other fashion.

Finally, as we saw in §5.11.2, the limits on the risks that it is reasonable to pursue in different activities can change according to what I there called the principle of proportionality. For example, the risks to which volunteer paramedics or fire fighters can be exposed in the course of protecting property, or safeguarding individuals from threats that are more distant in time, is often lower than the risks to which such persons can be exposed when the risks to others are greater and more immediate. So too, then, permissible research risks can be subject to a similar requirement of proportionality. When research is in early stages, the permissible level of residual risk to the basic interests of study participants should be lower than when those risks are necessary to ensure that results are more directly applicable to patient care or clinical practice.

6.4 Uncertainty as a Practical Test within the Integrative Approach

6.4.1 Uncertainty Regarding Basic Interests

Because the integrative approach rejects the two dogmas of research ethics discussed in the last chapter, it can fill out the template for the appeal to uncertainty (§5.4) in a way that is both conceptually and practically coherent. To see this, we must first articulate the practical test that is to be used to determine whether or not a particular clinical trial satisfies the second operational criterion outlined previously—special concern for basic interests.

To construct a practical test for the second operational criterion we need to know when it is ethically permissible to allocate a study participant to a given intervention and when doing so constitutes substandard care and therefore represents a violation of equal concern. The integrative approach uses the following definition of admissibility to construct this practical test.[5]

---

[5] More formally, let $I = \{1,...i,...n\}$ be the set of individuals with a particular medical condition for which there is a set of available treatment options $S = \{s_1,...,s_m\}$. Let U_i be the set of interventions from S to which individual i might be allocated within a particular clinical trial and let U_i^* be the set of interventions from S that are admissible treatment options for the individual i.

Uncertainty Regarding Basic Interests: A treatment s_j is admissible for individual i just in case there is either uncertainty among, or conflict between, expert clinicians about whether s_j is dominated by any other members of S as a treatment for individual i. For each individual in I, the care and protection afforded to that individual's basic interests falls within the threshold of competent medical care just in case each intervention in U_i is a member of U_i^*.

Uncertainty Regarding Basic Interests: For each individual with a particular condition (e.g., a health problem), the care and protection afforded to
that individual's basic interests satisfies the condition of equal concern just in
case every intervention to which that person might be allocated in a research
study is admissible. An intervention is admissible for an individual just in
case there is either uncertainty among, or conflict between, experts about
whether it is dominated by any other intervention as a means of safeguarding
the basic interests of that individual.

Notice that this practical test is formulated at the level of the individual
study participant. This addresses a concern raised by Miller and Weijer
(2006b) and discussed in §5.7.5, namely, that although medical experts
might be uncertain or disagree about the merits of a particular intervention for patients with a particular medical condition, they may not be uncertain about its merits for any particular individual. This might happen,
for instance, if that individual has a medical condition that is clearly
contraindicated, putting them at elevated risk were they to receive a particular treatment.

This practical test requires that each potential study participant can
only be invited to participate in studies that allocate them to admissible
interventions. In this respect, it is similar to the criteria of admissibility
recommended by Kadane and colleagues (1996). In that trial, a treatment
was deemed to be admissible for a particular participant just in case it
was judged to be the best treatment option for that individual by at least
one from among a set of expert clinicians. In this case, however, the expert clinicians were actually computer models that had been constructed
out of a careful elicitation process involving real clinicians. A less com-
putationally complex solution to this problem is for each participant
to be screened by several experts. If different experts who each prefer
one intervention over another for a particular medical condition regard
their favored intervention as admissible for this particular participant,
then it is permissible to allow that individual to be randomized to those
interventions.

The most salient difference between the concept of admissibility defined
here and the one articulated by Kadane and colleagues is that the integrative
approach limits the scope of these judgments to the basic interests of study
participants. Nevertheless, when this condition is met, each individual who
participates in a clinical trial is assured of receiving a package of medical

care that would be recommended for them by at least a reasonable minority of expert clinicians.

This practical test is also similar to Freedman's clinical equipoise, but here too there are some important differences. First, the moral force of this requirement is grounded, not in the individual physician's therapeutic obligation, but in the fundamental importance of the basic interests of individuals as both a target for the research enterprise and as a constraint on the way it is organized and operates. The judgments of particular experts, such as medical professionals when evaluating medical research, are used only to determine the practices, procedures, or interventions that represent the most effective means of safeguarding the basic interests of the individual in question. They do not play any role in grounding the normative foundation of the integrative approach.

Second, this practical test explicitly distinguishes agnosticism from a state of clinical conflict between experts (§5.6.3). The former obtains when individual clinicians have no ground for preferring one treatment from among the set of available options over any others as a treatment for that individual. This state might occur, for example, when a novel intervention begins to show sufficient promise in animal models and in early trials in humans that clinicians become uncertain about its net therapeutic advantage relative to existing interventions for some set of individuals. When this occurs, it may be permissible to initiate a clinical trial in which individuals for whom both of these interventions are admissible are randomized to one of them.

Clinical conflict exists when individual expert clinicians have definitive expert assessments that one intervention is preferable to the other options for a particular individual, but different experts prefer different interventions from this set of options for that individual. So, for example, one expert might regard high-dose chemotherapy with autologous bone marrow transplant (HDC-ABMT) for end-stage breast cancer as the best treatment option for a particular patient. A different expert may regard continuation of standard chemotherapy as preferable to this more aggressive intervention for the same patient. In this case, offering this person the option of participating in a clinical trial in which she might be randomized to either of these treatment options is ethically permissible since, no matter what the result of the randomization, this person is guaranteed to receive an intervention that would be recommended for her by at least a reasonable minority of expert clinicians.

6.4.2 Reconciling Social Value, Concern for Welfare, and Equal Concern: HDC-ABMT as an Example

The integrative approach provides a clear rationale for studies like the landmark trial conducted by Stadtmauer and colleagues (2000) that tested HDC-ABMT against standard doses of chemotherapy in patients who responded well to an initial 6–8 week course of induction chemotherapy. While some clinicians were passionate proponents of HDC-ABMT, others were skeptical that its benefits outweighed its significant burdens. In some cases, the degree of polarization may have been sufficiently high that members of the various camps regarded those who did not share their treatment preferences as violating the clinical judgment principle discussed in §5.7. Nevertheless, this study helped put to rest a decade-long debate about the relative clinical merits of HDC-ABMT, showing that it offered no advantage over standard of care (Mello and Brennan 2001).

For women in this trial, both HDC-ABMT and conventional doses of chemotherapy were admissible treatments because there was no consensus in the expert community that either one of these interventions dominated the other. In fact, the informed expert clinical community likely divided into two camps. The first would have recommended the more aggressive treatment to their patients. The second would have recommended conventional treatment to their patients. There might have been a third camp who, seeing this polarization, was uncertain about the relative merits of these therapeutic alternatives. But the integrative approach does not presuppose or require the existence of such a third group to justify conducting a well-designed clinical trial.

Without a randomized clinical trial, an informed and well-resourced patient with end-stage breast cancer might have sought a second opinion. Had they encountered clinicians from each of these camps, they would have been told that HDC-ABMT is their best option and also that it is not their best option. They would also have been told that conventional chemotherapy is their best option and also that it is not their best option. Faced with these conflicting recommendations, such a patient could arbitrarily decide to accept the recommendation of one of these groups or could have decided to flip a coin.

The opportunity to participate in a randomized, controlled, clinical trial presents patients in this situation with the opportunity to receive a modality of care that would be recommended for them by at least a reasonable minority of experts, but under conditions that facilitate valid inference about the therapeutic effects of these alternative interventions. In this respect, the clinical trial offers patients an opportunity to contribute to the common good without knowingly sacrificing their basic interests in the process.

Because this study satisfies the conditions outlined here it has a strong claim to satisfying the social value requirement. The knowledge it was designed to produce is necessary to improve the ability of health systems to safeguard and advance the basic interests of people with breast cancer. A trial designed to resolve conflict or uncertainty about how best to manage this fatal medical condition generates information that bridges a knowledge gap concerning how best to effectively, efficiently and equitably address an important health need of this community.

Trials that satisfy the conditions of the integrative approach also satisfy the principle of concern for welfare (§5.4 and §6.2.1). In particular, if it was consistent with concern for welfare for informed and conscientious clinicians to prescribe continued chemotherapy for a patient—to ensure that the patient received that modality of care with certainty—and for other informed and conscientious clinicians to prescribe HDC-ABMT, then it cannot violate concern for welfare to allow that same patient to be randomized to these interventions. Ensuring that no individual in the study is allocated to an intervention that is substandard, as defined here (§6.3.2), thus ensures that studies with a strong prima facie claim to producing socially valuable information are consistent with the requirement of concern for welfare.

Studies that satisfy these conditions are also consistent with the principle of equal concern. First, the risks to which participants are exposed have been reduced to those that are necessary to answer an important medical question (the first operational criterion). So, no participants are asked to bear a burden or to be exposed to a risk that is gratuitous or unnecessary. Second, the level of care and protection for the basic interests of each person in the study does not fall below what at least a reasonable minority of the expert medical or public health community would regard as the most beneficial method of response (the second operational criterion). So, no individual in the study is knowingly subjected to substandard care. Third, the residual risks to participants that are not offset by the prospect of direct benefit to a participant's basic interests are not greater than what it would be permissible for individuals to undertake in the course of a comparable social activity. In this respect, individuals who participate in research that meets these requirements are not treated with less respect or concern than the population of persons who do not participate in the study.

As a result, individuals could participate in this study secure in the knowledge that their basic interests would be respected and that their status as free and equal persons would not be denigrated in the course of study participation. Although which modality of care they receive is determined by a random process, the care that they in fact receive is not worse than what would be recommended for a person who opted not to participate in the study. In that sense, participants are not subject to a standard of care that is worse than what is available to other study participants or to patients outside of the trial.[6] Individuals who did not want to take up, as a personal goal, the project of determining the relative clinical merits of these interventions were free to refuse to participate. For those who saw answering this question as a worthwhile project to adopt, participation offered an avenue to advance the common good without compromising their status as free and equal.

What about the charge that as data from this study accrue, the states of uncertainty or conflict that justify its continuation are likely to evaporate long before the trial reaches statistical significance (Marquis 1983; Gifford 1986; Hellman 2002)? In the previous chapter I argued that this was a powerful objection against all views that locate the relevant uncertainty in the mind of the individual clinician. I also argued that although Freedman took the critically important step of moving the relevant uncertainty out of the mind of the individual clinician and into the larger expert medical community, his approach suffered from the fact that its normative foundations were still located in the moral obligations of medical professionals. For this reason, I want to give a short answer to this question here that I will then unpack and elaborate in more detail in the next section.

It is a strength of the integrative approach that the criteria for admissibility articulated in the practical test for the second operational criterion are tightly connected to the social value requirement. When there is uncertainty or conflict among experts about how best to safeguard or advance the basic interests of individuals, trials that are designed to eliminate this conflict or uncertainty have a strong prima facie claim to generating social value. Imagine now that an interim analysis of data was pre-planned. If the evidence generated by such a trial at this interim analysis is sufficient to create consensus about the superiority of one option over the other, then the trial will

---

[6] It is important to note that the equipoise requirement is often charged with myopically comparing the relative merits of interventions on offer within a clinical trial without taking note of the care that might be available outside of such a study (see Kukla 2007). So it is important to emphasize that the position outlined here avoids this problem by requiring that study participants not be treated worse than other study participants and other members of the community whose basic social structures the research is designed to strengthen. See §2.6.3 note 12 and chapter 9 for further discussion.

have served its social function and ought to be terminated. In other words, if the evidence is sufficiently compelling that conscientious and fully informed experts shift their expert medical opinion in favor of one option and against the rest, then the study has served its legitimate social purpose and should be terminated.

If, in contrast, only some fully informed and conscientious clinicians are convinced and a reasonable minority remain uncertain or would continue to make clinical recommendations that conflict with those of their peers, then we have moved from either a state of uncertainty to one of clinical conflict or we have reduced but not eliminated the conflict in informed and conscientious medical judgment. In that case, it is permissible to continue the trial since both of the interventions in question remain admissible.

When interim evidence is sufficient to alter the judgment of some clinicians, that alone is not sufficient to warrant stopping the trial. The question is whether, if the trial were stopped, other conscientious and informed experts would continue to recommend the different treatments in the trial to their patients. If so, then the conflict in expert medical judgment, and with this the diversity in actual treatment practices, would persist. As a result, stopping the trial makes no person better off, but it detracts from the social value of the study. Continuing the study ensures that the trial satisfies the social value requirement without requiring any individual to be allocated to substandard care.

Another way to state this is to say that the close connection between the social value requirement and the criteria for admissibility in the integrative approach help to ensure both that trials continue until they serve their legitimate social function and that the basic interests of participants receive the same degree of care and concern as is shown for individuals outside of research.

6.5 A Social Model of Learning, Uncertainty, and Disagreement

6.5.1 The Most Difficult Case: Response Adaptive Randomization

It is a theme of this book that some of the shortcomings of orthodox research ethics stem from the way it frames the core issues of the field as being situated within the relationship between individual researchers and individual subjects. The two dogmas of research ethics embody and reinforce this framing and, in doing so, they exaggerate the extent to which tensions within the research enterprise are taken to constitute moral dilemmas that require empowering some entity within this system to make tragic choices.

The integrative approach connects conflict and uncertainty in the relevant expert community with a normative standard for regulating research that is also social in nature. This symmetry allows for a closer connection between uncertainty and the social value requirement, on the one hand, and conflicting expert judgment and concern for welfare, on the other. We can illustrate the advantages of this connection by turning to what is likely the most difficult case for approaches to risk management that appeal to uncertainty, namely, studies that incorporate response adaptive randomization (RAR).

In most clinical trials, a decision is made at the time a study is designed about the proportion of participants who will be allocated to a novel intervention and the proportion who will be allocated to the comparator (which might be the current standard of care or a placebo control). This allocation is usually fixed, in the sense that it does not change throughout the course of the trial. If the chosen allocation is 50:50, then a fair coin (or its computational analogue) is flipped to decide which intervention to provide to each participant. More generally, trials with an equal allocation assign each participant a $1/n$ chance of receiving each of the n interventions on offer in a trial. In some cases, this allocation is fixed but unequal. So, for example, a trial might have a fixed 60:40 allocation in favor of the investigational intervention.

Generally, when trials involve a fixed randomization allocation (FRA), their sample size is calculated at the time the study is designed and then a specified number of participants are recruited and allocated to the interventions in the trial's various arms. It is common for data and safety monitoring boards (DSMBs) to take an "interim look" at the data to make sure that any effects observed in the trial to that point are not so dramatic that the trial should be stopped, either because some intervention is performing extremely well or extremely badly. These interim analyses have to be planned in advance and the power of the study to detect effects of a given size has to be adjusted accordingly.

Trials that use RAR differ from this model in several ways (Lin et al., 2016). In particular, a study might begin with an equal probability ($1/n$) of participants being assigned to each of the n interventions in its various arms, but after a predetermined number of outcomes are observed (a "block" of participants), the randomization allocation is changed. The proportion of participants allocated to the various arms in a trial is altered dynamically depending on the outcomes that are observed from blocks of patients. If more promising outcomes are observed in the arm in which participants receive intervention A, for example, then the probability that participants in the next block will be allocated to A is increased. If the trial has three arms, then the probability that they will be allocated to arms B or C will be lower than the probability of being allocated to A. The relative likelihood of being allocated to B or C might remain equal or it might also be altered in favor of one of those interventions (e.g., B) if it performs worse than A but better than C. The rate at which these proportions change is determined by a function that is pre-specified at the time the study is designed.

How the randomization allocation in a study using RAR changes will depend, in part, on the outcomes that are observed in each of its arms. One of the advantages of this kind of design is that interventions that do not perform well will have their allocation proportion reduced as the trial proceeds. Normally, some threshold will be specified in advance for dropping underperforming interventions from the study. For example, if its fraction drops below 10%, then it might be dropped from the study.

RAR is often an element of study designs that allow new interventions to be added to ongoing trials without having to design a new protocol to test this new intervention (Berry 2011; Lewis 2016; Saville and Berry 2016; Trusheim et al. 2016; Renfro and Sargent 2017; Angus et al. 2019). The flexibility of being able to drop or add arms within the same study protocol makes such designs particularly attractive to a variety of stakeholders as it offers the prospect of reducing delays associated with designing and receiving approval for new studies. For example, this is attractive for pharmaceutical companies because reducing delay can increase profits by increasing the amount of time the firm has exclusive right to sell a drug. It is also attractive to patients to the extent that shorter research timelines mean that new interventions might be available sooner rather than later.

6.5.2 The Virtue of Rational Expectation

Proponents of designs that incorporate RAR argue that they are more attractive for participants because dynamically updating the randomization allocation in light of observed outcomes allows trials to allocate more participants to interventions that are performing well (Meurer, Lewis, and Berry 2012; Lewis 2016)[7]. This increases the probability that a participant in a trial with RAR will receive a direct medical benefit from participating, relative to the probability of receiving such a benefit in a trial with a FRA. In effect, the proponents of RAR argue that it is superior to designs that use FRA on the following ground.

Rational Expectation: If in expectation a participant has a greater probability of being allocated to what turns out to be a superior intervention in study design F than in design G, it is rational for that participant to prefer design F to G.

6.5.3 Does Rational Expectation Violate
Concern for Welfare?

Critics argue that trials of this kind reveal a fundamental moral dilemma for research ethics because any design using RAR that satisfies rational expectation must violate concern for welfare and, with this, the principle of equal concern. The rationale for this claim is stated by Saxman (2015), although not quite in these terms. Phrased in the terms I am using here, the charge is that when the randomization weights are $1/n$ the study might respect concern for welfare and the principle of equal concern. But once evidence emerges that one intervention (e.g., A) produces better outcomes than the others, and randomization weights adjust in favor of A, then it violates concern for welfare to allow subsequent patients to be randomized to B or C.

---

[7] "Advocacy of adaptive designs is predicated on the belief that such novel designs will result in fewer numbers of subjects having to participate and receive an 'inferior' treatment during the research process" (Laage et al. 2017, 192).

This objection can be pressed further. If we assume that studies involving RAR satisfy the principle of rational expectation, then critics of this design can be seen as worrying that it purchases whatever gains in efficiency it offers, at the cost of violating the principle of equal concern. In particular, although more participants will be allocated to what turns out to be the most beneficial intervention (if there is one) in the trial, it is nevertheless the case, they claim, that a smaller proportion of study participants are knowingly allocated to arms of the trial that are believed to produce outcomes that are inferior to those that could be produced if they were allocated to A.

6.5.4 No Impermissible Gambles

Additionally, RAR faces a criticism that is often lodged against unequal randomization more generally, namely, that even in the best case such designs reduce the burdens on some participants by knowingly exposing other participants to care that is credibly believed to be inferior. But if it is wrong to allocate someone to intervention C with certainty, when A is available—to just give them C instead of A—then we cannot make it permissible to give that person C when A is available by reducing the probability that they will be given C. Doing this violates the following principle:

No Impermissible Gambles: If it is impermissible to directly give intervention C to a person (give it to them with probability 1) when some other intervention A is available, then it is impermissible to include C as an option in a design that would randomize that person to C with any positive probability when A is available.

The point of the exposition so far is not to defend the methodological merits of study designs that use RAR, but to formulate what looks like an extreme example of the objection we saw in the previous section. In other words, if we assume that proponents of RAR are correct when they say that it offers a range of methodological advantages over studies that use an FRA, then we appear to find ourselves immediately back in the jaws of an in-principle moral dilemma: if the study satisfies rational expectation then it appears to violate the principles of equal concern, concern for welfare, and no impermissible gambles.

6.5.5   Forcing Uncertainty into the Model of a Single Decision-Maker

Although the argument that RAR produces a conflict between the principles of rational expectation, no impermissible gambles, concern for welfare, and equal concern sounds like a novel objection, it hinges on a criterion for admissibility that is derived from the judgment of a single expert. The difference is that, in this case, the trial itself is regarded as the single expert whose views are used to represent the relevant uncertainty. It is useful, therefore, to explain why this perspective seems so appealing and what is wrong with it. In the next section I then show how RAR can be thought of as helping us to model a moderately idealized learning health system and that, when studies are designed on these terms, the apparent dilemma disappears.

The reason that studies that use RAR seem to pose a deeper problem for approaches to research risk that appeal to uncertainty is that it encourages the idea that we can regard the randomization weights in a trial as expressing the preference of the medical community for the best performing intervention. When the randomization weights are $1/n$, for each of the n interventions, then the trial appears to be indifferent between those n interventions. But once the weights shift in favor of one intervention, the trial is no longer indifferent. It favors one option over the others. In effect, the trial is treated as a meta-agent constructed by taking a weighted average of the opinions of the different treatment communities. In that sense, the critique of RAR seems novel and interesting because this meta-agent that the trial is treated as modeling is easily seen as occupying a privileged epistemic state such that its judgments ought to be normative for the practice community in a way that the judgments of ordinary individuals might not.[8]

This view is alluring because it appeals to the idea that rational inquiry requires an agent, it treats the trial as such an agent, and it treats the randomization weights as though they are that agent's degrees of belief about the relative merits of the interventions in question. This social agent is created by aggregating the judgments of the diverse experts in the community, combining them into a higher-order decision model. In essence, it assigns a weight to the likelihood that each expert is correct and then chooses in a way that maximizes expected value. This is a concrete example, in microcosm, of a larger view of scientific consensus that many find intuitively appealing,

---

[8] Leonard Savage attributed a similar view to Woodbury (Savage 1972).

namely, that the goal of scientific consensus is to take in the diversity of beliefs in the scientific community, assign them weights, and form a single all-things-considered model out of this diversity.

This view faces several problems. First, it is a version of the linear opinion pooling rule for combining individual judgments into a group or social judgment. But the social agent constructed by assigning weights to the views of the individual experts can make recommendations that radically diverge from the recommendations of all of the experts from which it is created. For example, each expert may regard certain events (the temperature in Beijing today and whether to use treatment A or B for a certain patient in New York) as probabilistically independent and, as a result, would not base treatment decisions on what he or she recognizes as an irrelevant event (no medical expert will decide the merits among rival treatments for a patient who resides in New York by asking what the weather is that day in Beijing). But these relationships of probabilistic independence are not generally preserved in the linear opinion pool. As a result, the "social agent" can change its treatment recommendations upon learning the weather in Beijing, even though no particular expert would do so.[9] It is not clear why any expert should see as normative a model that would change its treatment preference on the basis of information that is not regarded as relevant by any of the models from which it is constructed.

Second, we already assumed from the beginning that every expert knows that many other, equally well-credentialed and informed experts make treatment recommendations that conflict with their own. So, it is not clear why adding another expert to the mix (in this case, the expert created by aggregating the views of the community) should alter the fact that the original experts do not find the existing evidence sufficiently persuasive to alter their treatment practice.

Third, there is the problem that, given the impoverished nature of our understanding of the underlying causal structure of health problems, experts

[9] Genest and colleagues (1986) establish that in order to be "Externally Bayesian" the pooling rule has to be of the "logarithmic" form. For the purposes of the present argument, it is sufficient to see that one aspect of the Externally Bayesian condition is that when experts regard two events (A and B) as independent, this condition requires preserving the expert judgments that each event is irrelevant to the probability for the other ($P(A \mid B) = P(A)$), after pooling. Treating a trial as a social agent involves creating a social consensus model by taking weighted averages of different treatment communities. But weighted averages are a convex combination and, as Seidenfeld and colleagues (2010) show, a convex combination of expert judgments is not a logarithmic rule. As a result, the social agent discussed above cannot preserve the judgments of experts about which events are relevant to treatment decisions.

have a difficult time predicting which theories of disease or interventions are likely to be correct or best (Kimmelman and London 2011). In this environment there are significant dangers from group-think, the situation in which experts too quickly converge to the same view of a problem. If experts in a community too readily update their beliefs on the basis of what their colleagues regard as persuasive, then spurious results that are bound to happen as a matter of chance can cause such communities to prematurely adopt promising but ultimately false beliefs.

Communities with more diversity among experts are more productive in the sense that they are less prone to converging on false answers and more efficient at exploring alternatives. As a result, communities with this kind of diversity are better at locating effective solutions to pressing problems (Hull 1988; Solomon 1992; Kitcher 1995; Zollman 2010; Muldoon 2013).

The point for our present purposes is that we must be wary of research methods that impose consensus on conscientious and informed medical experts in cases where the available medical evidence is not sufficient to alter their medical practice. Experts who embrace different theories of disease pathology and intervention mechanism are likely to update their beliefs at different rates in the face of the same evidence. Reasonable, transient diversity among experts is not simply a descriptive feature of many actual scientific communities, but a normatively desirable feature that plays an important epistemological role in the health and fecundity of those communities (Zollman 2010). In light of this, trials must be designed with rigorous methods so that the evidence they produce is viewed as credible by reasonable experts. Although such experts may change their beliefs at different rates, the goal is to produce the evidence that these stakeholders need to alter their assessments of interventions or strategies and, ultimately, to improve clinical practice.

6.6 Modeling a Learning Health System

6.6.1 Reasonable Diversity of Conscientious and Informed Experts

It is important to recognize that RAR can be a useful part of a learning health system if it is an element of trials designed to model the transient diversity of reasonable experts without amalgamating their beliefs into a single, meta-model of uncertainty. Demonstrating how this can be accomplished makes it easier to see how the objection discussed in the previous section reflects the dogmas of research ethics that I have argued should be rejected. It also illustrates how the integrative approach provides concrete guidance for ensuring that studies can meet the social value requirement while continuing to adhere to the principles of respect for welfare, no impermissible gambles, and equal concern.

If studies are to provide evidence that will change clinical practice, then they must be designed in ways that reflect and address the reasonable diversity of expert opinion within communities of informed and conscientious experts. Consider again a case in which there are three interventions, A, B, and C for treating patients with a particular illness and that at least a reasonable minority of experts favor A, as a treatment for this condition, while other experts favor B, and still others favor C. According to the integrative approach, if experts from each of these groups would recommend their favored intervention for a particular patient (providing it to that patient directly so that there is no uncertainty about which intervention the patient receives), then it cannot violate the principles of respect for welfare or no impermissible gambles to allow that same person to be allocated to one of these interventions by a random process.

Imagine that names of the experts from each of these groups were placed into a hat. Individuals draw the name of an expert from the hat and that expert evaluates them and then recommends their favored treatment unless there are specific reasons to avoid this intervention for the person in question. In this situation, the probability that a patient would be treated by an expert from an A-favoring community would depend on the number of A-favoring experts in the bag, relative to B- and C-favoring experts.

Imagine further that after a name is drawn and the recommendation given, the name is returned to the bag. After a block of results are observed, every expert whose name is in the bag updates their beliefs. If the block of observed results favors A, then experts who favor A will favor it more strongly. Some experts who weakly favored B or C may now favor A, while others become uncertain about the relative merits of A versus their previously favored interventions. Some who more strongly favored B or C may continue to favor these interventions but less strongly than before. This process is repeated. If, at some point, the evidence against one intervention, C, is so consistent that the number of C-favoring experts drops below a specified threshold, then we might remove C-favoring names from the bag because we judge that they no longer represent a reasonable minority of experts. The key point is that as evidence emerges and the beliefs of these individual experts change, the relative size of the communities that favor each intervention will grow or shrink.

This model provides a framework for designing trials that use RAR so that they model a health system that is moderately idealized in this respect: the beliefs of the experts in these communities reflect the beliefs of fully informed and conscientious experts in the real world, with the idealization that when evidence emerges about the relative merits of a set of interventions, the experts update their beliefs about the relative merits of those interventions on the basis of that information. Because these experts reflect the diversity of reasonable and informed expert opinion in the real world, they should agree about when evidence favors one intervention over the others, but they may differ in how they respond to this information. If evidence that favors A emerges, experts who favored A will now favor it more strongly. Some experts who were uncertain may now favor A, but others may remain uncertain. Some who favored B or C may now be uncertain, but others may continue to favor B or C, only slightly less strongly.

On the model I am proposing, randomization weights in a study that employs RAR do not reflect the beliefs of any agent. Instead, they should reflect the relative proportion of experts who, in a moderately idealized community of experts, would recommend each intervention in the study. This approach captures the idea that if a trial were stopped after only the initial block of evidence, some experts in the actual medical community would continue to favor and to recommend B or C. As long as the community of experts who favor B or C constitutes at least a reasonable minority, then it remains permissible to randomize patients to these trial arms. It remains permissible because participants within such a trial are not provided with substandard care, as defined in §6.3.2—they continue to receive a level of care that would be recommended for them by at least a reasonable minority of expert clinicians.

The goal is for the trial to capture the extent of the uncertainty about, or conflict over, the relative merits of interventions in a way that reflects the diversity of real experts while ensuring that these experts update their judgments in light of emerging evidence. In this way, diversity should be reasonable—experts change their judgments in light of emerging evidence, although different experts may change their judgments at different rates. This is meant to exclude situations in which diversity persists because experts are unaware of evidence, because communities are wedded to tradition rather than scientific information, or because communities are in some other way impervious to evidence.

6.6.2 Reconciling Social Value, Concern for Welfare, Equal Concern, and No Impermissible Gambles

When studies model the beliefs of conscientious and informed experts and are designed to generate the evidence that such experts are likely to regard as credible, then they have a strong prima facie claim to social value. The reason is that they are designed to generate evidence that is likely to alter the practice of experts in the relevant medical community. Thinking of trials on the model I've described in this section, and designing them accordingly, helps to ensure that studies with social value continue until they generate the evidence necessary to alter practice in the expert clinical community.

Altering the randomization weights in this framework does not violate concern for welfare. From the fact that some particular expert is persuaded that A produces better outcomes than B or C it does not follow that all other conscientious and well-informed experts who see this same information will find it compelling enough to shift their treatment recommendation to favor A. If it is permissible for a patient to be treated in clinical practice by practitioners from clinical communities that each favor one of these interventions, then it follows that A, B, and C are all admissible treatment options for that patient. If it is consistent with concern for welfare for a patient to be directly treated with A or B or C (to receive that intervention with certainty from a conscientious and informed expert who regards it as best for the person in question), then it cannot violate concern for welfare if that patient is assigned to those interventions with any distribution of probabilities that sums to 1. Even if every clinician in these treatment communities has a strict preference over the available treatment options (nobody thinks the probability of success for each is 1/3), the condition of uncertainty over basic interests exists between these treatment options, and no set of randomization weights that sums to unity is impermissible. As long as the admissibility criterion outlined in §6.4.1 is satisfied, continued randomization is consistent with the principle of concern for welfare.

Altering the randomization weights in this framework does not violate the principle of no impermissible gambles. The criterion of admissibility defined here prohibits participants from being randomized to interventions that are substandard in the sense that they would not be recommended for that person by even a reasonable minority of experts. As a result, all of the gambles permitted by the integrative approach are morally permissible.

The arguments made here and in the previous section demonstrate that trials employing RAR can be designed on terms that are consistent with the principle of equal concern as long as they satisfy the conditions of the integrative approach. Stopping such a study when some particular expert or group of experts find its results persuasive is thus self-defeating if at least a reasonable minority of other conscientious and informed experts who look at the same information would continue to provide B or C to their patients.

6.6.3 More General Relevance of the Result

The model proposed here for dealing with RAR can be used to think about randomized clinical trials that employ a fixed randomization design as well. The only difference is when experts see the data on which they update their beliefs. In other words, we can think of a traditional FRA design as one in which a participant draws the name of an expert from the hat, the expert makes a treatment recommendation, and then the name is returned to the hat. This process continues until a predetermined number of patients have been treated by experts from the different groups. The predetermined number should be calculated on the basis of the strength of evidence that will be needed to alter practice in this moderately idealized learning health system. Once that number of participants has been treated, the outcomes are revealed and the experts that make up these treatment communities alter their beliefs. Rather than updating their beliefs on outcomes as they emerge in the study, experts update their beliefs once all participants have received the relevant interventions.

Here again, one key point is that such a study must be designed to detect effects that experts regard as meaningful, with sufficient power that the results of the trial can credibly be expected to change the practice of the experts in these communities. The main difference in studies that use RAR is that individual experts are given the opportunity to change their beliefs on the basis of evidence as it emerges from the trial. The proponents of RAR hold that, if properly designed, this form of adaptation is morally superior because it satisfies the principle of rational expectation. On average, fewer participants will be allocated to study arms that are ineffective or harmful than are allocated to such arms in a design that employs a fixed randomization scheme.

For our present purposes, the key point is that the use of RAR does not conflict with the key ethical principles I have outlined here. The model I have described in this section is useful because it illustrates how a social understanding of conflict and uncertainty avoids the errors of appeals of uncertainty that focus solely on the beliefs of a single agent. It is also useful for the way it highlights the connection between the criteria for admissibility and the transient diversity of expert beliefs in order to ensure that studies fulfill their social purpose and shift the practices of the informed and conscientious experts on whom community members rely to safeguard their basic interests.

6.6.4 The Limit of Reasonable Diversity

At this point it might be objected that the approach I have described here requires an account of when we should stop regarding a minority of the medical community as reasonable and view their treatment preferences as no longer a part of the standard of care. This is indeed an important and pressing problem. But it is one that we face whether or not we embrace the integrative approach. After all, the moral purpose of medical research is to alter clinical practice in ways that improve the ability of health systems to meet the basic interests of community members. When experts are not conscientious, when they do not continue their medical education or do not update their beliefs on the basis of evidence, then that is a problem for any approach to research and research ethics. Alternatively, when conscientious and informed experts disagree, we must resist trying to settle those disagreements by fiat. In some cases, minority opinions turn out to be correct and the received wisdom is wrong. The best practice is to use well-designed studies to generate the evidence that conscientious and informed experts use to change their beliefs and to make sure that studies are designed to generate that evidence.

It is an advantage of the approach I describe here that it highlights the importance of ensuring that the beliefs of the idealized communities reflected in any study design capture the enthusiasm of real-world clinician-researchers for the various interventions for a medical condition as well as the more conservative or skeptical views of other experts. Explicit decisions can then be incorporated into the trial about when a community's views should be regarded as no longer reflecting the practice of responsible medicine.

In other words, the integrative approach helps to align the design of trials with their social purpose of improving the capacity of health systems to effectively, efficiently, and equitably meet the needs of those they serve. It also ensures symmetry between the practices that are regarded as ethically permissible outside of a trial and the practices that are permissible within the trial. The key point is that the integrative approach preserves these symmetries—participants in clinical trials are not deprived of a level of care that would be recommended for them by at least a reasonable minority of experts, and studies that are designed to generate the evidence that such experts need to alter their practice have a strong, prima facie claim to generating socially valuable information.

6.7 The Integrative Approach versus Alternatives

6.7.1 Criteria for Evaluating Alternative Frameworks for Risk Assessment and Management

Up to this point the goal of the present chapter has been to articulate the key elements of the integrative approach to risk assessment and management and to show how it reconciles a set of ethical requirements that capture ethical concerns that have traditionally been treated as incompatible or irreconcilable. The rest of this chapter is aimed at clarifying the merits of this approach relative to the main alternatives.

When comparing the merits of alternative frameworks for evaluating and managing risk in research, three broad criteria are relevant. The first is their *normative foundation*: an acceptable framework for risk assessment should ground its key insights and requirements in values that stakeholders can recognize as legitimate for guiding and restricting their conduct in this domain. This justification should also provide a coherent standpoint of sufficient generality that it applies to the full range of cases that occur in research involving humans. If all else is equal, frameworks that achieve a greater range of applicability without recourse to ad hoc, ancillary principles should be preferred to frameworks that require the addition of such principles.

The second criterion is the *appropriate integration* or reconciliation of the distinct concerns to which any such framework must be responsive. As we saw in the previous chapter, in diverse communities where people are free to cultivate a wide range of life plans, different individuals are likely to have attitudes about the reasonableness of various risks that disagree or conflict with the attitudes of others. While some may be particularly averse to certain types of risk, others may be willing to accept quite significant personal risk for the prospect of advancing socially meritorious projects. An acceptable framework will need to promote socially valuable research, demonstrate respect for individual autonomy, and recognize the social value of undertaking risk in the pursuit of socially valuable ends, while providing credible safeguards to protect the rights and welfare of study participants. To the extent that this involves setting limits on the risks to which participants may permissibly be exposed in research, an acceptable framework should set such limits on the basis of reasons that all stakeholders can recognize as non-arbitrary restrictions on the pursuit of their own ends and projects.

A third criterion is *operational clarity*. As a branch of practical ethics, the guiding ambition of research ethics is to provide a framework for evaluating clinical research that can help stakeholders resolve reasonable disagreements in a way that is publicly accessible and defensible. As such, an acceptable framework should not only ground its requirements in a unified normative perspective, but it should (1) elucidate a set of operational criteria or markers that delineate the parameters or boundaries that separate reasonable from excessive risks and (2) articulate practical tests that deliberators can use in order to determine whether or not these operational criteria have been met in any particular case.

It is my contention that the integrative approach fares better on these criteria than the available alternatives. In §6.7.2 I address other approaches that, like the integrative approach, attempt to ground their framework in an appeal to uncertainty. In 6.7.3 I address approaches that reject an appeal to uncertainty and instead adopt a more consequentialist approach.

6.7.2 Other Appeals to Uncertainty and Component Analysis

It is a strength of the integrative approach that it is grounded in a unified moral and political foundation that is normative for anyone motivated to respect other persons as free and equal. In particular, in diverse communities, different individuals will develop different life plans within which various activities take on particular personal importance or significance. As a result, individuals in such communities may disagree about a range of issues, including the value of various life plans, the value of various risks in relationship to particular ends and the place of health and health-related values in their individual and shared conceptions of the good life. To ensure that the activities of social institutions, including those that regulate the conduct of research, are not asserting arbitrary social authority, the members of such communities require a social standpoint from which they can evaluate the extent to which both impositions of risk and limitations on permissible risk are socially justified and not morally arbitrary. This standpoint need not be one that individuals embrace as part of their first-order conception of the good or the good life, but it must be a standpoint they are capable of inhabiting and which they can recognize as morally authoritative for regulating social institutions.

The integrative approach constructs the required standpoint by appealing to the distinction between personal and basic or generic interests that grounds the generic interest conception of the common good. Although individuals may adopt particular life plans that have little in common or that conflict or diverge in fundamental ways, each person who embraces such a life plan is committed to its value and, therefore, to the value of the freedom and capabilities necessary to formulate, pursue, and revise a first-order life plan. Despite differences in dress, demeanor, or aspiration, each person who takes the time to reflect can recognize every other person as a moral and political equal in this sense: to the extent that each is committed to a life plan grounded in some conception of the good, each is committed to the value of being able to formulate, pursue, and revise an individual life plan.

This shared higher-order interest in being free to advance one's personal interests defines the "space of equality," the domain over which all community members have a just claim to equal treatment. It is from this social standpoint that the institutions of research ethics are evaluated. As a result, the integrative approach is sufficiently general in scope that it applies to research carried out by individuals who fill a wide range of social roles, from physicians to economists, psychologists, management scientists, public health experts, citizen scientists, and anyone else seeking to generate socially valuable information from studies that involve human participants. Other frameworks that appeal to the narrow duties of particular professions lack this generality in scope.

The integrative approach also provides a unified framework for integrating various concerns that arise in this domain. The egalitarian research imperative is to foster a system of social cooperation in which individuals can take up, as part of their personal life plan, the project of developing the knowledge needed to better safeguard the basic interests of community members without sacrificing their status as free and equal persons. The justifications for exposing people to risk, and for limiting the risks that volunteers can accept, are grounded in the same shared interest of every individual in having real freedom to formulate, pursue, and revise a life plan of their own.

As we saw in §6.6, the integrative approach is capable of reconciling the social value requirement with the principles of equal concern, concern for welfare, rational expectation, and no impermissible gambles. Ensuring that trials reflect and address the uncertainty or disagreement in a moderately idealized community of experts ensures that research initiatives have a strong prima facie claim to producing socially valuable information while prohibiting study participants from being subjected to substandard care. This creates the conditions necessary for free and equal people to see research as an avenue through which they can generate the evidence that stakeholders need to more effectively, efficiently, and equitably meet the needs of community members without compromising their moral or social standing in the process.

As we saw in the previous chapter, other frameworks that seek to manage risk by using the template for the appeal to uncertainty rest on problematically narrow moral foundations. In particular, views grounded in the moral obligations of individual physicians are incapable of reconciling the social value requirement with the principles of concern for welfare or equal concern. Clinical equipoise fares better because it adopts a social conception of medical uncertainty. But it lacks generality because it cannot use the same normative foundation—the clinician's fiduciary duty to her individual patient—to provide guidance about how to evaluate all study risks. Rather, purely research-related risks have to be evaluated using a risk-benefit calculation of a kind that is inconsistent with the clinician's duty of individual care.

Component analysis recognizes this limitation and attempts to overcome it by presenting a comprehensive approach to risk assessment in medical research. But this expanded scope—the ability to cover interventions delivered with "therapeutic warrant" and those delivered solely for research-related purposes—is purchased at the price of conceptual disunity.

In component analysis, the risks from procedures that are offered with one motivation are bounded by the clinician's fiduciary duty while the only constraint on purely research-related risk is that it be outweighed by the value of the information a study is designed to produce. To the extent that the interests of participants is the normatively basic consideration, this appeal to the motivation or warrant for risk is morally arbitrary—whatever the source of a risk, consistency requires that the health and welfare of individuals be valued in the same way in relevant cases. If the welfare of participants is the morally basic concern, it seems arbitrary to circumscribe risks from interventions motivated by the prospect of direct benefit to the individual by the physician's duty of personal care and to allow the risks that are grounded in scientific necessity to be largely unbounded (see also Wendler and Miller 2007; Rid and Wendler 2010).

This inconsistent concern for participant interests is compounded by the fact that if an intervention is deployed with therapeutic warrant it does not follow that the condition being addressed is of sufficient medical importance that it affects the individual's basic or generic interests. Treatments that target a range of mild medical conditions (such as small cuts or abrasions, bruising, swelling, rash, temporary nausea, muscle aches, headaches, or male-pattern baldness) are delivered with therapeutic warrant. So, consistency would require that proponents of component analysis should hold that withholding a known effective treatment for such a condition in the context of a clinical trial would be unethical. In that case, component analysis faces two serious problems. First, it seems inconsistent to prevent participants from accepting risks from foregoing access to a known effective intervention for a minor medical condition, while permitting them to be exposed to significant risks from procedures that are necessary to collect study data. Second, this looks like an unacceptably paternalistic restriction since, for example, baldness seems to be a paradigm example of a medical condition whose meaning and significance will depend almost entirely on the contours of an individual's life plan.

Proponents of component analysis claim that they are not committed to such a position since non-treatment is a medically permissible response to minor medical conditions such as male-pattern baldness. But this appeal to professional practice is either an inappropriate deference to arbitrary professional authority or it is an unexplained explainer. It is an inappropriate deference to arbitrary professional authority if the normative ground for permitting the withholding of an effective intervention is the brute fact that doctors find it acceptable not to treat this medical condition. In other words, if the normative basis of the appeal is to the preferences of medical professionals, as such, then it vests too much authority in those professionals since it empowers them to limit the decisions facing patients or study participants for reasons that are grounded solely in their preferences as professionals.

If, instead, the claim is that it is permissible for clinicians to leave baldness untreated because it is not a sufficiently significant health problem that it requires medical intervention, then we need an account of the severity or seriousness of medical conditions that is independent of the judgment of experts. But this is precisely what is lacking in views that appeal to the moral obligations of professionals for their normative foundation.

Differentiating standards of risk management on the basis of the warrant for deploying an intervention is also vulnerable to the charge of inconsistency from a different angle. In particular, the nature of the question that a study can answer is shaped by numerous variables including which interventions are provided to study participants out of the motive of therapeutic intent. If it is permissible to evaluate the risks of purely research-related interventions in terms of the value of the information the study is likely to generate, then it seems arbitrary to apply a different standard to other elements of a study that also impact the value of the information a study can produce. Since decisions about which diagnostic, therapeutic, or prophylactic interventions to provide to participants also affect the goal of producing scientifically sound and socially valuable information, critics argue that all aspects of a clinical trial should be assessed in terms of whether the associated risks are reasonable in light of the value of the information the study is likely to generate (Rid and Wendler 2010).

Proponents of component analysis have argued that there is a unified moral foundation underlying the different standards that are applied to these different components, namely, the importance of securing trust between study participants and the state (Miller and Weijer 2006b; Weijer, Miller, and Graham 2014). It is surely correct that a viable framework for assessing and managing research risks must be capable of securing social trust and I am deeply sympathetic to the claim that clinical equipoise should be thought of as an important mechanism for securing that trust. But within component analysis, this insight is swamped by the repeated claim that the central dilemma to be resolved is the reconciliation of the physician's duty to act in the patient's interest with the demands of clinical research and the assertion that "clinical equipoise does not adequately specify the doctor-researcher's duty of care to the patient-subject" (Miller and Weijer 2006b, 546). As I argued in the last chapter, if the fundamental dilemma concerns reconciling research with the therapeutic obligations of clinicians, and if purely research-related interventions are delivered without therapeutic warrant, then importing a separate risk standard for such interventions reflects an unresolved internal tension within this approach.

In fact, the problems we have been rehearsing in this section are simply a reiteration of what I called the dilemma of determinate duties (§5.10.1). Views that appeal to the professional's duty of care require a standard for limiting risks that has sufficient content that it can provide useful guidance for regulating research risks. The traditional, Hippocratic interpretation of the duty of personal care provides such independent and operationally meaningful content but at the cost of being overly restrictive and unjustifiably paternalistic. Adopting a less paternalistic conception of the duty of care has the advantage of bringing the content of that duty into better alignment with the way it is understood within clinical medicine. The problem, however, is that it purchases this alignment at the cost of its independent, operational content.

In contrast, the integrative approach focuses directly on the interests of study participants. When individuals face risks to their basic interests, or experience conditions that restrict, impede, or impair those interests, those individuals are placed at a disadvantage. This is a disadvantage not merely with respect to goals or ends that they happen to have insofar as they, for example, value being a member of a particular club or aspire to look like a particular celebrity, but with respect to their ability to pursue their personal interests, whatever they are, on an equal footing with others. The integrative approach uses the condition of uncertainty regarding basic interests (§6.4.1) to ensure that study participants are not knowingly deprived of the means of securing their basic interests in the course of research. This means that asking participants to forego interventions that are intended to treat only minor ills is consistent with respect for those people as free and equal because those conditions do not affect their ability to formulate, pursue, or revise a reasonable life plan. In contrast, when patients face risks that threaten their standing in this space, it is inconsistent with respect for their standing as free and equal to provide them with a level of care that falls below what at least a reasonable minority of experts regard as best for their condition.

Like clinical equipoise and component analysis, the principle of uncertainty regarding basic interests (§6.4.1) invokes the judgment of experts. Unlike those views, the integrative approach only appeals to experts to determine whether an independent moral standard has been met. In this case, the standard is grounded in the special moral status of a person's basic interests. The judgment of experts reflects the state of medical knowledge about how best to safeguard or advance those interests.

Additionally, the integrative approach strives for consistency in the assessment and management of risks not just within research, but across other socially valuable activities. To the extent that other activities pose risks to the health and welfare of individuals, we should strive for consistency with respect to the treatment of like cases. As I argued in §6.3.3, a society that prohibits its members from taking risks to their basic interests would be oppressively restrictive in its limitation of legitimate life plans. Research is a social activity in which there are special considerations that warrant special forms of oversight, such as prospective review before committees of diverse membership (see chapter 7), but these should not preclude individuals from freely and knowingly accepting a broad range of risks to their personal interests and a reasonable range of affirmative risks to their basic interests.

6.7.3 The Belmont Approach

In the previous chapter I argued that the second dogma of research ethics is the view that research with human participants is an inherently utilitarian undertaking. In light of the profound problems with attempts to fill out the template for the appeal to uncertainty that rely on parochial moral foundations, some have argued that we should instead jettison that approach entirely and simply embrace the utilitarian essence of research.

This alternative has some distinct advantages. First, it has the advantage of founding risk assessments on a compelling normative foundation. In the *Belmont Report* (1979), the National Commission asserts that considerations of risk in research are grounded in the value of beneficence. Beneficence is attractive as a normative foundation for a framework of risk assessment since it reflects a fundamental concern for the welfare of persons.

Second, this compelling normative foundation is also sufficiently general in scope that it can be applied consistently to all aspects of research with humans. In particular, beneficence gives rise to a general duty that is expressed by the rule "maximize possible benefits and minimize possible harms" (National Commission 1979, B.2). This concern for welfare thus requires consideration of both the risks and benefits that accrue to individual research participants as well as risks and benefits that accrue to society more broadly. As such, "beneficence thus requires that we protect against risk of harm to subjects and also that we be concerned about the loss of the substantial benefits that might be gained from research" (C.2).

By grounding questions of risk in the value of beneficence and embracing the language of maximization, the *Belmont Report* frames questions of risk as a kind of utilitarian optimization problem. Research risks are to be assessed and managed by quantifying the net impact of the potential benefits and risks to the welfare of individual study participants, quantifying the potential benefits to the welfare of the future persons who stand to benefit from the knowledge the study is designed to produce and then ensuring that the net gains to future persons are sufficient to outweigh any loss of welfare incurred by study participants. I will refer to frameworks that embrace this language of risk-benefit analysis as following the Belmont approach.

In the scholarly literature, the Belmont approach has been adopted and explicated within the non-exploitation approach (Miller and Brody 2002, 2003) and the net-risk approach (Wendler and Miller 2007; Rid and Wendler 2010), and it is one of the standards used in component analysis (Weijer 2000; Weijer and Miller 2004). As I argued in the previous chapter, proponents of the Belmont approach capitalize on the shortcomings of most frameworks that rely on a parochial foundation to fill in the content of the template for the appeal to uncertainty. Because those views appear to be the most natural and intuitive way to fill out the template and because they are riddled with deep problems, the Belmont approach appears to be the only coherent alternative.

At the end of the previous chapter, I argued that it is not necessary to think of research as an inherently utilitarian undertaking, and the main goal of the present chapter has been to establish how it is possible to reconcile the social value requirement with the principles of equal concern, concern for welfare, and no impermissible gambles. It is important to emphasize, therefore, that the utilitarian approach outlined in Belmont and refined by proponents of the net-risk and non-exploitation approaches is not somehow a necessary or privileged approach to risk assessment in this domain. Its connection to a long and well-developed moral tradition, and the appearance of technical and operational clarity adds to its allure. But I want to suggest that the downsides of this approach are considerable and that its merits are not as substantial as they appear once you begin to consider them carefully.

First, the Belmont approach brings with it the specter of conflict that we discussed in chapter 2 between the rights and interests of study participants and the invariably greater good that stands to flow to future persons from advances in science and social progress. The single clearest aspect of the Belmont approach is the explicit moral permission that it provides to trade the welfare of study participants for sufficiently large increases in the welfare of future people. The most obscure aspect of this approach is whether this permission can be reconciled with a commitment to respect study participants as free and equal persons and whether respecting something like the principle of equal concern is even morally desirable within such a framework.

If the research enterprise is to be organized on terms that are capable of securing the voluntary cooperation of free and equal persons, then these shortcomings of the Belmont approach are not trivial. That framework foregrounds precisely the kind of moral permission that was used to justify past cases of abuse without having clear and coherent internal resources for reassuring community members that the institutions of research with human participants are designed to respect their status as free and equal. The Belmont approach thus lacks adequate resources for providing clear, public assurance that no stakeholder in the research enterprise will be subject to domination, abuse, exploitation, indifference, antipathy or wrongdoing at the hands of others.

To take one example, proponents of the non-exploitation approach argue that researchers are not bound by the clinician's duty of personal care but, instead, by the duty not to exploit study participants. In explicating the content of this requirement, they hold that it requires the observance of the following conditions:

(1) that risks to subjects are reasonable,
(2) that the research has social value and
(3) scientific validity,
(4) that subjects give free and informed consent,
(5) that there is fair subject selection,
(6) independent review, and
(7) respect for persons.

If these conditions seem familiar it is because they have been put forth as capturing the consensus requirements for ethically acceptable research with human subjects (Emanuel, Wendler, Grady 2000). As such several features of this proposal are striking.

First, the first three of these requirements are not actually constraints that limit the pursuit of utilitarian goals in clinical research. Rather, they serve to define those utilitarian goals and to express necessary conditions for their achievement. As such, these requirements would be endorsed by any legitimate utilitarian theory, whether it includes a constraint against exploitation or not.

Second, the other constraints are not limits on risk, per se. Because risk assessments have to be made prior to seeking informed consent, the requirement in (4) does not directly curb or limit the extent of the potential sacrifices that can be *asked* of trial participants in order to advance the common good. If we think of informed consent as the primary bulwark for limiting the risks to which study participants can be exposed in exchange for increases in the greater good, then inevitable defects in that process will result in research going forward that undermines the warrant for trust in the capacity of that system to respect study participants as free and equal persons.

Similarly, fair subject selection prohibits bias in the selection of who can be approached with the option to take on research risk, but that does not provide criteria for determining when those risks pass a limit or a threshold for what is reasonable. Independent review is an important safeguard, but keep in mind that the topic under consideration is what framework for risk assessment and management should govern that independent review process. So, we cannot appeal to independent review as an independent check on the framework for risk that is supposed to be used in that very review process.

Respect for persons, at least within the non-exploitation framework, covers a variety of protections for privacy, confidentiality, and the provision of information both during the conduct of research and once it is completed. This value does require careful monitoring of participant welfare, and "if subjects experience adverse reactions, untoward events, or changes in clinical status, they should be provided with appropriate treatment and, when necessary, removed from the study" (Emanuel, Wendler, and Grady 2000, 2707). But the ongoing monitoring of participant welfare is consistent with an ex ante study design that imposes significant burdens and exposes participants to significant risks for the purpose of advancing socially valuable and scientifically sound research.

The only principle for determining how individual health or welfare can be traded off against gains in knowledge, and therefore the advancement of the common good, is the requirement that risks be reasonable. Risks that are not offset by benefits to individual trial participants are judged to be reasonable if and only if they are sufficiently offset by gains in the knowledge that the research is designed to generate. At the end of the day, once we look carefully at the constituents of this view, the only substantive constraint on research risks is that they be justifiable in utilitarian terms.

My first concern is thus that even if the Belmont approach is a feasible alternative, by foregrounding the permission to trade participant welfare for benefits to future persons, it lacks clear resources for ensuring that the research enterprise is configured on terms that respect the status of all stakeholders as free and equal persons. Since the integrative approach grounds both the moral mission of research and the limits on the demands it can make of stakeholders in the same fundamental respect for persons as free and equal, it is preferable as a framework for regulating research risk.

My second concern with the Belmont approach is that it has a veneer of elegance and simplicity that obscures deeper problems that have yet to be addressed in research ethics. First, since this framework is grounded in concern for welfare, the risks and benefits in question should relate to the welfare of those affected. The value of the information a study is designed to generate must be represented as a function of the welfare of the various people likely to benefit from the information that will be generated. Similarly, the burdens and risks to study participants should be represented as a function of gains and losses to welfare incurred through study participation. Once these two quantities can be represented, whether their ratio is acceptable will depend on some normative standard or trade-off function. Each of these issues is left to deliberators to address at a largely intuitive level.

However, it is not clear that it is even possible to make the kind of interpersonal comparisons of welfare that this approach requires if it is to be taken seriously as a decision rule. Consider first that *intrapersonal* comparisons of welfare are facilitated by appeal to the way care advances or detracts from goals, ends, or means that are organized and ordered by an individual's personal life plan, given the ideals and values that motivate and suffuse it. When we consider whether the risks that an intervention poses to one person are outweighed by the expected benefits of that intervention for that same person, our ability to quantify and compare each side of this equation is facilitated by an understanding of the larger life plan and life projects of that person. If the side effects of a medication make it more difficult for a patient to engage in activities that play a particularly central role in their individual welfare—in, for example, the subjective quality of their life or in their ability to function in ways that are central to defining projects or plans—then they may be willing to forego such care, or to undertake a less effective course of care without those specific side effects. As we saw at length in the previous chapter, in such patients, the optimal course of care, with respect to the patient's welfare, may be the course of care that is less effective or more burdensome when evaluated solely from the narrow standpoint of the patient's physical health. In contrast, other patients may have life plans in which their narrow health interests and the particular benefits and burdens of what is regarded as optimal clinical care from the standpoint of their narrow health interests dovetail with the contours of their larger life plans.

The key point is that each individual's larger life plan, and the conception of personal welfare that it helps to structure, creates a context in which different experiences and functionings can be compared and ordered because it is relative to that person's larger values, plans and projects that such experiences and functionings have determinate value. In other words, an individual's life plan creates the criteria or desiderata relative to which the benefits and burdens of various activities, including alternative courses of medical care, can be evaluated and ranked.

To make *interpersonal* comparisons of welfare, we have to compare the cumulative gains or losses to the welfare of one group of people to the cumulative gains or losses in welfare to another group of people (the population of study participants, on one side of the equation, and the larger beneficiaries of scientific progress, on the other side), all of whom may embrace different life plans. If we rely on the larger life plan of an individual to assign a determinate value to an experience or a functioning, then it is unclear how to make cross-life-plan comparisons of welfare. The life plan of each person may render welfare rankings or scores determinate and meaningful for that person, but cross-life-plan comparisons cannot be made relative to the contours and valuations of a single person's life plan.

Within economics, there is a history of skepticism about whether interpersonal comparisons of welfare are possible. Common sense as well as a long philosophical literature argues that we can make such comparisons because we often do make them. And these observations are sound, as far as they go. In particular, they are telling against a radical skepticism of the form that asserts that we cannot know anything about the welfare states of others because we have no way to compare them to our own. But the question, for our present purposes, is not whether interpersonal comparisons of welfare are possible in any sense, but whether they are possible in the sense required by the calculous of risk we are considering here. And at this level, there appears to be room for significant doubt.

In particular, Louis Narens and Duncan Luce (1983) have shown that common sense is correct in holding that such comparisons are possible at least in the sense that pairs of individuals can, over time, develop a shared representation of each other's utility function. As a result, the common experience of being able to compare the magnitude of impacts on the welfare of those close to us to similar impacts on our own welfare can be vindicated at a technical level. What it appears we cannot do, however, is extend that shared representation to accommodate the utility functions of additional individuals. Since the calculous of risk required in research ethics must extend beyond pairs of individuals to groups, the skeptical position appears to hold at that level.

Although the results presented by Narens and Luce have far-reaching implications, they do not constitute a proof that it is impossible to make any kind of interpersonal comparison of welfare of the form required in research ethics. So, it might be argued that it is still reasonable to consider such comparisons to be possible. But this raises a second concern addressed by Kenneth Arrow (1951).

Arrow's concern is this: if it is possible to make such interpersonal comparisons of welfare, then it matters whether there is a single, unique way of doing this. If so, then the problem might be clarified over time and given ever greater clarity and precision. But if, as seems more likely, there are many different ways of making such comparisons, then we face a further decision about which of those ways we should use for the purposes of regulating research. In particular, because these different ways of representing the relative values in question can support making different trade-offs, our choice of welfare metric can implicitly influence the substantive decisions we make when we use that framework. So, it is not sufficient to establish that such comparisons are possible. We need to establish either that there is only one way to make them, or that of the many possible ways to make them, one approach is ethically correct or superior to the rest.

To the extent that all of this work is left to the intuitions of stakeholders, the concern is that the variety of different ways of specifying the value of scientific information and of trading it off against the interests of individual trial participants are at least as vast as the imaginations of different deliberators. In other words, if it is possible to specify a metric for making such trade-offs, then there may be as many ways of doing this as there are different sets of weights that might be affixed to each kind of value.

Proponents of this or related approaches have dismissed these worries as a misguided desire for a kind of precision that cannot be had. Such issues ultimately boil down to matters of "judgment," they claim, and cannot be quantified (Miller and Brody 2002, 2003; Miller 2003). If we consider the role that risk assessments play in IRB deliberations, this is surely correct—there is no clearly worked-out utilitarian calculous in research ethics because stakeholders are not really making the computations that this kind of equation suggests. This is rather what Ruth Macklin has called a "pseudo-metric," a principle that is given a mathematical formulation but that is not part of any real formal system of assessment. In this case, the Belmont approach adopts morally troubling language that most clearly enunciates the permission of trading participant welfare for gains to the common good without any offsetting benefits that might come from the operational clarity of a precise formal system.

The integrative approach provides operationally meaningful guidance to stakeholders by setting clear criteria for making a prima facie claim to social value and then reconciling such research with a set of deeply compelling moral principles. Addressing uncertainty or conflict among experts about how best to advance the basic interests of community members helps to connect research questions with gaps in the ability of health systems to effectively, efficiently, or equitably meet important needs of community members. The importance of these needs is not cashed out in terms of welfare since welfare is a function of the substantive, first-order life plan of an individual. Instead, the importance of health needs is determined from the standpoint of an individual's shared, highest-order interest in being able to formulate, pursue, and revise a life plan of their own.

Whether smarter people than I can give more precise operational content to this distinction between personal and basic or generic interests remains to be seen. Until then, the integrative approach also rests on the informed and conscientious judgments of stakeholders. But, rather than enunciating the permissibility of sacrificing the interests of a few to promote the good of the many, this framework encourages stakeholders to design studies on terms that are consistent with respect for study participants as free and equal persons. The judgments regarding risks and burdens required by this framework can be guided, in particular cases, by the underlying rationale for this distinction and by features of risk that are likely to track this distinction. These features include whether a harm is likely to be transient, temporary, or reversible or whether it is likely to be permanent and irreversible; whether it results in a limitation or impairment of ability to function or whether it affects the capacity of a person to perform a wide range of functions that are implicated in the process of forming, revising, and pursuing a reasonable life plan of one's own.

6.8 Conclusion

The integrative approach articulates the conditions under which it is possible to jointly satisfy the core requirements of the egalitarian research imperative. That imperative asserts a moral responsibility on the part of community members to create a system of research with humans that is responsive to the basic interests of community members in two ways. First, this division of social labor must be organized around the public goal of generating the evidence that is necessary to bridge the gaps between the basic interests of community members and the capacity of the basic social structures of that community to safeguard and advance those interests. Second, as a voluntary scheme of social cooperation, the research enterprise must be organized on terms that respect the status of all community members as free and equal persons.

The integrative approach also articulates the terms on which the production of socially valuable information can be reconciled with a network of compelling ethical requirements including the principles of equal concern, concern for welfare, and no impermissible gambles. This demonstrates that an imperative to carry out research can advance the common good without dispensing with the rule of law, without empowering anyone to make arbitrary judgments about the rights and welfare of others, and without running roughshod over the integrity of the individual.

If nothing else, the arguments of this and the previous chapter illustrate the importance of rejecting the problematic views that structure the conceptual ecosystem of orthodox research ethics, including the two dogmas of research ethics discussed in the previous chapter. Understanding research as a social enterprise that serves a social purpose that is closely connected to the proper functioning of the basic social structures of a community (such as its individual or public health system) provides a solid foundation for ensuring that this cooperative enterprise is carried out on terms that its stakeholders can recognize as basically just.

7

A Non-Paternalistic Model of Research Ethics and Oversight

7.1 Introduction

The last three chapters introduced the egalitarian research imperative and provided a substantive defense of the claim that its core requirements can be reconciled in both theory and practice. One of the implications of the present work is that IRB review alone is not an adequate mechanism for ensuring that the diverse stakeholders in research act in ways that promote the egalitarian research imperative. In this chapter, however, I examine the role that prospective review of research before bodies of diverse representation can play in creating conditions necessary to advance the egalitarian research imperative.

In particular, I argue that research oversight should not be framed in paternalistic terms. Rather, the justification for research oversight, on the view I propose here, is to provide concrete and credible social assurance that the research enterprise constitutes a voluntary scheme of cooperation; that this scheme of social cooperation offers an avenue through which diverse stakeholders, often pursuing their personal ends and interests, can contribute to the common good; that this cooperative enterprise includes checks and balances designed to prevent it from being co-opted to unfairly advance the parochial ends of particular parties at the expense of the common good; and that in contributing to or participating in this scheme of social cooperation, stakeholders will not be subject to the arbitrary exercise of social authority including antipathy, abuse, coercion, domination, exploitation, or other forms of harmful, unfair, or disrespectful treatment.

Because these conditions are necessary to ensure the justice of this undertaking, providing credible social assurance that they are met establishes the warrant for public trust in, and support for, this enterprise. Since the egalitarian research imperative requires that the research enterprise be organized as a voluntary scheme of social cooperation, this credible social assurance

For the Common Good. Alex John London, Oxford University Press. © Oxford University Press 2022.
DOI: 10.1093/oso/9780197534830.003.0007

also provides the warrant for the personal support of diverse stakeholders including the participants who make their bodies available to science in the process.

It is my contention that both critics and proponents of orthodox research ethics mislocate the source of the need for research oversight by focusing on deficiencies in individual agents rather than potential conflicts or shortcomings in the structure of the *social system* in which they participate. The paternalism of orthodox research ethics locates the need for research oversight in defects of individuals—the inability of some community members to adequately protect their own interests in the research context is regarded as justifying a system of oversight whose moral mission is to limit the risks of research for all participants (Miller and Wertheimer 2007; Jansen and Wall 2009; see also Edwards and Wilson 2012). The purpose of research oversight, on the view I propose in this chapter, is not to remedy deficiencies in *agents*, but to address structural features of the *strategic environment* in which diverse agents, often pursuing a diverse set of personal or parochial interests, engage in a long series of interactions over an extended period of time.[1] This chapter thus builds on a theme that runs throughout this book, namely, the importance of adopting a fundamentally social understanding of the research enterprise.

An effective system of research ethics should foster the sustainability of this scheme of social cooperation by helping stakeholders resolve coordination problems that threaten its ability to advance the common good on terms that respect all participants as free and equal. We saw one such coordination problem in §5.8.5 with the claim that research represents a prisoner's dilemma. In §5.9.3 I demonstrated that this claim is false and that research participation has the structure of a stag hunt. In this strategic interaction, research participation is an option that is rational for an agent to choose so long as two critical conditions are met. First, participants must regard the information a study is likely to produce as sufficiently valuable that they are willing to take on and adopt participation, with its various risks and burdens, as a personal project. Second, participants must believe that it is sufficiently likely that enough people will participate that

---

[1] In particular, the position I defend does not presume that any community member lacks autonomy or the cognitive and affective capacity to advance his or her own interests. Nor does it presuppose that any researcher has nefarious intent. My argument does not make these presumptions because it does not require these claims to justify its core conclusions. Nor does the argument I make here preclude the participation in research of individuals who lack decision-making capacity.

the study or studies in question will produce the valuable information they are designed to generate. The more risks and burdens to participants decrease and the value of the information likely to be produced increases, the more attractive research participation will be for a greater number of people.

In §7.2 I argue that prior to the work of the National Commission, this coordination problem was resolved by the use of social authority to conscript captive or easily manipulated populations into research. The result was a system that was poorly aligned with each of the requirements of the egalitarian research imperative—not only was the moral equality of study participants denied, but peer review was insufficient to ensure that this professional discretion advanced the greater good rather than the more parochial interests of researchers.

I then argue that prospective review helps to solve two additional coordination problems that would otherwise plague unregulated research and frustrate the willingness of various parties to contribute to it. The first, discussed in §7.3, is a social dilemma known as the tragedy of the commons. In this situation, reasonable choices by diverse actors pursuing their individual interests wind up exhausting the store of public trust on which the research enterprise depends.

The second coordination problem, known as the lemons problem, is discussed in §7.5. In this situation, low-quality studies that are easier to field crowd out higher-quality studies that are more costly and time intensive to design and carry out. Oversight practices that help communities avoid this dilemma provide assurance that research participation is likely to contribute to an important public good.

Conceptualizing research oversight explicitly as helping to resolve these coordination problems corrects another significant deficit in orthodox research ethics. In §7.6 I argue that some of the backlash to research oversight stems from the perception that prospective review represents a paternalistic intrusion into an otherwise private transaction that primarily implicates the interests of researchers and prospective participants. This narrow framing obscures the larger social purposes that research serves, including its relationship to the ability of basic social institutions to advance the basic interests of community members. Rejecting paternalism and adopting a view of research oversight as fostering the twin branches of the egalitarian research imperative better aligns the rationale for research oversight with the important benefits that it produces.

The system of research regulation in the United States is far from perfect and the purpose of this chapter is not to defend red tape and bureaucracy. Rather, the point is that any effort to reform and improve this system must have a clear conception of the goals to be achieved and promoted and the problems to be minimized or avoided. I argue that prospective review advances important goals that are currently overlooked but that should be emphasized and strengthened. Understanding how prospective review before bodies of diverse representation helps to create a system in which free and equal persons can see research as a viable avenue through which they might advance the common good is essential to ensuring that reforms do not cast out the ethical baby with the administrative bathwater.

7.2 Democratizing and Legitimating Research as a Social Practice

7.2.1 Social Authority and Abuse

Although the reforms brought about in the 1970s by the National Commission were motivated and understood on protectionist grounds, some of the policies and institutions they engendered have effects that can be understood in quite different terms. In particular, they laid the foundations for a system of research that more closely approximates the ideal of a voluntary scheme of social cooperation.

The post-war period from the passage of the Public Health Service Act in 1944, authorizing the NIH to conduct clinical research, up to the founding of the National Commission for the Protection of Human Subjects of Biomedical and Behavioral Research in 1974, was a period of tremendous growth in research (Rowberg 1998). During that period, members of the various professions that drove the research enterprise could see themselves as committed to social advancement through freedom of inquiry and enterprise and view their choice of profession as an expression of democratic freedom (Katz, Capron and Glass 1972, 1–2). Scientific and medical research were noble undertakings directed at advancing an important social good, and pursuing a career as a researcher offered individuals an outlet to develop their talents and abilities while contributing to that end.

In contrast, research participation and research participants were not thought of in comparable terms. To meet the demand for research with human participants, the system of research in the United States relied heavily on captive populations and relationships of inequality. Although respect for study participants was desirable, it was regarded as unavoidable that some "already unlucky individuals" would have to be subject to "an arbitrary judg-ment" in order to secure to society its right to medical progress (McDermott 1967, 40). Given the perceived conflict between the rights of the individual and of society, many in the research community shared Walsh McDermott's frank assessment that it would be "unwise to try to extend the principle of 'a government of laws and not men' into areas of such great ethical subtlety as clinical investigation" (1967, 41).

That research prior to the reforms of the National Commission was predicated on exploiting highly unequal social relationships is exem-plified by the extent to which it was concentrated in institutionalized populations. Already at the trial of Nazi doctors at Nuremberg, for ex-ample, the defense had argued that, not only was there no explicit legal prohibition against conducting research on prisoners, but from the fre-quency of reports of such research in professional and popular media one must conclude that it "does not violate the basic principles of criminal law of civilized nations to carry out experiments on convicts" (Tribunals NM, 51).

Almost half a century later, the Advisory Committee on Human Radiation Experiments would put the matter this way:

> It is difficult to overemphasize just how common the practice [of using prisoners in research] became in the United States during the postwar years. Researchers employed prisoners as subjects in a multitude of experiments that ranged in purpose from a desire to understand the cause of cancer to a need to test the effects of a new cosmetic. After the Food and Drug Administration's restructuring of drug testing regulations in 1962, prisoners became almost the exclusive subjects in nonfederally funded Phase I pharmaceutical trials designed to test the toxicity of new drugs. By 1972, FDA officials estimated that more than 90 percent of all investiga-tional drugs were first tested on prisoners. (1996, 273)

Many of the perceived advantages of these populations stemmed from their being subject to institutional control. Their behavior, including intake of food, fluids, medicine, and their schedule, could be closely monitored and controlled. They could be sorted into uniform groups on the basis of characteristics such as weight, height, ethnic background, and so on, with little worry that they would be lost to follow-up.

Research on these populations was also largely hidden from public view. As a result, researchers had only to justify their conduct to their peers and to the authorities that operated host institutions. To the extent that researchers were viewed as responsible for advancing the greater good, or as being members of professions that had a special prerogative to advance the greater good, they could count on a certain amount of discretion from their peers, and perhaps even from the public, over the rights and welfare of research participants. To the extent that research brought economic benefits to host institutions, or a sense of prestige that often attaches to the scientific enterprise, researchers could count on a fair degree of accommodation and deference from facility administrators.

Finally, researchers could also count on a certain social leniency about subjecting institutionalized or otherwise marginalized populations to practices or procedures that would be questioned or repudiated if used on more fully enfranchised citizens from more "sympathetic" social groups. In other words, it was easier to deny the moral and political equality of populations that were already regarded as "lesser," in some morally important respect. Convicts, the disabled, the poor, and racial minorities were subject to severe social prejudice that downplayed or denied their humanity and often conceptualized them as consuming social resources without providing an offsetting social contribution. Against such background presumptions, harmful, demeaning, degrading, or otherwise disrespectful treatment could be "redeemed" in the eyes of the public by the idea that research offered an avenue through which otherwise "burdensome" populations could make a social contribution.

In his exposé of widespread ethical problems in research, Henry Beecher worried that the increased resources and institutional pressures to carry out research "may be greater than the supply of responsible investigators" (1966, 1354). For Beecher and others (Lasagna 1971), the surest path to ensuring ethically responsible research was a more concerted investment in the character and virtue of the individual researcher. But, as we will see in more detail momentarily, this perspective ignores the extent to which these individuals interact in a strategic environment—a environment in which they face a range of incentives—that encouraged conduct that was inconsistent with respect for the basic interests of research subjects. It also ignores the extent to which the institutions of scientific research placed relatively few constraints on the extent to which researchers could advance a wide range of interests at the expense of the rights and welfare of study participants.[2] In some cases, these were interests, such as publication, promotion, notoriety, and other forms of individual success, that a more virtuous researcher might refrain from advancing in ways that would exact such harsh sacrifices from participants. But Beecher's position ignores the extent to which this environment permitted, if not encouraged, researchers to make arbitrary judgments against individuals, not from selfish motives, but from the otherwise virtuous motive of advancing scientific and social progress.

Revelations of abuse at places like Tuskegee and in the exposé of Henry Beecher drove home the extent to which the *institutions* of scientific research constituted a social arena in which researchers were vested with considerable discretion and study participants could be subject to the arbitrary, and sometimes debilitating and lethal, exercise of social authority. Deception, coercion, avoidable suffering, injury, and death were concrete and visceral horrors. But they reflected the potential for excess inherent in the largely unregulated exercise of social authority.

7.2.2 Unnecessary Risks and Inadequate Social Value

The system of research in the United States prior to the work of the National Commission was objectionable, not only because it failed to reflect basic concern for the rights and welfare of study participants, but because it lacked adequate assurance that the social authority of key stakeholders was exercised in ways that were necessary for social progress. For example, Tuskegee lasted forty years; it left behind a legacy of deception, manipulation, and harm. If the researchers involved in this study were to argue that these wrongs and harms were justified by society's right to social progress, they would have to demonstrate that this study actually contributed to that goal. But this research produced no great bounty of scientific progress. In its final report, the Ad Hoc Advisory Panel charged with evaluating this research noted numerous scientific and ethical shortcomings of the study, including the absence of an explicit study protocol. As a result, they concluded:

[2] Calabresi (1969) is one of the few early commentators to note that research with humans was subject to few systems of social control and oversight, and that the absence of these systems of control threatened trust in that activity. He also recognized that informed consent was likely to play only a limited role in rectifying those shortcomings.

However, the conduct of the longitudinal study as initially reported in 1936 and through the years is judged to be scientifically unsound and its results are disproportionately meager compared with known risks to human subjects involved. Outstanding weaknesses of this study, supported by the lack of written protocol, include lack of validity and reliability assurances; lack of calibration of investigator responses; uncertain quality of clinical judgments between various investigators; questionable data base validity and questionable value of the experimental design for a long term study of this nature. (US Public Health Service 1973, 7–8)[3]

Overshadowed by larger debates about whether the perceived utilitarian goals of science could ever justify the sacrifice of individual autonomy and welfare was the hard fact that what actually occurred at Tuskegee could not be justified in these terms. In other words, even if we were to grant, for the sake the argument, that egregious harms to participants can be justified if they are necessary to generate sufficient social value, the Tuskegee syphilis study could not be justified on such terms because it failed to yield any meaningful scientific advances.

Similar concerns could be raised about other cases of research abuse. In his exposé, for example, Beecher questions the value of some of the studies he identifies or whether such knowledge could have been procured through less harmful, less demanding, or less disrespectful methods.[4] But if the discretion invested in researchers is intended for the public purpose of advancing medical progress, these defects cast grave doubt on the ability of stakeholders in this endeavor to hold one another to account, both for respecting the interests of study participants and for using their discretion and authority to advance meritorious social purposes that could not be advanced through other means.

Peer review and the open publication of research were insufficient safeguards because they would only expose behavior that was regarded as deviant or objectionable against the background social norms that were shared

---

[3] For more general concerns about the way this report frames the ethical issues raised by the Tuskegee study, see Brandt (1978).

[4] In their long study of the research conducted on institutionalized children at the Willowbrook State School, Rothman and Rothman note that at the same time that Saul Krugman was infecting children with hepatitis to differentiate its different types, another scientist, Baruch Blumberg, was unlocking similar results in laboratory research. As they conclude, "those with a utilitarian bent, who might be prepared to give Krugman leeway with his means because his ends were important, will have to consider that, however accidentally, we would have learned almost everything we needed to know about hepatitis B in the laboratory" (Rothman and Rothman 1984, 267).

within the expert medical and scientific community. They were insufficient checks against conduct that was widespread and driven by norms and social dynamics that applied across the profession.

7.2.3 Curbing the Arbitrary Exercise of Social Authority

The reforms of the National Commission are easily seen as grounded in and guided by the goal of protecting the welfare and autonomy of study participants. But these protectionist reforms changed the strategic environment in which research was conducted. Prospective review before bodies of diverse representation effectively repudiated the broad discretion vested in researchers. Gone was the idea that research subjects could be treated as "soldiers for science," whose autonomy and welfare could be unilaterally abrogated by researchers in order to advance the frontiers of scientific progress.[5]

Without the socially sanctioned authority to conscript or to dominate large populations of institutionalized people, the increasing demand for scientific evidence as a foundation for responsible medical practice and as an engine for innovation would have to be met by engaging a larger proportion of participants from more enfranchised groups. However, these reforms also repudiated the unilateral discretion of researchers to determine the acceptable level of risk in research and to withhold information, to actively deceive participants, or to otherwise manipulate people into research participation.

Instead, researchers would have to submit to bodies of diverse representation protocols that explain how risks to participants have been minimized, how remaining risks are reasonable, and then detail a plan for communicating this and additional information to prospective study participants or their surrogates in order to secure their free and informed consent. The adequacy of risk assessment and information disclosure would now be assessed relative to norms that would reach beyond common or accepted practices among a narrow class of professionals.

Although these reforms may have been understood in protectionist terms, my contention is that they had the effect of moving the social institutions of

---

[5] The term "soldiers of science" is used by James H. Jones (2008) to describe the reasoning of the US Public Health Service when it prevented the men who were the unknowing participants in a scientific study from attempting to join the US military to fight during World War II. Rather than being soldiers in the military, if these men were to be put in harm's way, it would be as soldiers of science.

medical and scientific research into better conformity with civic republican ideals that have deep roots in American political life.[6] In particular, these ideals include the importance of freedom from arbitrary interference and the important role of law and social policy in reducing the prospect that citizens will face socially sanctioned domination at the hands of more powerful parties.[7]

Prospective review provides public assurance that antipathy or disregard of the welfare and the rights of research participants is not an acceptable element of the practice or institutional structure of research with humans. Repudiating the permissibility of exposing participants to unnecessary or unreasonable risk is a means of curbing the arbitrary exercise of social authority within important social institutions.

In §5.11, I distinguished two models of research participation embodied by Pat and Sam. The reforms of the National Commission moved away from a model in which researchers had the socially sanctioned authority to treat participants on the model of Pat, as conscripts whose autonomy and welfare interests could be set aside and subordinated to purposes that they need not share. Instead, substantive constraints on research risks and an informed consent process that requires an accurate depiction of the goals of a study, the risks and burdens associated with participation, and a clear statement that participants can withdraw at any time helps to better approximate a context in which study participants are treated like Sam. This is a context in which more enfranchised populations, with a wider range of social resources and opportunities, can see research as an avenue through which they can contribute to a social good. Just as a researcher would have to persuade colleagues of the merits of a study in order to secure their collaboration and participation as investigators, they would have to approach their compatriots as autonomous persons like Sam in §5.11.2 and explain the nature, purpose, and merits of a study in order to secure their free and informed consent to participate.

---

[6] On the link between regulation relating to the FDA and civic republican values, see Carpenter (2009).

[7] Compare to Philip Pettit's articulation of the civic republican conception of freedom and equal standing: "Being unfree consists in being subject to arbitrary sway: being subject to the potentially capricious will or the potentially idiosyncratic judgment of another. Freedom involves emancipation from any such subordination, liberation from any such dependency. It requires the capacity to stand eye to eye with your fellow citizens, in a shared awareness that none of you has the power of arbitrary interference over another" (1997, 5).

I have been careful to say that the reforms of the National Commission helped to better approximate an institutional setting governed by respect for participants as free and equal persons. Foreclosing the reliance on captive populations in research did not foreclose shifting to other populations, including poor or disenfranchised populations, whose autonomy could be influenced through offers of various types of benefit. Nor did it correct for the harm to groups whose medical needs have not been subject to careful investigation as a result of protectionist norms (Dresser 1992; Kahn et al. 1998).

Rather, the point of these remarks is to highlight aspects of the current system of research oversight that are responsive to important parts of the egalitarian research imperative so that these aspects can be preserved and strengthened. This is also helpful to the extent that it demonstrates that the egalitarian research imperative is not completely incompatible with core structures and practices in research ethics, even as we identify aspects of those structures and practices that are in need of reform.

7.3 Preventing a Social Dilemma: The Tragedy of the Commons

7.3.1 The Standard Formulation

In the previous section I argued that reforms instituted in the 1970s, including prospective review before committees of diverse representation, helped to alter the strategic environment in which research takes place. Better approximating a voluntary scheme of social cooperation among free and equal participants likely facilitated the ability of the research system to absorb a dramatic increase in the supply of resources and to better satisfy the demand for research participants. To illustrate how this could happen, it is important to understand some of the forces that conspire to make the unregulated practice of human research prone to coordination problems that threaten the interests of all stakeholders to the research enterprise.

The "tragedy of the commons" refers to a dilemma that arises from a lack of coordination among individuals who rely on a shared resource (Hardin 1968). In particular, multiple agents recognize that they all depend on a shared resource for survival and therefore that it is in their individual and collective long-term interest to maintain the viability of this resource. Nevertheless, when each acts on his or her own initiative, rationally pursuing his or her own goals or objectives, all wind up depleting that resource.

Here is a simplified version of the problem. A community of herders shares a large pasture where they graze their animals. Each recognizes that their livelihood and continued survival depends on maintaining sufficient grasslands to support their herd. Periodically the herders have the option to grow their herd by keeping and raising the offspring of their livestock. Larger herds bring several rewards to their owners including greater economic wealth and elevated social status. Herders who opt to raise larger herds capture more social goods for themselves. They may benefit in nonrelational ways, to the extent that they are better able to meet their needs, and in relational respects, to the extent that they garner greater social status and competitive advantage. Each therefore has a strong individual incentive to increase the size of their herd.

The problem is that larger herds also consume more of the grasslands. Each herdsperson reasoning in the same way increasing the size of their individual herds eventually leads to overgrazing. In part, this is because the immediate benefits of adding new animals to the herd accrue directly to the individual whereas the stress on the pasture is spread out among all community members. Eventually the carrying capacity of the pasture is exceeded, the grass cannot recover quickly enough to support demand, and the pasture is ruined.

7.3.2 The Tragedy of the Commons in Research

How is this relevant to research with humans? I will state the analogy briefly and then provide a more detailed discussion. To make the analogy clear, researchers are the herders and their "flock" is the number of morally questionable studies that they decide to carry out, or put into the "field." The common resource that such studies consume is the social support, cooperation, and trust of stakeholders that make the research enterprise possible. In an unregulated market, researchers can garner competitive advantage by putting more questionable studies into the field, and the risk of exhausting the reservoir of public support is spread across the group. Unconstrained in the pursuit of their individual goals, researchers in this environment ultimately reach a tipping point where the density, or the perceived density, of questionable studies in the field exhausts the fund of social support for their activities.

If this analogy sounds strained, consider how it maps onto some of the prescient concerns that Henry Beecher enunciated in 1966. Beecher argued, in effect, that American medicine was close to such a tipping point:

> I should like to affirm that American medicine is sound, and most progress is soundly attained. There is, however, a reason for concern in certain areas, and I believe the type of activities to be mentioned will do great harm to medicine unless soon corrected. It will certainly be charged that any mention of these matters does a disservice to medicine, but not one so great, I believe, as a continuation of the practices to be cited. (1966, 1354)

Beecher's article was driven by a concern that unethical studies were becoming increasingly common. He claims that he was able to identify 50 cases of unethical research and that merely following the references of these studies led to 186 additional likely examples with "an average of 3.7 leads per study." A sample of 100 studies from a major medical journal in a single year produced 12 that appeared to be unethical.

As a cause of the rise in the unethical behavior he carefully documented, Beecher pointed to several factors. First was the "sound and increasing emphasis of recent years that experimentation in man must precede general applications of new procedures in therapy, plus the great sums of money available" for research. These factors created both pressures and opportunities for ambitious investigators. Second, Beecher worried about the way these pressures and opportunities shaped the incentives facing young investigators. As he noted, "medical schools and university hospitals are increasingly dominated by investigators. Every young man knows that he will never be promoted to a tenure post, to a professorship in a major medical school, unless he has proved himself as an investigator" (1966, 1354–1355).

The pathway to personal and career advancement in medicine wound its way through the corridors of medical research. In the face of demand for results and the requirements of prolific productivity for promotion and tenure, Beecher lamented that "there is reason to fear that these requirements and these resources may be greater than the supply of responsible investigators" (1966, 1354).

Finally, Beecher like others in the research community was aware that social mores around research with humans were changing. The twenty-two examples outlined in Beecher's article included studies in which known effective treatment was withheld from participants, cases in which participants who experienced life-threatening or debilitating side effects from medication were challenged with the medication again to confirm the source of the adverse effects, and numerous cases in which subjects were unaware that they were involved in a research study. In some cases, death rates from the withholding of known effective therapy were announced in the study results themselves, and in other cases Beecher was left to estimate these himself. Beecher worried that if the values of society relative to research were changing, then what researchers might regard as the costs of doing business would be met with horror and revulsion in the eyes of the public.

In addition to the human toll of these studies, it was unclear that the harms, deception, and disrespect associated with this research was somehow necessary to procure leaps in understanding that would be unattainable without such sacrifice. Rather than a necessary and unavoidable tithe to scientific progress, the human hardship and suffering appeared to be simply a convenience for researchers pressed for time and eager to publish.

As we noted in §2.4.3, it is stunning that Beecher did not have to cull through some secret and arcane tome of clandestine activities to find studies with questionable ethical aspects; he merely had to attend with a sensitive eye to the published medical literature. Beecher feared that the volume and frequency of such studies was increasing and, with this, so was the prospect that the public would rouse from its normal routines and turn a spotlight onto the otherwise private and hidden world of research with human participants. Beecher feared that the revelations that the public would find in doing so would undermine public trust in, and public support for, the institutions of scientific advancement in the United States.

Ultimately, Beecher's fears were well founded. The National Commission and the rule-making and institution building that it engendered effectively imposed outside oversight on the research enterprise. Although it may have been conceived of in protectionist terms, my claim is that the unregulated practice of research in the United States created a strategic environment in which there were strong pressures and individual incentives to push ethical boundaries, that these pressures could affect the conduct of even the most well-meaning and publicly oriented researchers, and that one of the most important benefits of prospective review before bodies of diverse representation is the way that it effectively curtails these pressures. To make this case, we need to be more precise about some of the dynamics that give rise to these strategic problems and how prospective review resolves them.

7.3.3 Trade-Offs and Incentives

Part of the dynamic that can lead to the exhaustion of the reservoir of public support and social trust stems from the fact that it can be costly for researchers or sponsors to properly manage tensions between generating socially valuable information, respecting the welfare interests of participants, and ensuring respectful treatment. At almost every level, basic aspects of clinical trial design are suffused with ethical decisions between the burdens and risks to the rights and welfare of participants and the size, speed, and inferential power of a trial (Goodman 2007). Efforts to reduce the burdens and risks of research on study participants can increase the time it takes to run and complete a study, the number of personnel required to implement a trial, and, ultimately, the cost associated with answering the research question. This means that efforts to conduct more respectful, less burdensome, and less risky research can frustrate researcher or sponsor interests by inflating costs and delaying timelines. Even when taking more time or using more careful methods can produce socially valuable information without imposing unreasonable risks or burdens on study participants, the costs in time and resources of implementing such methods may conflict with the parochial interests of researchers who face promotion deadlines, grant deadlines, or anxious investors.

Similarly, choice of control represents a case where the narrow health interests of trial participants may be in direct tension with the inferential power of a trial (Temple and Ellenberg 2000). If we assume that all else is equal, testing a new drug against a placebo alone might produce clear data about whether the drug is superior to the comparator of merely interacting with a clinician without receiving effective medical care. In cases where effective treatment or prevention measures exist, however, there are strong ethical grounds for providing all participants in the trial with existing measures to protect their health. This does not preclude the use of a placebo-controlled trial design, since that design can be implemented on top of a baseline of care that includes effective prevention measures for all trial participants (Senn 2001). It does, however, raise the cost of the trial significantly by increasing the number of people who have to participate in order for the trial to generate statistically significant results (Potts 2000; Leon 2001; Freedman, Weijer, and Glass 1996).

A similar tension arises from other design features. Consider the difference between two approaches to measuring the efficacy of a prevention intervention, such as a vaccine. In one case, researchers randomize participants to receive a vaccine candidate or a placebo and then wait for participants to be exposed to the relevant pathogen. They then have to estimate the efficacy of the investigational intervention by comparing infection rates among the two groups. But they could also take the more direct approach of administering the prophylactic measure to a small number of people and then directly exposing them to or "challenging" them with the relevant pathogen (Miller and Grady 2001). Challenge studies of this kind could enroll far fewer people, practically eliminate ambiguity about who was exposed to the pathogen, and more effectively control for other features of recipients or their environment that might confound trial results.

When the infection in question is relatively benign, like the common cold, the consequences of these trial design features for the rights and welfare of participants will be less momentous than in cases of more severe conditions such as Ebola or HIV.[8] Similarly, how demanding such studies are on participants will depend on whether there are effective rescue interventions available to treat those who become infected and whether participants can be exposed to an attenuated form of the pathogen that is more likely to result in only mild sickness. Such preparatory work itself takes time, since isolating and replicating an attenuated version of a pathogen can be difficult. As a result, decisions about how to investigate the safety and efficacy of prevention measures initiate a cascade of decisions that have profound implications for both the burdens and risks to participants as well as the costs and duration of the study and the way those factors implicate researcher interests.

The process of searching for and implementing a study design that minimizes risks to participants while optimizing the scientific and social value of the information collected can be costly for researchers. In particular, it can be costly in terms of the time that it takes to search through feasible alternative designs and to evaluate their relative merits. It can also be costly in the sense that added safeguards may require additional expense, whether in terms of personnel hours, providing closer monitoring, additional testing, or

---

[8] For revelations of the lengths that researchers from the US Public Health Services were willing to go to in order to infect research subjects with syphilis in the 1940s, see Reverby (2011).

additional interventions that reduce risks to individual participants. Designs that require a larger sample size or more time to reach statistical significance can also be costly to researchers in terms of the expense of recruiting more participants and the delay in finding study results.

Informing participants about, and making a credible effort to ensure that they comprehend, both the importance of what is being studied and the full range of ways it may affect their health and welfare will always be an expensive proposition. It consumes time and resources and it may slow the pace of recruitment. In contrast, strategies that involve omission, euphemism, or outright deception may appear to be convenient, cost-cutting measures.[9]

7.3.4 Two Asymmetries

Another part of the dynamic that creates the potential for a tragedy of the commons in research with human participants stems from two important asymmetries related to risks and benefits in this context. First, there is an asymmetry in the *ex ante* and *ex post* assessment of a research study. Researchers can evaluate a study from the ex ante perspective—they understand the protocol that is to be initiated before it is carried out. They make and assess probabilistic judgments about the likelihood that relevant benefits or adverse events will materialize in practice or that problems will be uncovered and brought to the attention of the public. Without prospective review, the public is constrained to evaluate research ex post—they only see what was done in practice and thus only detect problematic conduct if it materializes in the form of adverse events.

The problem is that there might be many studies that involve unreasonable or objectionable practices when assessed from the ex ante perspective but the public will only be aware of the few that actually result in serious adverse events ex post. Additionally, there will be studies that are carefully designed with thoughtful precautions that result in serious adverse events just as a matter of bad luck. For this reason, evaluating studies solely from the ex post standpoint makes it difficult for the public to know whether the occurrence of an adverse event represents an unavoidable incident in an otherwise

---

[9] The prospect that informed consent would delay research, inconvenience researchers, and cause avoidable anxiety in research subjects is a recurring theme in research scandals of the post-World-War II era. For an excellent case study see Arras (2008, 73–79).

sound system or the overt manifestation of a system in which many unwarranted risks are being taken on a routine basis.

Second, there is an asymmetry in the costs and benefits to researchers of making such gambles. In a system without prospective review, researchers who scrupulously inform subjects of risks and benefits or who use trial designs that reduce burdens on participants voluntarily and unilaterally increase their own costs. Moreover, without prospective review, investing time and resources in this aspect of research is unlikely to be salient or visible to stakeholders such as participants or the public. Scrupulous researchers thus bear the costs of implementing these safeguards, but without prospective review there is no direct mechanism for rewarding them for doing so. At the same time, using resources in this way may put such scrupulous researchers at a competitive disadvantage relative to their peers. Researchers who do not incur these costs may be able to stretch scarce resources further and use their cost savings to bolster the depth or breadth of their research portfolio.

Two additional factors may reinforce these asymmetries. First, researchers work in a competitive environment. They compete for grants, personnel support (such as collaborators, post-docs, and lab assistants), institutional advancement, and professional honors. Second, even without such competition, researchers are likely to be biased in favor of their own projects. They would not pursue a research agenda if they did not regard it as important or worthwhile. As a result of their personal investment in and commitment to their particular research program they may overestimate the degree to which its advancement warrants or justifies subjecting others to particular risks or burdens.[10]

Different researchers may be motivated by a mixture of these factors, and these social and competitive forces may affect some researchers more than others. Nevertheless, these dynamics create the context in which rational researchers will be led to increase the representation in their research portfolio of studies that push the envelope in one or more of several directions. They might push the envelope in terms of the burdens placed on participants in the hope of generating benefits for society. They might push the envelope

---

[10] Indeed, one of the factors that enabled the Tuskegee syphilis study to persist over a forty-year period was the commitment of public health researchers to the idea that understanding the natural history of the disease was of fundamental importance. This professional curiosity persisted even after this information lost any clinical value it may once have had. Moreover, those involved in the study maintained its importance even after it was clear that the study itself had little or no social value. See Jones (1993, 2008).

by reducing costs that would be associated with implementing feasible protections for the rights and welfare of study participants. Or they may push the envelope by using speedy recruiting practices that leave participants uninformed, foster misconceptions about therapeutic potential, or amount to outright deception.

Each researcher knows that when one of these gambles goes wrong, the public is confronted with a case of serious harm or wrongdoing that consumes some of the warrant for the reservoir of social cooperation and trust on which all researchers rely. It is unlikely, however, that any single revelation will exhaust this reservoir of trust and any strategic advantage enjoyed by taking such gambles accrues directly to the individual researcher.

7.3.5 Public Support: A Tipping Point

As I indicated earlier, Beecher worried that the incentives in American medicine were prompting young researchers to increasingly engage in practices that would jeopardize the social standing of research and the public cooperation needed to meet increasing demand. We are now in a better position to understand the variety of ways in which such a tipping point might be reached. This includes increases in the volume of questionable research but it also includes changes in the values that the public uses to evaluate that research and whether they continue to evaluate it from an ex post perspective, or they shift their scrutiny to the ex ante standpoint.

First, the number of ex post scandals could increase because the number of gambles taken by each researcher increases. This would be a situation in which a majority of researchers are led to push certain boundaries. This might happen because failure to do so puts researchers at a competitive disadvantage, thereby increasing the social pressure on all researchers to cut corners.

Second, even if some researchers refuse to compromise their high standards, a tipping point might be reached if a smaller proportion of researchers increases the rate at which they field studies that push the envelope. If a smaller number of researchers are able to increase their rate of productivity by cutting corners and taking gambles, then the total number of objectionable studies would increase.

Both of these dynamics can be influenced by factors mentioned by Beecher. Faculty with more secure institutional positions may have the time and resources to field studies that better approximate an optimal balance of scientific rigor, social value, and respect for study participants. If the requirements for promotion and tenure place greater emphasis on research productivity, then competition among many investigators for coveted professorships can lead ambitious scientists to press the envelope in the hope of increasing their productivity and producing the results necessary to advance through the ranks.

Alternatively, as funding for research grows, this increase in the supply of opportunity can create a greater demand for professionals to move onto the investigator track. Increasing the number of investigators can increase the overall number of studies and the dynamics outlined earlier can shape the trajectory of the research they produce.

Third, the probability that a tipping point will be reached is not solely a function of the number of questionable studies put into the field. Whether a tipping point is reached can be influenced by changes in the degree of public scrutiny given to the research enterprise. This means that at one point in time, a society might be willing to tolerate a fairly high rate of morally objectionable research so long as that research is hidden from view. Even if the rate of problematic research remains constant, increasing the frequency or the intensity of public scrutiny might produce a public perception that research involves sufficiently questionable practices that it is no longer worthy of social support or public trust.

Alternatively, even if the rate of questionable studies and the rate of public scrutiny remain constant, changes in the norms that are used to evaluate research can result in a public backlash. If, at one point in time, broad segments of the public regard certain classes of people as inferior or socially expendable, then the public might tolerate a fairly high rate of morally questionable research as long as it is sequestered in such marginalized groups. But if public sentiment changes in ways that result in greater recognition of the shared humanity, moral worth, and moral equality of once marginalized groups, then even a fairly low rate of questionable research in such populations might be sufficient to trigger public outrage.

Finally, a sudden shift in focus of the public from ex post problems to ex ante decisions would have a cascading effect since the number of ex post problems likely obscures a much larger number of studies that employed similarly questionable practices but were fortunate enough not to produce high-profile adverse events. If revelations of abuse garner greater scrutiny from reporters and public officials who then inquire more aggressively into the ex ante decisions of researchers, an otherwise "sustainable" rate of ex post revelations of abuse could be revealed as masking a much higher rate of studies that rest on objectionable ex ante decision-making, creating the perception of a deep and pervasive rot at the core of a vaunted profession.

It is likely that a mixture of all of these factors was responsible for the public outrage that precipitated the formation of the National Commission. The social demand for medical progress and the availability of funding and opportunity it produced increased the status of research and drew more professionals onto the investigator track, and competition and changing metrics for advancement and career evaluation created incentives to avoid costly delays in productivity. Research practices that were once widely accepted were increasingly out of step with changing social values that reflected and facilitated greater capacity to resonate with the humanity of marginalized groups. In a context in which the distribution of power and social authority were increasingly subject to public scrutiny, greater attention was given to a social activity that previously received public attention primarily to trumpet some important medical or scientific achievement.

As in the case of grazing animals, once the tipping point has been reached everyone suffers, not just those who gambled and lost. This is because, when the public is constrained to evaluate research from the ex post perspective, they cannot distinguish scrupulous researchers who bear the costs and burdens of designing studies that respect participant welfare to generate scientifically sound and socially valuable information from those who do not. As a result, it is in the long-term best interests of all parties to find a way to coordinate their individual decisions so that such a tipping point is never reached.

7.4 Benefits of Prospective Review

7.4.1 Eliminating Asymmetries between
Ex Ante and Ex Post Perspectives

One of the benefits of the current system of prospective review before committees of diverse representation is that it helps to resolve some of the dynamics that give rise to the tragedy of the commons. By requiring researchers to submit protocols for review before they are initiated, prospective review evaluates all studies from the ex ante standpoint, eliminating the asymmetry between ex ante and ex post standpoints. This means that researchers are no longer the only parties privy to the way their research manages tensions or conflicts between the health interests of study participants and the scientific and social value of studies. Now those decisions can be scrutinized before they are put into practice. Review boards can flag the imposition of gratuitous risk, unreasonable risk-benefit ratios, studies that use sloppy research methods or that are not sufficiently relevant to an important health or social problem.

This in turn creates a more resilient system in that when bad outcomes occur, or when there are breaches of the public's trust, it is unlikely that public investigation will reveal widespread and systematic disregard for the rights and welfare of community members (Moss 2007). This was illustrated by the TGN 1412 study in which six participants in a phase I trial experienced life-threatening adverse effects after receiving what was expected to be a sub-clinical dose of a novel immunomodulatory drug (Suntharalingam et al. 2006). The disclosure of these severe adverse reactions fueled speculation about unethical research practices. But as one critic of the expanding scope of IRB review concedes:

> However, the impact of these events on confidence in clinical and experimental research has clearly been contained by the evidence of good faith regulatory review: in a situation where research participants were not well able to make judgments for themselves, the regulatory systems had provided a check. The adverse outcome could be explained as entirely untoward and not reasonably foreseeable, precisely because the investigators had not been judge and jury in their own cause. The known risks had been described to the participants and they had voluntarily accepted these. The regulatory institutions have functioned to supply legitimacy to the institutions of biomedical science. (Dingwall 2008)

In other words, prospective review creates a public assurance that the studies put into the field reflect responsible balancing of these core values and allows the public to better distinguish studies that cut corners and which may or may not produce adverse effects in practice from studies that result in serious adverse events even though from the ex ante standpoint they did not cut corners or evidence antipathy, disrespect, or disregard for the rights or welfare of participants.

7.4.2 A Check on Self-Serving Assessments

Prospective review before committees of diverse representation also reduces the likelihood that judgments about how to balance risks and burdens to participants against social benefits will be based on biased judgments of a narrow class of professionals. Recall that as concerns about the ethics of the Tuskegee syphilis study were building within the US Public Health Service, a scientific review committee was convened in 1969 to review the study (Jones 2008). The vote of this body to allow the study to continue was in sharp contrast to the public reaction to its eventual revelation in the popular media. The presence of non-researchers and lay members of the public on boards that conduct prospective review is intended to provide a check on the potential for professional prejudice and to give voice to community values.

In practice, there is significant evidence that community members often do not constitute a strong, independent check on proposed research. As such, there is significant room to strengthen and improve the role of community members on such committees. But it will be difficult to improve the IRB review process if it continues to labor under a faulty and overly parochial conception of its ultimate rationale and social purpose.

7.4.3 Risk of Delay Changes Incentives

It is important to emphasize that many of the aspects of IRB oversight outlined previously do not need to be perfect in order to improve the conduct of researchers. This is because the knowledge that protocols must be submitted for review itself changes the incentives that researchers face. For instance, researchers do not know whether the lay person on the IRB will assert a strong voice and play a leading role in public oversight or largely go along with the consensus of the rest of the board. They do not know whether the board will pay careful attention to the social value of a study or restrict their assessments more narrowly to the verbiage on the informed consent form. But researchers do know that if their protocol is returned because it is morally objectionable, they will suffer a costly delay. As a result, even if IRBs vary in these practices and even if researchers know this, the incentive to avoid delays associated with lengthy revisions to rejected protocols provides strong incentive for researchers to write protocols that reduce the probability of being returned for significant revision.

As a result, the public criteria that IRBs use to evaluate research and features such as the presence of a public voice on the IRB likely exert their most powerful influence by changing the incentives that researchers face when they are *designing* their studies and writing their protocols. Knowing that their research will be reviewed by committees of diverse representation and assessed on specific criteria—including whether unnecessary risks have been eliminated, remaining risks are reasonable, and the adequacy of the proposed procedures for informing prospective participants of the nature of the study and its incumbent risks—creates an incentive for researchers to search for study designs that more closely approximate the optimal balance of those criteria.

The knowledge that protocols will be assessed relative to their risk-benefit ratio and the quality of their procedures for informed consent creates an incentive for researchers to spend the time and resources necessary to more closely approximate an optimal ratio of risks and benefit. The reason is that, in a system with prospective review, the efforts of scrupulous researchers who dedicate time and resources to promoting social value, scientific rigor, and respectful treatment are no longer invisible. Reviewers can see the lengths to which investigators go to achieve these goals and they can reward the scrupulous by approving their protocols expeditiously and penalize the careless or the unscrupulous by requiring revisions in order to demonstrate a more careful concern.

The fundamental point is that the public knowledge that protocols will be reviewed on these terms creates an upstream incentive for researchers to conform to the norms they expect the IRB to enforce. This public expectation reduces, and possibly eliminates, the competitive advantage that would otherwise be gained from pressing the envelope either in terms of trying to reduce costs by lowering protections for participants or trying to increase the social value of a study by demanding larger sacrifices from them.

One of the upshots of the argument in this section is that despite its protectionist and often paternalistic justification, prospective review before committees of diverse representation helps to facilitate aspects of the egalitarian research imperative. In particular, it helps to approximate a context in which free and equal people can voluntarily participate in research as an avenue for advancing the common good. It does this imperfectly, and indirectly, by incentivizing researchers to ensure that risks in research are not gratuitous, that they are required for meritorious research, and that study involvement will be carried out under conditions of respect.

IRBs are limited in their ability to influence the full range of stakeholders who make decisions that shape the way research is conducted. Nevertheless, my contention is that we should jettison the paternalistic justification for prospective review and, with this, its protectionist stance and instead more explicitly align IRB review with the requirements of the egalitarian research imperative. The goal of these reforms is to more explicitly and directly shape the incentives for researchers to ensure that proposed studies contribute to the production of a public good while respecting the status of participants as free and equal.

7.5 Quality Assurance and the Lemons Problem

7.5.1 The Standard Formulation

If research participation has the strategic structure of a stag hunt, as I argued in §5.9.3, then the willingness of individuals to participate in studies hinges on reducing the risks and burdens associated with participation to the point where participants can see them as a reasonable and unavoidable cost required to advance a valuable personal or social goal. Resolving the tragedy of the commons that plagues an unregulated system of research advances this goal by reducing the risk and burden side of this equation.

When IRBs view their purpose and justification as paternalistic in nature, they frequently view questions regarding the social value of research as beyond their purview. Nevertheless, I now want to demonstrate how prospective review before committees of diverse representation has the effect of helping to solve a problem that reduces the quality of research and that can, as a result, erode support for the research enterprise. This is the so-called lemons problem (Akerlof 1970).

The dynamic of the problem is easily understood with an example from commerce. Some used cars are "cherries" and some are "lemons." The cherries don't have major defects, they run well, and with routine upkeep they will be reliable transport. In contrast, the lemons are plagued with problems. They require extensive maintenance and are ultimately expensive and unreliable transport.

The "problem" results from three factors: asymmetric expertise and information, asymmetric cost, and uncertainty about outcomes. The asymmetric expertise and information stems from the fact that the dealer has the knowledge and the means of ascertaining the true state of the car whereas the buyer often lacks the relevant expertise and has limited opportunity to evaluate the car. Moreover, the buyer is almost entirely dependent on the dealer for information about the car.

The asymmetry in cost refers to the fact that it costs a dealer more to procure a cherry than a lemon. Uncertainty about outcomes refers to the difficulty that consumers face in ascertaining whether a used car is actually a lemon, even after purchase. The car may work fine for a while before problems emerge, and it may take an extended period before it is clear that it suffers from extensive problems.

The result of these factors is that consumers have a difficult time ascertaining ex ante who is selling cherries and who is selling lemons. This is because all dealers extoll the virtues of their products and talk up their value and reliability. They also charge roughly the same price for the same make and model car. Because consumers cannot tell ex ante who is selling cherries and who lemons, they cannot direct their consumption behavior so as to reward only reliable dealers. As a result, vendors who purchase lemons and sell them at cherry prices realize a larger profit margin than vendors who procure the more expensive cherries and sell them at the same price. Those who sell lemons thus achieve a competitive advantage that allows them to crowd out those who sell only cherries, and this puts pressure on the latter to introduce some lemons into their inventory.

The result of this dynamic is that markets with these features are prone to poor-quality products. Because consumers cannot reliably detect cherries or lemons in any particular case, they shun such markets and, if left unchecked, the fear of being taken advantage of chills participation and the market withers. Those who inhabit such markets, used-car dealers in this case, are also stigmatized and lose some of their social status.

7.5.2 The Lemons Problem in Research

Each of these factors is present in an unregulated research "market." Asymmetric knowledge and information are ineliminable features of scientific research. Researchers often possess expertise that is highly specialized and a comparable proficiency with the specific subject matter of a study may be limited to a relatively small group of experts. Participants and other stakeholders, including the institutional actors who are the ultimate consumers of the information produced by research, may lack comparable scientific expertise. Study participants often fall far below the level of acumen, education, and literacy of other stakeholders, but of researchers in particular. These parties may thus vary in their degree of familiarity with the substance of a research study and in the intellectual and social resources they can bring to bear in order to enrich their understanding. As a result, they are heavily, if not exclusively, dependent on researchers for relevant information and explanation.

Similarly, as discussed in §7.3.3, there are asymmetric costs to preparing protocols and implementing studies that are "cherries." In other words, it takes more time and resources to plan and conduct studies that generate high-quality, socially significant information without exposing participants to unreasonable risk while securing the free and informed consent of an adequate number of participants.

Finally, uncertainty about outcomes is an inherent feature of most research with humans. The "outcomes" here include whether a study will result in serious adverse events and whether it provides a reliable answer to a question of social importance. Participants and other stakeholders will not have this information at the conclusion of a study and if the results are not published they may never have access to them.[11] If the study results are published, many participants may not seek out this information or be able to evaluate scientific publications on their own. Even those who seek out and digest this information will not know whether the results that are published address the question that the trial was designed to answer, or whether the study has been re-described in order to enable the publication of findings that were incidental to the original hypothesis. As a result, participants and other stakeholders in an unregulated environment are largely unable to

[11] For a discussion of cases in which trial data were not published, or were published only years after studies were completed, see Fauber (2012).

assess whether their participation or support contributes to well-designed, socially relevant science.

In an unregulated market, participants are also unlikely to be able to assess "outcomes" that relate to the regard that was shown for their rights or welfare. That is, participants are unlikely to know that they were deceived about the nature of the study, or about what was done to their persons or to their private information. They are unlikely to know that they were exposed to excessive risk, either because bad outcomes don't materialize, or because individual participants are not in a position to ascertain whether their bad outcomes are exceptional cases that happened in the face of reasonable precaution, or an easily foreseeable consequence of the study design or the lack of reasonable precaution and protection.

In this environment, because potential research participants are unable to distinguish researchers who implement high-quality, socially valuable studies that respect participants' rights and welfare from those who do not, they cannot reward the former with participation and penalize the latter by staying away (London, Kimmelman, and Emborg 2010). Participants therefore enroll in both types of studies alike. As a result, low-quality studies flourish and to the extent that they are cheaper to implement, they will gradually crowd out higher-quality studies, which are usually more costly and time intensive. The diversion of resources to such trials, however, represents a poor use of scarce social resources that yields a lower return on investment than would be expected in a market in which protocols are subjected to prospective review before committees of diverse representation (Carpenter 2009).

As participants and the public in general become aware of the differential in quality among studies in an unregulated market, distrust in the market builds. This awareness of differential quality can come about through several routes. One is via a dynamic described in §7.3.5. As ex post revelations of abuse prompt scrutiny into ex ante research decisions, the public becomes aware of the asymmetric nature of their relationship to researchers and the degree to which researchers have taken advantage of the potential for the betrayal of trust latent in that dynamic.

Another dynamic, however, may arise from revelations of the frequency of poor-quality science. When an area of inquiry absorbs public funds and resources but fails to bear significant fruit, it draws public scrutiny. Revelations that studies in this area suffered from methodological flaws that compromised the value of the data they generated feed concerns about the social return on investment from support for the research enterprise and speculation that researchers are benefitting from such investment without taking due care to ensure that their work advances the common good through high-quality scientific inquiry (London, Kimmelman, and Emborg 2010).

7.5.3 Benefits of Prospective Review

Prospective review before committees of diverse representation can reduce this kind of quality assurance problem. Independent assessment of the study rationale, the relevance of the question to uncertainty in the medical community (see chapter 6), the reasonableness of risks in relation to anticipated benefits, and the steps taken to reduce burdens on participants serve to reduce the frequency of ethically problematic studies. This, in turn, increases the probability that social resources are allocated to studies that reflect respectful treatment with responsible limits on risk.

As a result, even if IRBs do not explicitly evaluate research in terms of their social value, altering researcher incentives in a way that reduces the proportion of low-quality studies submitted for review has the indirect effect of raising the overall quality of research. To the extent that resources that would have been allocated to lower-quality research are instead directed to higher-quality studies, this promotes and improves the value of a community's investment in research.

Again, even if IRBs are not the best venue for ensuring that research is aligned with and advances the health priorities of communities, promoting a more explicit focus on the social value of research during IRB review would more directly promote the overall value of research. Even with an imperfect focus on social value, independent review can improve the average quality of studies available to potential participants and the likelihood that research participation will represent an avenue for contributing to a socially important discovery.

Rather than casting prospective review of research as an intrusion into the private affairs of researchers and participants, grounded in a paternalistic concern for the welfare of the latter, the view I am defending here treats prospective review as a mechanism for resolving coordination problems within an activity that serves a sufficiently important social purpose that there is a social obligation to promote its proper functioning. Resolving these coordination problems contributes to the proper functioning of research by providing a credible social assurance that participating in research offers a means of advancing the common good without exposing participants to indifference, neglect, abuse, or other forms of domination or unfairness.

The mismatch between the value of prospective review and its public justification or rationale is a source of profound instability at the foundations of research ethics. The system of research oversight instituted in the wake of the National Commission emphasizes protectionist goals grounded in benevolent paternalism. Its most significant value, however, need not be understood in these terms. That is, despite this public rationale, I have argued here that prospective IRB review has the effect of resolving a set of dynamics that give rise to two social dilemmas in an unregulated system. Resolving these problems helps to elevate the quality of research while providing credible public assurance that the institutions of social progress are not also instruments of domination that routinely abrogate the rights and interests of participants. The result of this mismatch is a system that has the effect of preventing tragic outcomes that all stakeholders in this enterprise want to avoid while generating resentment and anger from those same stakeholders in the process.

7.6 The Paradox of Cooperative Resentment

7.6.1 Misalignment between Value and Justification

If the analysis I have presented here is correct, then features of the conceptual ecosystem of orthodox research ethics are responsible for a profound tension at the foundation of the field. On the one hand, orthodox research ethics treats research as a series of optional, private undertakings, disconnected from the larger social purposes of a just social order. As I argued in chapter 2, this view of research fortifies the bulwark of protections for the rights and interests of study participants because of the widespread perception that linking research to morally weighty social goals would invariably justify abrogating the rights and interests of study participants.

On the other hand, I have argued in this chapter that the system of prospective review instituted in the wake of the National Commission has had the effect of creating a system of research that resolves coordination problems that are likely to plague unregulated systems. Telegraphing to researchers that protocols will be assessed by committees of diverse representation who will evaluate the quality of their procedures for securing informed consent, whether they have eliminated gratuitous risks, and whether remaining risks are reasonable in light of the importance of the information a study is likely to generate, has the indirect and admittedly partial and imperfect effect of improving research quality while providing social assurance to study participants that in contributing to this enterprise they will not be subject to antipathy, exploitation, domination, or abuse. The net effect of these reforms was to create a system of research that could absorb increasing demand for research at the same time that it prohibited researchers from drawing disproportionately on institutionalized populations that had been the primary source of fodder for research in the immediate post-war period.

However, because this system of research oversight operates on terms that are disconnected from the social benefits that it provides, few of the stakeholders who benefit from this system appreciate its value. To the extent that orthodox research ethics frames research as a series of discrete interactions among private parties, the rationale for social interference in their private transactions hinges on the proposition that study participants lack the ability to secure their own interests in this domain. Yet, as researchers and study participants participate in a system that promotes interactions of respect and freedom from domination and abuse, they increasingly see IRB requirements, couched in paternalistic and often protectionist terms, as unwarranted intrusions into private interactions and as unjustified restrictions on individual liberty and academic freedom.

7.6.2 Fostering the Appearance of Arbitrary Interference with Private Purposes

Ironically, perhaps, the success of scientific research has produced a zeal for access to novel therapeutic candidates on the part of patients who suffer from conditions that are not well treated by current methods. When patients and their advocacy groups push for access to novel treatment modalities, paternalistic concerns about the overreaching of researchers seem out of place. If participants are eager to access novel interventions and willing to accept the risks and if researchers are happy to have these intrepid patients as partners in inquiry, the protectionism of IRBs seems self-defeating.

However, the parochial focus on the desires of study participants obscures and eclipses the social role of research in generating information on which a wide range of stakeholders rely to discharge important moral and social responsibilities (§4.7). Participants seeking access to novel interventions and researchers eager for career advancement may be happy to move forward with research that advances their personal interests. But if such studies do not generate information that subsequent researchers, clinicians, patients, and policy makers need in order to properly evaluate and use novel interventions, then such studies can represent the co-optation of research by stakeholders who advance their parochial interests.

For example, even if participants are willing to face the prospect of serious adverse events, the emergence of serious harms in a trial can derail promising research programs by altering the assessments other stakeholders make about the prospects for success of such a program (London, Kimmelman, and Emborg 2010). If study sponsors view adverse events as limiting the value of an intervention, they may invest their resources elsewhere. Serious adverse events may dampen the interest of subsequent researchers who prefer to investigate strategies that have a more benign adverse event profile. Because research is a stag hunt (§5.9.3), if serious adverse events arise in an early-phase trial then it may be more difficult to recruit sufficient numbers of participants in subsequent studies.

But the most intense animosity for IRB review comes from those who view it as curtailing their academic freedom. To judge from the rash of recent law review articles, it is a miracle that research with human subjects in the United States continues to draw breath under what is portrayed as the asphyxiating heel of the rent-seeking,[12] creativity-stifling,[13] jack-booted bureaucrethics that is the current system of research ethics oversight and review. IRBs have been accused of perpetrating "probably the most widespread violation of the First Amendment in our nation's history," resulting in a "disaster, not only for academics, but for the whole nation" (Columbia Law School 2009). One member of the President's Council on Bioethics went so far as to assert, "There has been no greater damage to academic freedom in the

---

[12] See Mueller (2007) for the clearest "capture-theoretic" account of research ethics regulation. Mueller argues that the one clear benefit of increased regulation has been "jobs, jobs, jobs" for the research ethics "industry," going so far as to wonder "if there may not be nearly as many ethics reviewers, regulators, and staff as there are researchers," and referring to the research ethics enterprise as a "pyramid scheme" (820–821).

[13] "Trying to unravel the mystery of the social sciences' survival in the face of IRB encroachment is a challenge replete with paradoxes and illusions. The exercise demands that we probe the convergent logics of two mutually exclusive things that must somehow co-exist: creativity and regulation." Later, these authors assert that the survival of any creative research at all must itself be attributed to complicity of researchers with these organs of censorship: "That any creative research at all has survived under the IRB system, distorted as we believe it has become, must be attributed to the dynamics of consensual censorship between investigators and IRBs" (Bledsoe et al. 2007, 597, 628).

United States in my lifetime. And my lifetime encompasses McCarthy and it encompasses political correctness, both" (Schneider 2009). Locked in the bureaucratic "iron cage" of IRB oversight, critics charge that researchers have been transformed into a vulnerable, exposed population, subject to domination (Bledsoe et al. 2007, 608, 610), resulting in a denial of benefit to some study populations that has been likened to "Tuskegee in reverse" (Malone et al. 2006).

Assessing the burdens of IRB review, critics point to a loss of creativity, spontaneity, academic freedom, and squandered time, as well as money and even lives lost (Whitney and Schneider 2011). When it comes to the benefits of research oversight, they simply gape in outraged silence. We are told that "it is clear that the constraints imposed on academic inquiry have not been accompanied by an increase in public benefits" (Mueller 2007, 810) and that "there is no empirical evidence that IRBs have any benefit whatsoever" (Hyman 2007).

If these allegations are true, then we are living in a truly Orwellian dystopia in which "the problem is with the ethics industry, not the researchers" (Mueller 2007, 832). According to critics, IRBs restrict the liberty of researchers and participants, consume scarce social resources, and impede the ability of more nimble and knowledgeable agents to produce important social goods. If research ethics and the mechanisms of regulation and oversight it has spawned have had such disastrous effects on the one social enterprise fundamentally dedicated to seeking truth and producing new knowledge, then we should all grab torches and pitchforks and take to the streets.

What critics would have us do once we have assembled an angry mob, however, is somewhat unclear. Some critics regard IRB review as having a proper place in biomedical research and simply want to rein in what they regard as its uncritical and unnecessary expansion into areas such as the humanities and the social sciences. Others want to overturn the whole regulatory edifice, end the inquisition, and found a social renaissance by returning to the heady days of individual virtue and unsupplemented professional ethics.

Although I believe that radical critics of research regulation in the United States are mistaken, the questions they raise go to the foundations of research ethics and, like the discussion of Wertheimer's principle of permissible exploitation in chapter 3, they reveal a deep tension at the heart of orthodox research ethics. In both of these cases the protectionism of research ethics is challenged on the ground that it is ineffective at best and counterproductive at worst.

7.6.3 The Egalitarian Research Imperative as a More Stable Foundation

My claim is that the discordance between the beneficial effects of research oversight and the public justification offered on its behalf creates a kind of paradox. All individual researchers prefer the situation in which they have the greatest personal freedom and discretion over their work, but implementing such a system results in an outcome that everyone wants to avoid. Conversely, a regulatory system that avoids the tragic outcome benefits all stakeholders: researchers benefit from continued social support, participants benefit from safer studies that provide an avenue in which to advance the common good, community members benefit from the fruits of sustained scientific inquiry into questions of social significance, and sponsors benefit either by advancing valuable science in accordance with their social mandate or by generating profits through the creation of interventions that improve welfare. Nevertheless, this system produces discontent among these various stakeholders because it is presented as a public intrusion into private interactions to curb individual freedom and discretion in order to protect people who, within this system, chafe at the demeaning allegation that they are in need of protection or that they are bent on turning participants into scientific cannon fodder.

Where the costs associated with this system are clear to many stakeholders, its benefits are far less salient. I have been arguing that this is partly the result of a mismatch between the benefits this system actually produces, and the justification orthodox research ethics offers on its behalf. But this is also due to the fact that those benefits accrue most directly at the *system level* while orthodox research ethics focuses myopically on the discrete interactions of private parties.

To see the benefits of prospective review we must adopt the kind of social perspective I am advocating. This social perspective is essential to a coherent and comprehensive research ethics. The current discussion illustrates this by showing how prospective review resolves fundamentally social problems of coordination among a wide range of actors. Such problems cannot even be articulated within a research ethics that is myopically focused on the discrete interactions described in individual study protocols.

Moreover, the benefits of prospective review not only accrue at the social level, but they become most clear only in comparison to alternative ways of organizing research as a cooperative social enterprise. Because this aspect of research ethics is, at least in part, an exercise in what economists call *mechanism design* (§3.7, chapters 6 and 8), the only way to assess the merits of one set of institutions and rules for organizing this social activity is to compare it against an alternative set of institutions and rules (see also §7.7).

When research is severed from larger social purposes, and the moral epicenter of the field is located in the private interactions between researchers and participants that are described in individual study protocols, the paternalistic justification for research oversight enflames the sensibilities of political liberals who tend to view liberty as a right to be left alone. Severing research from larger social purposes and treating it as a set of goals and ends that are adopted by individual actors creates a conceptual ecosystem in which the core values of the field—beneficence and respect for persons—can be marshalled against the discipline's own self-conception. In other words, prospective review appears to infringe the rights of both researchers and participants to engage in private transactions for mutual benefit.

I have argued here that prospective review before bodies of diverse representation helps to resolve coordination problems that would plague an unregulated system. Resolving such problems is a legitimate use of state authority when those problems plague institutions that are part of a just social order (Galston 2004, 3, 125). Even if from a traditional liberal perspective we might say that prospective review may represent an infringement on the liberties of the parties whose conduct is regulated, this infringement is justified by its contribution to the proper function and long-term sustainability of the research enterprise and by the importance of that enterprise to a just social order.

This point is easily formulated within the civic republican tradition, where resolving coordination problems is not an instance of domination or illegitimate use of state authority to the extent that that authority tracks the larger interest in advancing the common good (Pettit 1997, vii, 68; 2004). Although the many parties that contribute to the research enterprise may have personal or parochial interests that are frustrated by prospective review (e.g., unfettered discretion over study design, unfettered pursuit of profit, unfettered access to investigational medicines), subordinating the pursuit of those parochial interests to the common good is not an instance of arbitrary interference because resolving these coordination problems helps the parties to achieve goals that they recognize—it "track[s] their interests according to their ideas" (Pettit 1997, 68). This includes providing credible public assurance that the research enterprise represents a form of social cooperation that will advance the common good. It also includes public safeguards that ensure that stakeholders in this enterprise can advance their parochial interests, but only on terms that are consistent with promoting the common good. This includes prohibitions against subjecting other parties to this scheme of social cooperation to harmful, demeaning, or disrespectful treatment.

Trust in the long-term sustainability of the institutions that ensure the alignment of the parochial interests of various stakeholders with the common good is also important as a means of encouraging individuals to see the research enterprise as an avenue through which they can also pursue some of their own parochial interests on terms that respect the status of others as free and equal. When the public has confidence in the quality of research and feels secure in the expectation that their rights and interests will be respected, they will be more likely to view research participation as a reasonable avenue through which to contribute to the common good.

7.7 Challenges of Measurement

7.7.1 Incentives Affect Which Protocols Are Written

The analysis presented here also explains one reason why it may be difficult to point to empirical evidence of the benefits of IRB review. The benefits of prospective research review before committees of diverse representation accrue at a system level. Instituting the system of regulation and oversight changes the *strategic environment* in which researchers act. In an unregulated environment, researchers might be "rewarded" for attaining a competitive advantage over their peers by pressing the envelope of risk or skimping on research safeguards for participants. In a system in which they must submit protocols for prospective review, researchers face significantly different incentives. The regulatory environment thus shapes which studies are pursued, how studies are designed, and the degree of regard shown for participants. Objectionable studies that would be carried out in the unregulated environment are less likely to be submitted for IRB review because researchers know that they are less likely to be approved, or that they will require protracted revision. As a consequence, studying the effect of IRB review on protocols that are actually submitted is only capable of capturing the *incremental benefit* (if any) of IRB review on protocols that *already reflect the influence of the regulatory regime*.

As a result, it could be true both that actual IRB review adds little or no (incremental) value to protocols that are reviewed and that the system of prospective review before committees of diverse representation is better for all stakeholders than an unregulated system. Such a situation would occur, for example, if the reason that IRB review adds little *incremental* value is that researchers have become relatively efficient at designing research studies that are likely to meet high ethical standards. This efficiency could come about because researchers internalize the relevant moral norms and act on them or because those who do a better job of simulating what will happen to various versions of a protocol once submitted for IRB review are less likely to face costly delays caused by protracted revisions. Regardless of which of these two mechanisms accounts for this efficiency, it does not follow that it could be preserved if we dispense with IRB review. The reason is that the incentive to become more efficient at designing trials that align with important social values hinges critically on the prospect that protocols will face review before bodies of diverse representation.

Here again, then, is something of a paradox. The prospect of having to submit a protocol for prospective review before a committee of diverse representation creates an incentive for researchers to become highly efficient at designing studies that will pass evaluative muster. In the real world, IRBs have to deal with researchers of varying degrees of experience and competence at navigating IRB review. It is likely that IRBs will spend considerable time attending to protocols submitted by researchers unfamiliar or inexperienced with IRB review. If all researchers were ideally rational and knowledgeable, however, almost all protocols would be submitted in a form that would be acceptable with, at most, minor revisions. In this environment, IRBs would be able to quickly approve most protocols and their actual review would add little incremental value.

Dismantling the system of prospective review, however, would change the incentives that even ideally rational and competent researchers face, and it would result in the production of studies that would be unlikely to pass prospective ethical scrutiny. We will never be able to measure the value of submitting such protocols for IRB review, however, because which protocols are produced itself depends on which system of oversight we implement.

7.7.2   IRBs and the Incentive to Make Work

The last point from the previous section deserves further examination because it may explain a behavior that some critics of IRBs have pointed out. That is, actual IRBs may want to feel like they are adding significant value to the system. But on the model outlined here, the most significant value might come from *the effects on researcher behavior of implementing a system of prospective review* and not necessarily from the incremental benefit of actual IRB review. As a result, IRBs that are fortunate enough to see protocols from experienced, competent, and ethically scrupulous researchers may nevertheless search for increasingly minor issues on which to focus out of a desire to feel like they are making a positive impact. Researchers who have become highly efficient at meeting high scientific and ethical standards in the design and implementation of their research will nevertheless find themselves having to address minor issues in their protocols. A central challenge, then, is to figure out mechanisms by which IRBs can remain sufficiently vigilant to detect significant problems with submitted protocols without becoming hyper-focused on minor details in order to manufacture the perception that they are making a difference.

7.7.3   Strategic Environment and Individual Virtue

If the analysis presented here is correct, then it should also drive a stake through the heart of a view with a long pedigree in research ethics. This is the view that the best way to safeguard the research enterprise is by investing in the character of the individual researcher. Although Beecher was prescient in warning that American medicine was nearing a tipping point, and although he was a proponent of informed consent, he argued that "a far more dependable safeguard than consent is the presence of a truly *responsible* investigator" (1966, 1355). Beecher's claim that "the more reliable safeguard provided by the presence of an intelligent, informed, conscientious, compassionate, responsible investigator" (1966, 1360) was echoed by others. As Louis Lasagna (1971) eloquently puts it:

> I submit that the successful development of such an ethical conscience, combined with professional skill, will protect the patient or experimental subject much more effectively than any laws or regulations.

> I have previously said that for the ethical, experienced investigator no
> laws are needed and for the unscrupulous incompetent no laws will help,
> except to allow the injured subjects to obtain compensation or to punish
> the offending scientists (109).

The impotence of regulation in comparison to the importance of moral
virtue (or vice) in individual investigators remains a theme that is echoed in
contemporary critics of IRB review.

The arguments I have articulated here are agnostic about the specific
motives or dispositions of character of researchers. It is perfectly consistent
with the dynamics outlined here that the public reservoir of social trust in
the research enterprise could be exhausted by the cumulative activities of
benevolent, smart, well-meaning, rational researchers. It is difficult to over-
state the importance of this fact, as it illustrates one of the fundamental
shortcomings of efforts to preserve the public trust by investing solely or
primarily in the character of individual investigators. Namely, not all bad
things are done by bad people, and extremely bad consequences (e.g., the
exhaustion of public trust) can result from the uncoordinated activities
of individual agents rationally perusing activities intended to advance the
common good.

7.8 Safeguarding a Unique Public Good: Beyond IRBs

7.8.1 Connecting Research to a Just Social Order

Rejecting the paternalistic focus and justification for research oversight
in favor of the framework articulated here has several advantages. First, it
promotes a better alignment between the goals of research oversight and the
criteria for a just research enterprise. I argued in chapter 4 that the egalitarian
research imperative is grounded in the importance of a set of basic interests
that all persons share, the role of the basic social institutions in a community
in protecting and advancing those interests, and the unique ability of the research enterprise to produce information necessary to bridge gaps between
the basic interests of community members and the ability of the basic social institutions in their community to safeguard and advance those interests.
Ensuring that the research enterprise produces information that constitutes
this public good is thus necessary to ensure the justice of this undertaking. If

this division of labor is to function as a scheme of voluntary cooperation that respects the status of its participants as free and equal, then there must also be concrete and credible social assurance that this undertaking advances the common good without knowingly compromising the basic interests of any stakeholder in the process.

The legitimate role of research regulation and oversight is to provide this credible social assurance in order to secure and promote the kind of broad-based and sustainable social support that is necessary to maintain a voluntary scheme of social cooperation among people who are respected as free and equal. To do this, research ethics must be configured to prevent four types of problems we have seen in this chapter: antipathy, disrespect, lack of social value, or unfair division of social labor.

The current system of research ethics is easily adapted to guard against problems of antipathy and disrespect, at least insofar as these values apply to study participants. Antipathy refers to a manifest lack of concern for the health, welfare, and broader interests of research participants. This includes exposing study participants to risks that are unnecessary or in some other way gratuitous. Disrespect refers to a failure to respond to the moral status of a person by treating him or her as a mere means to the ends of some other decision-maker. Deception, manipulation, coercion, and unfair treatment represent relationships in which some parties deprive others of their right to exercise their agency in the pursuit of their own considered values, free from unwarranted or unjustified interference from others. This includes the ability of study participants to understand the options that are available to them, to make an informed choice from among those options, and to be free from undue influence in the process.

But the value of respect does not apply solely to study participants. It includes the interest of many other parties to the research enterprise in having credible assurance that their support—whether in the form of money, time, effort, institutional space, or their contributions to the scientific evidence base on which research builds—is not being sought under false pretenses or used to support ends that serve only the parochial plans and interests of some other stakeholder.

This aspect of respect is tied to the other failings that research oversight should seek to avoid. When research lacks social value then it is unlikely to make a meaningful contribution to the ability of a community's basic social systems—such as its health care systems—to understand, protect, and advance the basic interests of community members. When participants, funders, host institutions, and other stakeholders support research as a means of generating valuable information, but that research lacks social value, then their support is misdirected and their efforts and resources are squandered.

Alternatively, an unfair division of social labor occurs when a group of stakeholders contribute to a joint enterprise for the purpose of generating a public good but more advantaged parties are able to co-opt the collaboration so as to advance their personal or parochial interests at the expense of the common good. When stakeholders support research to advance the common good, but that research lacks social value because it has been co-opted to advance the parochial ends of one stakeholder, then it is not merely that other participants are disrespected. The party who co-opts this system acts unjustly, diverting resources and cooperative undertakings away from their legitimate social purposes that are grounded in the prior moral claims of community members (§4.8.2).

7.8.2 Oversight of a Wider Range of Stakeholders

Second, embracing the vision of research oversight that I have outlined here underscores the limited role of IRB review in ensuring that research advances the common good. In particular, IRBs have limited ability to influence how priorities for research are set and for determining whether they create a general portfolio of research that is likely to expand the capacity of a community's basic social structures to advance the basic interests of its members effectively, efficiently, and equitably. They also have limited ability to influence downstream actions that are necessary to ensure that the knowledge produced in research is actually incorporated into the operation of these basic social institutions.

If the argument of the present work is sound, then research ethics should reconceptualize the role of IRB review along the lines I have sketched here and undertake the challenge of identifying new mechanisms for ensuring accountability from the wider range of stakeholders who participate in and influence the conduct of research with humans.

As we will see in the next chapters, the limited scope of IRBs came into stark relief when research began moving in higher volumes into low- and middle-income countries. In particular, it was ironic that prominent guidance documents stated that international research must be responsive to the health needs and priorities of host communities when research ethics in its domestic incarnation was largely silent on how health priorities should be defined and how research should align with them.

PART III

THE HUMAN DEVELOPMENT APPROACH TO JUSTICE IN INTERNATIONAL RESEARCH

8

Avoiding Justice: Research
at the Auction Block

8.1 Introduction

International research reveals fault lines in the foundations of research ethics produced by the tectonic friction between two metaphorical continents. One metaphorical continent represents orthodox research ethics in its domestic application in high-income countries (HICs) like the United States. Here, the principle of justice is, at best, woefully underdeveloped and, at worst, the subject of an almost principled aversion (e.g., §1.2.7, §2.5). Instead, the central focus is on ethical issues that can be most easily represented as falling within the confines of the IRB triangle. The other metaphorical continent is the domain of research conceived or funded by entities in HICs but carried out in low- and middle-income countries (LMICs).

On this second metaphorical continent, issues of justice rise to prominence and it becomes more difficult to shoehorn the relevant ethical issues into the narrow confines of the IRB triangle. In part, this is because it is difficult to ignore histories of unfair extractive relationships between HICs of the global north, many of whom are former colonial powers, and LMICs of the global south, many of whom are still dealing with the legacy of colonial rule. At a more practical level, disparities between the communities that sponsor and often drive the agenda for international research and the communities that host such trials calls into question background assumptions that are often taken for granted in the domestic context. With different burdens of disease from different sources of morbidity and mortality that must be addressed within different infrastructures and social systems, it is difficult to ignore the potential for disconnect between the questions international trials are designed to answer and the health priorities of host countries. As a result, issues about the relationship between research, local health needs, and health system capacity lie at the very heart of international research.

For the Common Good. Alex John London, Oxford University Press. © Oxford University Press 2022.
DOI: 10.1093/oso/9780197534830.003.0008

To address these issues, as we saw in §2.5-6 and §3.2.2, documents that provide guidance about the ethical conduct of international research include a series of requirements that address a group of stakeholders that are not typically the focus of discussion in domestic research. For example, at least some of the key stakeholders most directly able to influence whether research in low- and middle-income settings is responsive to the health needs and priorities of host communities fall outside of the IRB-triangle. These actors include international non-governmental organizations, foreign and domestic governmental authorities, and the agencies or entities that sponsor research. Similarly, whether a novel intervention will be made reasonably available to host communities after studies are concluded depends on the decisions and the conduct of a range of parties outside the IRB triangle, such as regulators, study sponsors, host governments, international organizations, or philanthropies that might help to fund access. Moreover, decisions or agreements that affect one or more of these issues might be made before stakeholders within the IRB triangle have been identified (before it is clear which team will carry out a research initiative or which communities will participate in the research) and some of their provisions will have to be effectuated by regulators, government officials, study sponsors, and others, after studies have been completed.

I have argued in previous chapters that research ethics in its domestic incarnation should embrace the relationship between research and the larger purposes of a just social order. Giving justice a more significant role in research ethics would, in effect, eliminate this tectonic friction by providing a unified foundation for a single framework of research ethics that can be consistently and coherently applied to domestic and international research. The next chapter shows how what I call the *human development approach* to international research can ground core requirements of international research in requirements of the egalitarian research imperative.

In this chapter, I examine the prospects of an alternative approach to reducing this tectonic friction that seeks, instead, to remain agnostic about larger issues of justice. It focuses on a process for ensuring that the microlevel transactions between the parties within the IRB triangle are fair and non-exploitative. This view aspires to eliminate what it views as a cumbersome mix of requirements on international research with their expansive scope in favor of a framework of procedures that render considerations of fairness more manageable within the confines of orthodox research ethics.

In §8.2 I lay out the core claims of the *fair benefits approach* to international research (Participants 2002, 2004), including its use of collaborative partnership and transparency to ensure the fairness of the discrete transactions between study participants and researchers.

In §8.5–6 I argue that, despite its considerable appeal, this approach is deeply flawed. At best, it is underdeveloped at both a foundational and a practical level. At worst, I show that, as the view has been described, it serves to increase the efficiency of market forces that are likely to reduce the share of benefits that host countries secure from international research, driving a race to the bottom. Additionally, it is unlikely that the outcomes of this procedure will satisfy the criteria that its proponents require of fair agreements. In this sense, this view risks creating a kind of ethical Trojan horse in which a veneer of fairness and respect cloak the extent to which it allows powerful entities from HICs to advance their interests largely unconstrained.

Ultimately, I am concerned that the appeal to procedures as an alternative to substantive conceptions of justice embodies a romantic, pre-economic conception of procedures. An important lesson from the literature on procedures in economics—the area referred to as mechanism design—is that similar procedures can result in radically different outcomes and that the process of designing and selecting relevant procedures is often highly influenced by substantive values, including judgments about the appropriateness of their outcomes and the moral acceptability of the baselines from which the various stakeholders interact.

I conclude by arguing that it is more difficult than it might seem to remain agnostic about questions of justice in research ethics. Avoiding an explicit and systematic analysis of important background issues of social justice and, instead, hewing closely to the established values of research ethics does not represent agnosticism about issues of justice; instead it represents the tacit acceptance of what Brian Barry calls "justice as mutual advantage" (1982, 219–252). As a result, those who approach this topic wanting to remain agnostic about controversial issues may find themselves formulating the basic problem in a way that tacitly presupposes a particularly anemic theory of justice.

This chapter also illustrates how norms that govern the review and approval of research initiatives shape the strategic environment in which stakeholders interact. Creating a system of norms that focuses on individual transactions and benefits from research that are not directly related to the value of the information that research generates for host communities is likely to perpetuate an extractive system that deprives the most burdened populations of LMICs of the unique public good that can flow from research as a scientific activity. This public good is the information that local stakeholders require to expand the capacity of their basic social systems to effectively, efficiently, and equitably safeguard and advance the basic interests of that community's members.

8.2 Fair Benefits and the Procedural Alternative[1]

8.2.1 Exploitation as an Unfair Level of Benefit

The fair benefits approach begins from a premise that is widely shared, namely, that one of the most central ethical issues in international research is to avoid situations in which more powerful parties from HICs take unfair advantage of LMIC communities. Also, like numerous other accounts, this view treats unfair advantage taking as synonymous with exploitation. But proponents of this view argue that it is a mistake to see the cumbersome list of requirements elaborated in international guidance documents as necessary conditions for avoiding exploitation.

Their argument rests, in part, on Wertheimer's account of exploitation (Wertheimer 2008). On that view, exploitation is a property of micro-level interactions between individual parties to a discrete transaction. Although exploitative relationships can result in net harms to the exploited party, this need not be the case. It is an advantage of Wertheimer's view that it recognizes that agreements can be freely and knowingly undertaken and mutually beneficial while still being exploitative. In particular, even within a voluntary and mutually beneficial transaction, Party A exploits party B if party A receives "an unfair level of benefits as a result of B's interactions with A" (Participants 2004, 19). In this view, whether researchers and sponsors exploit study participants and their communities depends on whether the share of the benefits that these parties receive from hosting particular research initiatives is fair.

[1] Much of the material in §8.2–8.7 originally appeared in London, A. J., & Zollman, K. J. (2010). Research at the auction block: problems for the Fair Benefits Approach to international research. *Hastings Center Report*, 40(4), 34–45. It is revised and reprinted here with the generous permission of Kevin Zollman.

Additionally, proponents of this view follow Wertheimer in arguing that fairness is not ultimately an issue of "what" benefits host communities receive but of the "level" or amount of benefit (Participants 2004, 20). If this premise is accepted, then it follows that no particular benefit is a necessary condition for avoiding exploitation. Instead, exploitation is about how much benefit parties receive from a transaction. For this reason, proponents of this view argue that all types of benefits that might flow from research, not just access to the investigational agent, must be considered in determining whether the benefits are fair (Emanuel 2008, 724–725).

8.2.2 Standards of Fairness

To identify exploitative relationships, we require a standard of fairness, now to be understood as a specification of the amount of benefit received by each of the parties to a discrete, micro-level transaction. But proponents of this approach also lament that:

(a) "Currently, there is no shared international standard of fairness; reasonable people disagree" (Participants 2004, 23).

Additionally, different individuals and different communities can have different valuations of the diverse benefits that might be on the table at any time. As a result, they go on to assert,

(b) "Most importantly, only the host population can determine the value of the benefits for itself" (Participants 2004, 23). Therefore
(c) "Ultimately, the determination of whether the benefits are fair and worth the risks cannot be entrusted to people outside the population, no matter how well intentioned" (Participants 2004, 22; 2002, 2134).

The claims in (a), (b), and (c) are quite strong and they provide the justification for the assertion that "the population being asked to enroll determines whether a particular array of benefits is sufficient and fair" (Participants 2004, 22).

These claims bolster the view, also adopted from Wertheimer, that fair distributions of benefits are defined by the results of free and informed transactions untainted by force, fraud, or deception. As they put the matter:

(d) "[A] fair distribution of benefits at the micro-level is based on the
level of benefits that would occur in a market transaction devoid of
fraud, deception, or force, in which the parties have full information"
(Participants 2004, 20).

Free agents with full information in a market devoid of force, fraud, and deception would evaluate the bundles of resources they can secure from alternative transactions and then choose according to their values. This reflects
the sovereignty of host community values and the importance of a deep respect for their freedom and values.

Rather than specifying that host communities must be provided with a
specific type of good, proponents of the fair benefits approach hold that a
fair distribution is determined by requirements on the relative amount of
benefits that relevant parties receive.

Benefits must increase with burdens: "As the burdens on the participants
and the community increase, so the benefits must increase" (Emanuel 2008,
725; see also Gbadegesin and Wendler 2006, 251; Participants 2004, 22).

Benefits must increase with benefits to others: "Similarly, as the benefits to
the sponsors, researchers, and others outside the population increase, the
benefits to the host population should also increase" (Emanuel 2008, 725;
see also Gbadegesin and Wendler 2006, 251; Participants 2004, 23.)

Benefits must track relative contributions: "The level of benefits that a
community should receive to ensure a fair deal depends on the community's
contribution relative to the contributions of all other parties that are involved in the research project, including sponsors, investigators, subjects,
and other communities" (Gbadegesin and Wendler 2006, 251).

Against this background, proponents of the fair benefits approach have
been staunch critics of the reasonable availability requirement on the
grounds that it does a poor job of avoiding the problem of exploitation.
First, in early-phase research, for example, or unsuccessful late-stage research, there is no intervention to make available to communities. In such
cases host communities bear any costs or burdens of participation without
receiving any offsetting benefits. Second, they argue that it is overly paternalistic to require host communities to accept, and perhaps even to pay for,
the fruits of a particular research study when there may be different benefits

that those communities would prefer (Participants 2004, 20; Weijer and LeBlanc 2006). Finally, reasonable availability is rejected because it doesn't track the criteria for fairness listed in the previous paragraph: "Reasonable availability fails to ensure a fair share of benefits; for instance, it may provide for too little benefit when risks are high or benefits to the sponsors great" (Participants 2002, 2133).

One particularly important implication of this reasoning is that if what matters is not the kind of benefit host communities receive but the amount, then if host communities are not interested in the information or the interventions that a study is designed to generate, and if it is not obligatory to provide post-trial access to the study intervention, then it is difficult to justify requiring cross-national studies to be aligned with or to focus on the urgent health needs or priorities of the host community. That focus itself appears to be overly narrow and perhaps also overly paternalistic because it focuses only on one way in which research can be responsive to interests of host communities (Wolitz et al. 2009).

8.2.3 Collaborative Partnership

The fair benefits approach relies on two additional principles to produce outcomes that are fair. The first is called *collaborative partnership*. At the level of concrete action, researchers and host community members are to engage in a collaborative process of negotiation in which host communities and researchers agree on a specific division of benefits. Freed from the constraints imposed by international guidance documents, host communities are free to negotiate for studies that are responsive to their health needs and for post-trial access to novel interventions. But they are also free to negotiate for a different package of benefits, such as help in cleaning their water supply, constructing a road, or vaccinating their children.

Collaborative partnership is thus intended to be more responsive to a wider range of needs and preferences among host community members and to take advantage of the special knowledge and insight of host community members about how best to advance or improve their condition or circumstances. In light of the strong claims in (a), (b), and (c), it also reflects deference to autonomy of individuals in LMIC communities to make decisions for themselves about the conditions that would justify research participation.

8.2.4 The Principle of Transparency

Collaborative partnership may help to ensure that agreements are mutually beneficial and therefore consistent with the requirements of beneficence. But Wertheimer holds that mutually beneficial transactions, freely entered, can still be exploitative. In part, that is because agreements in the real world can suffer from deficiencies that would not be present in a market in which all parties have full information and the transaction is free from fraud, deception, and abuse. Proponents of the fair benefits approach are particularly concerned about this problem in the international context. As they put it:

(e) "A population in a developing country is likely to be at a distinct disadvantage relative to the sponsors from the developed country in determining whether a proposed level of benefits is fair" (Participants 2004, 23).

The principle of transparency is supposed to structure the process of bargaining and negotiation in a way that approximates, as closely as possible, the conditions of such an idealized market. This involves creating a publicly accessible database of all benefits agreements between various research sponsors and host communities. This repository is supposed to be maintained by an independent party, such as the World Health Organization, with the expectation that various groups such as researchers, sponsors, governments, and potential host communities will have access to the data. In fact, their view requires that the database be advertised to potential host communities so that they can evaluate the various packages of benefits that have been exchanged in the context of other research projects.

How is this database supposed to ensure that agreements are fair? First, it reduces informational asymmetries between the host country and the researcher. This is required because fair outcomes must reflect agreements that would be struck under the condition in which the parties have full information (d).

Second, satisfying the requirement of full information is supposed to reduce the likelihood of fraud or deception by giving potential host communities access to information regarding a wide range of factors such as the costs of various aspects of research and the full range of benefits that might flow from a research project.

Third, seeing what other communities received in the past should allow communities to assess the competitiveness of a proposed division of benefits. This, in turn, can be a point of negotiation in their determination of whether a proposed package is worth accepting.

Fourth, proponents of the fair benefits approach also claim that the principle of transparency is supposed to advance a regulative as well as informational goal. In particular, their approach has been criticized for not recognizing the extent to which inequalities in bargaining power will allow researchers and sponsors to exact hugely disproportionate benefits from the agreements reached in this process (London 2005). In response, proponents of the fair benefits approach have argued that:

(f) "The criticisms seem to miss the fact that the fairness of agreements is not determined just by bargaining. The purpose of the transparency principle is to provide an external check that independently assesses the fairness of agreements" (Emanuel 2008, 725).

(g) "Such information will facilitate the development of "case law" standards of fairness that evolve out of a number of agreements" (Participants 2004, 24).

It is this regulative goal that is referred to in (f) and (g) in which the database of prior agreements and the case law that it engenders function as an external check on fairness.

Ultimately, the principle of transparency is supposed to ensure that collaborative partnerships produce fair agreements by counteracting some of the informational defects that separate real-world negotiations from more idealized markets. As a regulative tool that can be used by international organizations, it is also supposed to correct for imbalances in power by ruling out offers that do not provide a sufficiently larger share of benefits to count as fair.

8.2.5 Problems with Consistency?

The fair benefits approach has considerable allure, in part, because it appears to offer something for everyone. But a core question is whether this broad appeal reflects the merits of a view that coherently integrates different perspectives into a single framework or a vaguely articulated set of requirements that appeal to different constituencies but which, ultimately, cannot be reconciled.

Regulators and IRBs may be attracted to the prospect of reducing thorny questions of justice and fairness to terms that can be manageably addressed within the confines of the IRB triangle. This approach seems to embody the minimalist approach to questions of justice latent in the *Belmont Report* in which issues of justice are reduced to a function of beneficence and respect for persons (§2.5.3). However, it has the added attraction of recognizing the extent to which even voluntary and mutually beneficial agreements might reflect imperfections of real-world agents and, in this sense, fall short of fairness. So, it situates the minimalist's appeal to beneficence and autonomy within a more idealized context of full information and freedom from force, fraud, and deception. It thus holds out the promise of replacing the cumbersome mix of requirements enshrined in international documents with a single, seemingly much more manageable process.

Other stakeholders might be attracted to the fair benefits approach because they think that it will allow host communities to capture a much larger share of the benefits from international research. These parties might be attracted to the idea that benefits to host communities will increase with burdens and with benefits to others, and will track relative contributions. When LMIC communities host research that has the potential to generate hundreds of millions, if not billions, of dollars in revenue, then they might believe that host communities will be guaranteed to receive fairly substantial benefits in return for hosting the research. This prospect might be seen as justifying or rendering unproblematic the prospect that such research may focus primarily on HIC health needs or be designed to vindicate interventions that are unlikely to be used on a widespread basis in LMICs.

One question, then, concerns how the process of collaborative partnership and the transparency principle are to be structured so that they represent the conditions of an ideal market (d) while ensuring that agreements distribute resources in proportion to burdens, benefits to others, and relative contributions. In §8.4 we show that these two ideas are in fundamental tension and that ideal market transactions are unlikely to result in agreements that satisfy these conditions.

Other stakeholders may be attracted to the idea that LMIC communities must be the ultimate arbiters of what counts as a fair bargain as seen in (a), (b), and (c). They like the extent to which the fair benefits approach empowers LMIC communities to decide for themselves which agreements

are worthwhile in a context free from force, fraud, and asymmetric information. But this strong commitment to the evaluative sovereignty of host
communities might conflict with the substantive criteria for fair agreements
if host communities are willing to accept a bargain in which the distribution
of benefits does not vary according to one or more of those criteria.

In contrast, others might like the extent to which regulators or agencies
like the WHO are empowered to play a regulative role in preventing LMIC
populations from being offered unfair agreements, as reflected in (f), (g).
These parties like the extent to which the bargaining power of researchers
can be checked or constrained by outside parties who have the practical
ability to police these agreements and ensure their fairness. But if outside
regulators have the power to prevent mutually beneficial bargains that host
communities are willing to accept under conditions of full information, devoid of force or fraud, then this seems to impinge on the strong commitment
to the sovereignty of host community values in (a), (b), and (c).

Other stakeholders may like this approach because reducing inefficiencies
in the market for research (d) and removing cumbersome requirements such
as responsiveness and reasonable availability will allow firms from HICs to
carry out a much wider range of research in LMIC communities. Offshoring
research will result in considerable cost savings for firms and allow them to
leverage supply and demand to capture almost all of the benefits from such
transactions. Lowering the costs of research will, in turn, allow savings to
fund more studies, thereby improving the overall rate of research.

Which of these assessments is correct? Well, it is difficult to say and, as a
general point, that is itself part of the problem. We know so little about how
the process of negotiation is supposed to be carried out that it is difficult to
know how the market ideal in (d) is supposed to be reconciled with the dis-
tributional criteria for fairness. We know so little about how the database will
influence this that it is unclear how to reconcile it with the strong claims in
(a), (b), and (c).

8.3 Collaborative Partnership Is an Auction

8.3.1 Simultaneous, Iterated Bidding

How might the fair benefits approach be carried out in practice? We start
from the idea that, ultimately, the focus of negotiations concerns how to

divide the surplus value generated by research. Since this view is clear that the ultimate question is not "what" benefits are divided, but how much each party receives, this effectively focuses deliberations on the price that a community regards as fair for hosting a study, which is the cost to the researcher. We assume that every study has an expected surplus (the expected profits minus the cost of conducting the research), and that some of this surplus can be transferred to the LMIC host community. We also assume that there are some costs associated with hosting the research, and no community will agree to host research where its share of the surplus is less than its expected costs.

Consider first the situation in which researchers are free to negotiate simultaneously with as many interested parties as they like. In this case, researchers inform potential host communities about the various costs, risks, and potential benefits associated with a particular research initiative. After consulting their constituent members, each community proposes a basket of benefits that it would be willing to accept in return for hosting the initiative. Assume further that researchers are then free to inform each community of what the others are asking—as required under the principle of transparency and by the ideal of a competitive market. This would allow each community to compare a given level of benefit to what they perceive as their cost for hosting the research. At some point one community will be willing to accept a level of benefit that is less than what it would cost another community to host the initiative. At that point the latter community will withdraw from the negotiations. Other communities will consider whether the current "bid" is above their cost and, if it is, they will lower their bid. At some point negotiations will reach a level at which only two communities have a cost that is below the current offer. Negotiations will continue until the bid reaches the cost of the second-place community. That community will not lower its offer and the community with the lowest cost will reduce its bid accordingly. After this point there will be no more offers. The community with the lowest cost thus pays a fraction more than the cost of the second-place bidder. The division of benefits that results from this process will be such that the eventual winner gains the difference between its own cost and the cost to the second cheapest host community.

The process just described has the structure of a first price, open cry auction—those familiar to most of us from live and internet auctions. Instead of bidding larger amounts of money to purchase a commodity, potential host communities try to make themselves more attractive venues for research by lowering the share of the surplus value generated by the research that they are willing to accept in return for hosting a research initiative. Negotiating this way allows researchers to choose the venue with the lowest costs, in effect, maximizing the surplus that they can expect to receive from the bargaining process.

It might be objected that this is not the kind of negotiation process that proponents of the fair benefits approach had in mind. However, nothing in the fair benefits approach prohibits this form of negotiation. In fact, this form of negotiating is consistent with the few features of this approach that its proponents do stipulate. That is, in this scenario researchers are negotiating directly with individual host communities about how much benefit each is willing to accept as a fair return to collaboration. It closely approximates the full information requirement for ideal market transactions by giving each community the chance to adjust their assessment in light of the current bid of other communities. Each community determines which offers they are willing to accept and if a community regards a proposed split as unfair, it is free to refuse. Likewise, the benefits from any agreement accrue directly to the eventual host community.

If the fair benefits approach wants to rule out using this kind of negotiating procedure, then it needs to be much clearer about either the way that procedure should be conducted, or about the properties that it should satisfy and how those properties rule out this kind of approach. Nevertheless, it is true that proponents of the fair benefits approach do not describe a process of repeated negotiation between communities, and although they stipulate that all parties must have access to the database of previous agreements, they do not state that each community must be aware of what other contemporaneous communities are willing to accept.

8.3.2 One-Shot Bidding

So, we might imagine instead a process of negotiation in which researchers engage in a deliberative process with each community and then each has one opportunity to inform researchers of the amount they regard as a fair return. This eliminates the repeated process of negotiation or bidding and, in turn, eliminates the condition of perfect information that each community had in the previous scenario about the cost structure of other communities.

Unfortunately, as long as each community knows that there are others that are interested in hosting the research, and each community knows that they have only one chance to submit an offer, then, on average, the outcome will be the same as the first price, open cry auction. That is because negotiations of this type also have the structure of an auction; in this case it is a first price, sealed bid auction. Variants of this kind eliminate the situation of perfect information, but not the incentive to make educated guesses about the cost structure of other bidders. Bidders simply have to base their negotiation strategies on those guesses. Sometimes they miscalculate and get less than they would in an open cry auction, other times they get lucky and get more; on average, however, the outcomes will be the same.

There are many ways in which these two processes of negotiation may differ. But the irrelevance of these differences is established by a powerful and elegant formal result, now well known as the "revenue equivalence theorem." What this theorem proves is that, given a particular set of constraints, the average amount paid in an auction (here interpreted as the amount of the surplus kept by the researcher) is the same (Myerson 1981; Riley and Samuelson 1981). On average the researcher will keep all of the surplus minus the average value of the second lowest cost.

The assumptions required for the revenue equivalence theorem to hold require very little from the structure of the interaction.[2] There must be an imbalance between supply and demand (modeled as multiple cites vying to host a single research initiative). Individuals who are bidding cannot enjoy taking risk for its own sake (although they may be willing to take risks). The structure of the process by which research is awarded must be such that the person who bids the lowest receives the research, even if they pay an amount different from their bid. If a community has the highest possible cost for hosting research, they must expect not to get any surplus. There are some restrictions on what communities believe about each other's costs, and all of this must be known by all parties.

Notice that many of the features we commonly associate with auctions are not required for the outcome to be equivalent to the outcome of an auction. The high bidder need not pay her bid, or even the bid of the second highest

---

[2] We state these assumptions and defend their relevance to the fair benefits approach in Appendix A to London and Zollman 2010 available at: https://www.cmu.edu/dietrich/philosophy/docs/london/london-research-auction-supplement.pdf or from the author by request.

bidder. Bids can be made simultaneously or sequentially or any combination of the two. The result holds for an astonishing variety of ways of permuting the process of negotiation so that it differs from both first price, open cry or one-shot bidding auctions.

8.3.3 Modified One-Shot Bidding

For instance, in an effort to remove some of the strategic element to the competitive bidding process, each community might engage with researchers in a process of deliberation knowing that, at the end of that process, there will be one chance to submit a bid and that although the lowest bidder will still win, that bidder will receive an amount of the surplus that is equivalent to the bid of the second lowest bidder. This is known as a second price, sealed bid auction. The strategic element to the bidding is removed but the result remains the same. The researcher expects to receive the same amount of the surplus as in the other cases: almost all of it.

8.3.4 Commitment with the Option to Relocate

In fact, a negotiation process where there is not simultaneous competitive bidding can still function like an auction over time. Perhaps, for instance, host communities are first chosen on the basis of factors such as existing relationships, convenience, and ease of conducting the research. Assume, however, that at the completion of the study researchers have the option of locating subsequent studies elsewhere. As long as there are multiple potential host communities for each proposed research initiative then communities with a lower cost structure have an incentive to approach researchers, or their sponsors, in an effort to host a subsequent research study. As long as there is a realistic possibility that researchers will relocate, then the threat of being underbid in the future puts pressure on host communities to reduce their costs and, with this, the amount of benefit that they seek in return.[3]

---

[3] For a brief overview of repeated auctions see Klemperer (2004, section 1.10.3).

8.3.5 The Result of the Auction

Auction-like structures do an excellent job of realizing in practice the features of the ideal markets in (d) that are central to the fair benefits approach. What do these outcomes look like in practice?

Suppose that the anticipated benefits of a research project can be assigned a monetary value and that a particular project is expected to generate $10 million in surplus. To model the results of this bargaining process, we assign each host community a cost for hosting this initiative by randomly drawing a number between $100,000 and $1 million. If we randomly assign costs in this range to two host communities and carry out the auction process over and over, the average split will be $700,000 for the host community and $9.3 million for the researcher. The average cost for the winning host community is $400,000 so the average profit is $300,000. If there are three communities, the average profit drops to $225,000 (a $550,000 / $9,450,000 split). If there are nine, the profits are a meager $90,000 (a $280,000 / $9,720,000 split).

What if we retain all of these assumptions, but we assume that instead of $10 million dollars in surplus that the study is expected to generate $10 billion dollars? In this case, the payouts to the host community remain the same. The additional profits are absorbed entirely by the sponsor.

What if research does not impose such steep costs on host communities? If we assume, as in the previous example, that the expected profit is $10 million, but the costs to host communities are in the range of [$0, $100,000] then with two bidders the expected profit for the host community is $33,333 (a split of $66,666 / $9,933,334). For three bidders the expected profit drops to $25,000 (a split of $50,000 / $9,950,000), and if there are nine potential hosts the expected profit drops to $10,000 (a split of $20,000 / $9,980,000).

Notice now one respect in which this approach can have some counterintuitive consequences. Suppose that the costs for host communities are as described in our first example, somewhere in the range of $100,000 and $1 million. Now suppose that altruistically motivated researchers want to help defray the costs that host communities might incur from hosting a research project. So they lobby the research sponsor to use more of their own personnel, defraying personnel costs, or to bring in a mobile laboratory, defraying infrastructure costs. This altruistically motivated act would in fact work against the interests of host communities and would capture a potentially sizable increase in profit for the research sponsor. This is because defraying costs to host communities reduces the range of potential hosting costs, thereby decreasing the distance between the cost of the winner and the cost of the second highest bidder. If costs could be reduced to the range of our second example, between [$0, $100,000], then the benefits to host communities would decrease to those listed in the second example. In other words, with three bidders the host community's expected profit drops from $225,000 to $25,000 and with nine bidders it drops from $90,000 to a paltry $10,000.

8.4 Fair Benefits Cannot Achieve Its Own Benchmarks for Fairness

8.4.1 Participant Benefits Don't Increase with Burdens to Participants

This very brief modeling exercise allows us to answer some important questions that we raised in §8.2.5. For example, would the outcomes of this process satisfy the principles that benefits to host communities must increase with burdens and with benefits to others, as well as track relative contributions? Under auction-like structures it is unlikely that any of these desiderata will be satisfied.

The first principle from the fair benefits approach requires that the benefits to the host community must increase as the burdens to participants and the larger community increase. Under auction-like structures, however, the benefits that the host community receives (its profit) are not a function of the burdens that the research imposes on participants or the larger community. Sure, as costs for potential host communities rise, the size of the split that the host community receives will have to be larger in order to offset those costs. But "benefits" here are modeled as the share of the surplus that host communities receive that is over and above their costs. This is determined by the difference between the costs of hosting the research in the winning community and the costs of the community with the second lowest costs, and by the number of communities that are party to the negotiations.

Another way of putting this point is to say that trials that are more expensive cost more to conduct. But it does not follow from this that host communities will receive more benefit from this higher cost. Low-risk or less burdensome studies for rare conditions may reward host communities with sizable profits while high-risk or more burdensome studies for conditions that are quite common may produce minuscule profits for host communities. Our point is that under auction-like structures, the burdens that research participants or host communities bear do not directly influence the share of the benefits that they receive from hosting a trial. If outcomes of this process satisfy this condition, it will be as a result of happy coincidence and *not as a result of the structure of the negotiation process itself.*

8.4.2 Participant Benefits Don't Increase with Benefits to Others

The second principle states that the share of the benefits that host communities enjoy should increase as the benefits increase for other stakeholders, such as sponsors, researchers, and others outside the population. Under auction-like structures, however, the degree to which others profit from a community's participation is basically irrelevant to determining how the surplus is divided. In particular, if we hold fixed the costs of hosting a trial and the number of bidders, then it doesn't matter if the projected profit is $2 million or $20 billion dollars—the expected profit of the host community does not change. If the host community can expect to receive $20,000 of benefit in the first case, that is what it can expect to receive in the latter. It is therefore important to recognize that auction-like structures function in a way that makes it unlikely that outcomes will ever satisfy this condition.

8.4.3 Participant Benefits Don't Increase with Contributions

The third principle says that the benefits to host communities ought to be proportional to the community's contribution relative to other stakeholders. Unfortunately, the proponents of the fair benefits approach have not given us a clear account of what they mean by a "contribution" here. It should be clear from the previous analysis, however, that under auction-like structures, it is difficult to see how we could understand the contribution of the host community relative to those of researchers, sponsors, and others in a way that would make it relevant to determining the share of the benefits that host communities receive. Even if there are only two communities in the world that could host a particular trial, the magnitude of the benefits that the eventual winner receives will be a function of the difference between its cost and the cost of the other community. If the trial can be conducted with few costs, and the costs of the two communities are fairly close to one another, then the host community could expect to receive fairly meager benefits.

The upshot of this analysis is that there is little reason to believe that the process at the heart of the fair benefits approach will produce outcomes that satisfy the minimal conditions of fairness that the proponents of this view themselves endorse and certainly use as grounds for rejecting other views.

8.4.4 A Race to the Bottom

This brief modeling exercise also demonstrates the potential for the fair benefits approach to result in a race to the bottom when implemented in practice. And, just so the point is clear, the process of negotiation does not have to be structured as a first-price, open cry auction in order for this result to obtain. The structural features that create the incentive for host communities to lower their bids are present even in the sequential case where researchers locate their study in a particular community but have the option of relocating for subsequent studies.[4]

Several additional factors increase the likelihood of a race to the bottom. First, as international research becomes increasingly mobile host communities may realize that they need to restrain their requests for benefits or risk having researchers relocate (Petryna 2007). This is because the outsourcing of clinical trials has effectively created a market for companies whose purpose is to match research initiatives with potential host communities (Petryna 2007; McManus and Saywell 2001). These contract research organizations (CROs) seek profits by reducing research costs and more efficiently matching research with host communities. These companies therefore have a powerful incentive to increase the size of their "portfolio" of potential communities that might host various research initiatives. This, in turn, makes the prospect of relocation very real for host communities. It also creates a market environment where host communities are more clearly competing with one another to secure access to research.

---

[4] In fact, we argue in Appendix B to London and Zollman 2010 that even some fairly restrictive and unrealistic requirements aimed at equalizing the bargaining power of researchers and host communities would be unlikely to prevent a race to the bottom. This appendix is available at: https://www.cmu.edu/dietrich/philosophy/docs/london/london-research-auction-supplement.pdf or from the author by request.

The operation of CROs is thus making the marketplace for hosting research more competitive. Even if host communities are not bidding against one another each time they host a trial, the fact that the CRO can find a community that might be willing to host a similar study for less provides an incentive to reduce the size of the surplus that host communities seek to retain for themselves now.

What about the principle of transparency? It might come as a surprise to learn that it will do nothing to hinder the race to the bottom. This is largely because the race to the bottom is actually facilitated by the full information requirement of ideal theory that this principle is supposed to approximate.

Additionally, using the data from the repository of past agreements as a way to advertise research to eligible LMIC communities (Participants 2004, 23), would serve to increase the number of potential host communities by bringing new "buyers" into the market. Potential host communities could see what others have received in the past and enter the market armed with the information that they need to make competitive bids. After all, if one knows that researchers located an ongoing study in one place for some cost X, and one knows that one's community could host that research for considerably less cost than X, then one has an incentive to approach the researchers, their sponsor, or their CRO in an effort to host their next initiative. Even if the proponents of this approach do not intend the database to be used as a marketing tool to bring new host communities into the market, CROs have a powerful incentive to use it this way.

Rather than averting a race to the bottom or setting a floor for the benefits that host communities receive, the principle of transparency may actually place a ceiling on benefits as communities are forced by competition to seek less in return for hosting studies.

8.5 An Independent Check on Fairness?

8.5.1 Pure versus Imperfect Procedural Justice

One might object that this characterization of the fair benefits approach is overly pessimistic because we have left out the regulative aspect detailed in (f) and (g) (Emanuel 2008, 725). In this interpretation, the role of regulators might be to prevent a race to the bottom or to ensure that outcomes satisfy the principles that benefits to host communities must increase with burdens and with benefits to others, and must track relative contributions.

This objection dramatizes deep ambiguities within the fair benefits approach because it calls into question exactly what kind of procedural approach it is supposed to be. At some points, it sounds like it is supposed to be a *pure procedural approach*. Under a pure procedural approach, an outcome or a state of affairs is regarded as fair if and only if it is the result of a particular procedure. That is, the fairness of an outcome consists in the fact that it was arrived at or produced by a particular procedure. This view supports following (d) in defining fair outcomes as whatever "would occur in a market transaction devoid of fraud, deception, or force, in which the parties have full information" (Participants 2004, 20).

But, if the race to the bottom is prevented by a regulator imposing some constraints on which *outcomes* are acceptable, the fair benefit approach is not a pure procedural approach. How do we determine which restrictions should be imposed by the regulator? It cannot be from this *procedure*, since the regulator must now impose outcomes on the parties that differ from those that were arrived at by the relevant procedure.

At other points, the fair benefits approach seems like it is supposed to be an *imperfect procedural approach*. In an imperfect procedural approach, the special value of the procedure lies in its ability to produce, imperfectly, but more or less reliably, outcomes that are fair according to some independent standard or criterion of fairness. On this view, then, the fairness of the outcome is constituted by something other than its relationship to a particular process.

One such criterion requires that outcomes meet the conditions that benefits to host communities increase with burdens and with benefits to others, and that they track relative contributions. Moreover, the claim that "Reasonable availability fails to ensure a fair share of benefits; for instance, it may provide for too little benefit when risks are high or benefits to the sponsors great" (Participants 2002, 2133) seems to imply that satisfying at least the first two conditions is a necessary requirement for avoiding exploitation.

In light of the analysis presented here (§8.3-6) it is doubtful that proponents of the fair benefits approach can consistently endorse the more purely procedural criterion expressed in (d) and the more substantive criteria about the distribution of benefits relative to burdens and benefits and contributions. The reason is simply that transactions in a market of full information devoid of force or fraud are not likely to produce outcomes that approximate those substantive criteria.

8.5.2 Incompatible Criteria for Fairness

There are two possibilities for eliminating the incompatibility between the pure procedural and imperfect procedural aspirations of the fair benefits approach. One is to argue that fair outcomes should at least approximate the principles that benefits to host communities must increase with burdens and with benefits to others, and they must track relative contributions. In that case, we now need a detailed account of the procedures that will be used to enable researchers and host communities to negotiate in such a way that they are likely to arrive at outcomes that approximate these conditions. We have argued that on a number of plausible ways of making operational the conditions outlined in (d), these outcomes are unlikely to hold. If the job of ensuring that these principles are met is supposed to fall to regulators, then this would require a significant diminution of the expansive role of host community autonomy expressed in (c). On this new proposal, regulators, not host countries, would decide if a bargain is ultimately fair. Moreover, their decision would be based on a substantive view of fairness. In particular, host communities might be willing to accept some mutually beneficial offers that regulators would prohibit on the grounds that they are unfair (since they deviate from the substantive criteria regulators are empowered to enforce).

While this is a tenable position, it is very different from the original presentation of the fair benefits approach since it dispenses with the strong claims outlined in (a), (b), and (c). This new position would require defense on substantive, rather than procedural grounds and an account of the procedure for negotiation that will approximate these outcomes. It is worth noting that the same argument that support Wertheimer's defense of the principle of permissible exploitation (§3.3–4) would challenge the consistency of this position.

A second alternative would be to stick with the market norms outlined in (d) and to jettison a commitment to the principles that benefits to host communities must increase with burdens and with benefits to others, and they must track relative contributions. Now, the role of external regulators would be to make sure that actual agreements approximate those that would have been reached in the ideal market. In this case, we need a more precise specification of what constitutes the idealized market. For instance, is the ratio of buyers to sellers in the idealized market the same as in the actual one? If it is the same, then we are back to the discussion of §8.3-4. That is, not only will the principles that benefits to host communities must increase with burdens and with benefits to others, and must track relative contributions, not hold, but regulators will not provide an external check on the bargaining process, other than ensuring that there was no deception, fraud, or concealment.

Interestingly, if the ratio of buyers to sellers in the ideal market is not the same as the actual one, then regulators might play the role of adjusting bargains to reflect this ideal ratio. Although this is also an interesting proposal, it would require additional, substantive arguments to (a) specify the ideal ratio and (b) justify using *this* feature to determine a fair distribution of benefits as opposed to some other view of fairness.

8.6 Pure Procedural Justice Revisited

Perhaps we have underestimated the appeal of the fair benefits approach as a pure procedural approach to issues of fairness in this context. After all, collaborative partnership is a compelling ideal. What is there not to like about the idea that researchers and host communities should engage each other as "partners," "collaborating" to advance shared ends, in a way that is respectful of the autonomy of the host community and its distinctive values and ends? The relationship of moral equality implied by collaborative partnership also strikes a welcome contrast to ethical imperialism or the inequalities of the "white man's burden." Since the values of respect for autonomy and beneficence are the bioethics equivalent of mom and apple pie, perhaps we should follow them wherever they lead and simply call those outcomes "fair."

This sounds good. The problem is that endorsing these values does not entail that everyone who endorses them conceives of them in the same way. Nor does it entail that one has a set of procedures that are faithful to these values in practice. Both of these problems afflict the fair benefits approach.

The view contains within it several competing conceptions of the sense in which sponsors and host community members should be treated as equals in their "partnership." One ideal is grounded in the norms of the market. All parties should be equally free to make binding contracts in light of full information, free from fraud, coercion, and deception. Within those constraints, there is nothing unfair about participants using inequalities in urgent needs, endowments, and the like to their strategic advantage.

In contrast, different ideals of equality and partnership undergird the principles that benefits to host communities must increase with burdens, with benefits to others, and track relative contributions. Here, ideals of equal respect for welfare, partnership, and agency are conceived of in ways that differ from ideal market norms because they constrain the way that collaborators can use inequalities in endowments or urgency of needs to their strategic advantage.

The problem is not simply that these different ideals lead to incompatible outcomes, but also that the incompatibility of these outcomes reflects substantive differences in ideals of respect for others as moral equals.

Before we can know whether we should follow the procedures of the fair benefits approach wherever they lead us, therefore, its proponents need to (i) specify a consistent set of ideals that these procedures are supposed to track or embody, (ii) justify the claim that these are the relevant ideals, and (iii) demonstrate that their procedures for realizing these values in practice are faithful to those ideals, properly understood. Our claim is not that this can't be done—it is that there appear to be several, potentially incompatible, ways of doing this, and each represents a significant departure from the original ambitions of the approach.

For example, sticking with their claim in (d) that "a fair distribution of benefits at the micro-level is based on the level of benefits that would occur in a market transaction devoid of fraud, deception, or force, in which the parties have full information" (Participants 2004, 20), proponents might simply embrace the claim that auction-like structures represent the best way to ensure that real-world negotiations satisfy these conditions. If this process results in highly disproportionate divisions of benefits and if LMIC communities wind up receiving a lower level of benefits than they would have received under reasonable availability, then this simply shows that such outcomes are not exploitative, not that the fair benefits approach is somehow faulty.

If proponents want to move in this direction then they should drop the misleading language of collaborative partnership. After all, there is a sense in which online auction sites like eBay respect the autonomy of participants and treat them as morally equal. But nobody is confused into believing that whether they get the item at the end of that process depends on the reasons that they offer to their "partners" in some collaborative, deliberative interaction. This is because there is a more important sense in which auctions, and markets in general, are designed to harness the power of *competition*, not collaboration. More importantly, they would then need to provide substantive arguments to justify what would at least now be explicit claims about the status of research as a commodity and market norms as the relevant criteria of fairness.

8.7 Models and Empirical Assumptions

At various points in our analysis critics might object that we have relied on questionable empirical assumptions. For instance, we note that even if researchers are committed to conducting research in a particular community, others that could host future research projects at a lower cost have an incentive to recruit researchers away. But it might be objected that hosting a trial can give that community an advantage over other communities and make it more likely that they could retain future research initiatives while still increasing the benefits that they receive. So, things might not turn out as badly as our model predicts. Perhaps this is the case with other features of our model as well.

Several responses to are in order. First, our analysis is intended to illustrate the importance of providing stakeholders with some framework for assessing the normative claims that one makes on behalf of a proposed procedural approach. This framework should clarify for stakeholders how the proposed procedures are likely to behave, given realistic assumptions, and it should help stakeholders understand the variables that will determine how the approach performs in actual practice. Proponents of the fair benefits approach have not done this. We have tried to fill this gap. If proponents of the fair benefits approach have a different model to propose, they are welcome to elaborate it. But it is not a vindication of their approach, as it has been articulated to date, to leave our model and its general conclusions unchallenged and simply to hope that something will happen in actual practice that will avert its predictions from coming to pass.

Second, one advantage of articulating a model of the form that we provide is that it makes such questions more tractable by bringing into focus the set of factors or variables that are relevant to the model's predictions. In this case, for example, whether researchers are likely to relocate can depend on the extent to which the relevant stakeholders view research as just another form of economic exchange. Research sponsors, after all, are under constant pressure to cut costs and to make their basket of resources stretch farther. We suspect that, if anything, the Fair Benefits Approach contributes to the view that research is an economic opportunity that is rightly governed by market norms. As such, the widespread endorsement of this view might reduce the inhibitions of various stakeholders to relocate research when doing so can be justified on economic grounds.

Third, in all cases, the probability that researchers will relocate in the future hinges on whether other communities can make themselves more attractive hosts. It would be a mistake to understand this claim as somehow imputing crude or insensitive motives to researchers. This reflects one of the recurring themes of this work, namely, that the motives of various parties may matter much less than structural features of the social system in which those parties are constrained to act. The myopic focus of orthodox research ethics screens out the larger, social dynamics that influence the terms on which research is carried out. Researchers may have deep commitments to host communities, but they may not be able to live up to those commitments if they are under pressure from sponsors or others to relocate in order to cut costs. In fact, we have shown that the way that a particular system is structured can have such far-reaching consequences that it can create situations in which altruistically motivated acts have unintended, deleterious consequences (§8.3.5).

Nothing in our analysis presupposes that stakeholders have unsavory motivations. Nevertheless, it is important to recognize that there are armies of well-paid professionals who make their living analyzing systems and figuring out how to maximize the returns of their firms. "Gaming the system" may be frowned upon in some forms of "collaborative partnership," but in the market, the ability to work the system to one's advantage is regarded as a virtue rather than a vice. Since market norms play such a pervasive role in the fair benefits approach, these concerns are centrally relevant.

One implication of the analysis presented here is that the fair benefits approach could easily function in practice as a kind of ethical Trojan horse. Ambiguities and inconsistencies at the conceptual level make it attractive to a broad range of stakeholders, each of whom has a different view of how to understand and reconcile its core commitments. But when it is carried out in practice, this view may simply entail that LMICs are free to "collaborate" in research that advances the health interests of HIC populations while HIC sponsors are free to use their considerable bargaining power to capture almost all of the benefits generated by such collaborations.

We have also argued that in order to clarify the normative content of their position, proponents of this approach cannot avoid engaging substantive issues of fairness and justice. In this regard, both proponents and critics of the fair benefits approach need to pay greater attention to a move that the fair benefits approach uses to shape the terms of the debate, but for which we can find no explicit argumentation. Recall that Wertheimer treats exploitation as a micro-level concern. It is a property of discrete interactions between individual actors and it is supposed to be independent of broader background concerns about rights and justice. As we mentioned earlier, the key issue on this view is not which benefits are received, but how much. This in turn motivates the view that whether a particular research project is aligned with and focused on the health needs of the host community is less relevant (if it is relevant at all) than the question of whether they receive a sufficient level of benefits in return for hosting the study. And this leads to a view that effectively treats research as a commodity whose distribution is rightly governed by market forces.

But even if one were to agree, for the sake of argument, that Wertheimer's view of exploitation is the correct view of that concept, this does not establish (1) that the most fundamental or important ethical issues in the context of international research are those that occur at the micro-level, (2) that researchers (as opposed to other stakeholders such as governments, nongovernmental organizations, or funding agencies) should be seen as the primary duty bearers in this context, or (3) that researchers should be treated essentially as private parties with no prior obligations that are relevant to the exchange.

As we saw in §3.7, questions about the funding, regulation, and conduct of international research are issues of institutional design. But concerns about the fairness of *institutional systems* cannot be accommodated within Wertheimer's account of exploitation since his view applies only to the discrete interactions of individuals and not to the operation of institutions. Once again, the myopic focus on discrete interactions between a narrow set of stakeholders is insufficient to capture the way that the incentives that these actors face are structured by the rules and norms of larger social systems.

8.8 Why Minimalism about Justice Is Problematic

8.8.1 Allowing Power to Define the Space of Equality

In research ethics, the desire to avoid controversial commitments and pro-tracted debates about justice motivates what I have called a minimalist approach to this principle. It is minimalist in the sense that it offers a thin conception of justice in which the real evaluative work is done by the more well-defined and well-understood values of beneficence and respect for persons. Part of the allure of the fair benefits approach is that it purports to offer a procedure that can be used in the face of disagreement about difficult questions of justice to ensure that research agreements are voluntary, mutu-ally beneficial, and fair.

Despite appearances, this approach does not avoid entanglements with controversial conceptions of justice. Instead, its conditions together rep-resent an example of what Brian Barry calls "justice as mutual advantage" (Barry 1989). In seeking to avoid the controversies associated with thick conceptions of justice, the minimalist approach covertly elects a particular account of justice to govern international research initiatives without explic-itly having to defend this approach as a particular conception of justice.

In justice as mutual advantage, the parties to a transaction bargain to en-sure that each is made better off as a result of the interaction. The require-ment that acceptable bargains must provide each party with a net benefit, even if agreements must be reached under conditions of full information devoid of force and fraud, is perfectly consistent with agreements in which the distribution of those benefits is hugely disproportionate. This is in part because the way benefits are distributed reflects inequalities in the power of the bargainers.

Justice as mutual advantage does not deny that, from the moral point of view, equals should be treated equally. But it allows equality to be defined, often implicitly, by the capacity of individuals to help or harm others. Those who are equally situated in their capacity to help or to harm receive equal treatment while those in a less advantaged position receive proportionately worse treatment. Lopsided agreements between parties of unequal power are not only to be expected but track the underlying inequalities that define the space of equality.

Allowing inequalities in power to legitimate inequalities in entitlements effectively accepts Hobbes's view that "the value or worth of a man is, as for all other things, his price, that is to say, so much as would be given for the use of his power; and therefore is not absolute, but a thing dependent on the need and judgment of another" (Hobbes 1985, X, 16). Far from agnosticism about justice, this position tacitly embraces the view that the value or worth of a person is a function of their use value to a potential bargainer seeking to maximize her own share of the surplus of cooperation. Disease and lack of access to medical care effectively function as valuable commodities whose use value to researchers or sponsors from HICs gives some a place at the bargaining table. The more widespread a particular condition of sickness and disease, the less power individuals or communities of individuals with that condition have since those who hold out for more can be replaced by those willing to accept less.

Individuals and communities who lack the "good fortune" to suffer from a condition that is of interest to scientists and companies in HICs have no seat at the bargaining table. Their plight is of no use value to researchers and so they are consigned to die in silence because the power differential in their case is so great that they cannot either help or harm potential collaborators. As Barry notes in a discussion of principles of reciprocity or fair play in general, while they specify terms that cooperative endeavors must meet in order to be fair, they do not "say that it is unfair for a practice that would, if it existed, be mutually beneficial, not to exist" (Barry 1982, 231). In other words, when justice is framed as a fair exchange, it does not recognize any obligation to engage in cooperation where cooperation does not yet exist.

This has a profoundly distorting effect on our approach to LMIC health needs. Those who care about the plight of disadvantaged people simply because they are fellow human beings are forced to resort to eloquent attempts to portray rampant sickness and disease as a threat to global prosperity or national security—to the affluence and security of more powerful parties who already have a seat at the bargaining table (Heymann 2000). Highlighting the potential for disease to cross borders and to transgress socioeconomic, racial, and ethnic boundaries represents a way of pleading the case for the plight of groups who might otherwise not be recognized as having moral standing. In effect, this tactic seeks to make the plight of the least advantaged salient by emphasizing its instrumental importance to the people who are tacitly treated as really mattering, the more powerful groups whose interests might be impacted by unchecked disease that flows from conditions of deprivation.

Focusing primarily on transactional fairness also encourages a piecemeal and ad hoc approach to the needs of LMIC communities for two reasons.

First, it allows decisions about research priorities, which strategies to pursue and where research should be conducted to be determined by the nearly unchecked discretion of the stronger party. Second, it allows the stronger party's interests to dictate the terms on which bargains can be carried out. As a result, there are no grounds internal to this view on which to object to interactions with LMIC communities that are initiated by and structured entirely around the needs and interests of HIC firms or entities. Nor are there grounds, inherent to this approach, to differentiate between the types of need that research might address, whether research addresses root causes of problems or is orthogonal to the priority health concerns for host populations.

8.8.2 Screening Out Morally Relevant Information

Avoiding broader questions of justice carries with it a larger risk to which the parochialism of orthodox research ethics is already prone. Focusing narrowly on micro-level transactions between a narrow set of parties screens out as irrelevant some of the very questions that lie at the heart of justice, understood as a value of social institutions.

First, this approach treats the status quo as the relevant moral baseline against which possible actions are to be evaluated. Against this baseline, the only actors whose conduct is relevant to assessment are the parties to the specific micro-level transaction under consideration. These assumptions cast international research initiatives in terms that fit easily within the conceptual ecosystem of orthodox research ethics. But, in doing so, they risk begging the very questions that make such initiatives so morally fraught.

Second, this narrow frame effectively excludes as irrelevant the character and quality of past relationships of extraction and domination that might have contributed to social conditions of poverty and deprivation in which sickness and disease flourish. But past relationships of injustice, or the failure to discharge important social responsibilities can give rise to obligations to provide more or better than what is reflected in the status quo.

Finally, this narrow frame treats the relationship between the health needs of individuals and the broader social, political, and economic context that structure and shape those needs as morally unproblematic. But the health of individuals and their ability to influence their own health status is fundamentally shaped by the way basic social structures promote or frustrate the capabilities of, and the range of opportunities open to, the individuals whose lives they govern. Abstracting the health needs of a community from this larger context therefore excludes the information necessary to evaluate the extent to which important rules, practices, and social structures influence those needs.

Treating the organization of the basic social institutions of a community as given elides the distinction between cases in which populations suffer because of the failures of less-than-decent social structures and cases in which decent social structures are overwhelmed by natural disasters. This obscures some of the grounds on which individuals in the host community might have a legitimate claim against one another, or against their own government to better conditions. It also obscures the grounds on which the influence of third parties, such as foreign governmental and corporate entities, on the community's basic social structure might generate obligations to go above and beyond the status quo.

How power is distributed, the terms on which social authority is exercised and the purposes for which shared social resources are expended are issues that fall under the purview of a theory of justice (Freeman 1990). These questions structure the context in which research transactions take place and that determine who has the ability to negotiate for particular ends, on particular terms. But they also have a profound impact on other fundamental aspects of human agency and experience that provide far less arbitrary grounds for claims to equal consideration from the moral point of view.[5]

When we approach the problem of assessing potential collaborative research initiatives from this broader perspective, therefore, we must at the very least leave conceptual room to consider whether the interests that are frustrated or defeated by less-than-decent social structures are so fundamental as to generate a duty on the part of others to assist them.[6] In the next chapter I argue that claims of justice limit how research can be organized within national boundaries and how it can permissibly be organized when it reaches across national boundaries.

---

[5] On different efforts to define the space of moral equality and for a defense of a particular version of the capabilities approach see Anderson (1999).

[6] This point is dramatized by proponents of the so-called interest theory of rights. For example, Raz (1984, 195) argues that "'x has a right' if and only if x can have rights, and other things being equal, an aspect of x's well-being (his interest) is a sufficient reason for holding some other person(s) to be under a duty." See also Nussbaum (1999, 236).

9

Justice and the Human Development Approach to International Research

9.1 Introduction

The previous chapter illustrates how efforts to avoid difficult questions of justice in research ethics have not succeeded. At best this aversion has built up an unresolved "tectonic friction" between the way that orthodox research ethics deals with domestic research in high-income countries (HICs) and the set of issues and stakeholders that are salient when research is funded and conducted by entities from HICs but carried out in populations from low- and middle-income countries (LMICs). At worst, rather than preserving agnosticism about potentially controversial issues, the field's general aversion to questions of justice and reliance on other foundational principles of bioethics and research ethics has resulted in the default acceptance of one particularly narrow conception of justice from a much larger space of possible alternatives.

In this chapter I argue that the best way to eliminate this tectonic friction is to reconstruct the foundations of research ethics on terms that reflect the requirements of the egalitarian research imperative. The lesson to learn from recent debates about the ethics of international research is not that we need to purge international frameworks of appeals to requirements that are grounded in justice and that implicate a wider range of stakeholders. It is that we need to recognize justice as the first virtue of social institutions, acknowledge that research with humans is a scheme of social cooperation involving a wide range of stakeholders that both calls into action and feeds into important social institutions, and we need to hold both domestic and international research to the requirements of the egalitarian research imperative. I refer to the resulting view as the *human development approach to international research*.

Although the human development approach deals specifically with international research, it is important to emphasize that it extends into

For the Common Good. Alex John London, Oxford University Press. © Oxford University Press 2022.
DOI: 10.1093/oso/9780197534830.003.0009

the international context the egalitarian research imperative outlined in chapter 4, the integrative approach to research risk in chapter 6, and the non-paternalistic approach to research oversight in chapter 7. In §9.2 I provide a brief overview of the key claims of the human development approach. I then elaborate and defend particular aspects of this view in more detail. In §9.3 I show how this approach situates research within a larger project of human development that is focused on ensuring that the basic social structures of a community function to secure the fair value of the basic interests of community members. Then in §9.4 I argue that this position supports a duty to promote research that fulfills this social mission.

Within this context, the duties of responsiveness and post-trial access operate at two levels. At the system level there is a duty to shape the incentives of the research system so that it promotes the conduct of research aimed at generating the knowledge needed to expand the capacity of basic social institutions in LMIC communities—including their systems of individual and public health—to more effectively, efficiently, and equitably meet needs that represent development priorities for that community's members. Post-trial access ensures that this knowledge and the interventions, practices, and procedures that it supports are incorporated into the basic social institutions of the host community. At the level of research review these requirements should be enforced to prevent powerful parties from advancing their own interests at the expense of the common good of LMIC communities.

In §9.5 I argue that only the local de jure standard of care allows studies to advance the common good while respecting the status of participants as free and equal persons. To substantiate this claim I show how this interpretation of the standard of care dovetails with the requirements of the integrative approach from chapter 6 and how alternative interpretations of the standard of care can fail to track the requirement of social value or the principle of equal concern. This chapter then closes with some comments about the challenges associated with linking the conduct of research to philosophically contentious positions about domestic and international justice.

9.2 Overview of the Human Development Approach

The human development approach to international research is a framework for organizing and evaluating research that crosses national boundaries or that takes place within a single nation but involves funders, researchers, or other actors from other nations or from extra-national entities such as governmental or non-governmental international organizations. It is particularly relevant to research that takes place in LMIC communities that is funded, organized, conducted, or otherwise influenced by entities from HICs.

This framework is grounded in the same concern for the basic interests of persons that defines the basic interests conception of the common good and that motivates the egalitarian research imperative. It holds that in every community, individuals have a just claim to basic social structures that are organized around and function to secure the common good of that community's members. On the basic interest conception of the common good, this means that community members have a just claim to basic social institutions that function to secure for all community members the fair value of the basic intellectual, affective, social, and physical capacities they need to formulate, pursue, and revise a life plan on terms that are consistent with equal regard for the interest of their compatriots to do the same.

Because the basic social structures of most communities fall short of the requirements of justice, the members of every community have a claim on one another and their social authorities to support a larger program of human development. This is a multisectoral process of promoting and reforming the terms on which their basic social structures function so as to more closely approximate the requirements of a just social order for all community members. This includes a claim on local authorities to use existing knowledge and resources to advance the basic interests of that community's members. Internationally, residents of affluent countries, government officials, and stakeholders in private and public organizations also have a duty to contribute to this process of human development in LMICs.

In both domestic and international cases, the human development approach holds that the obligation to promote human development extends to a duty to discharge the egalitarian research imperative. This involves helping LMIC communities to create a certain division of social labor among one set of basic social institutions that has as its ultimate goal the improvement of a related set of basic social institutions. In particular, this is a division of social labor in which stakeholders and institutions employ the distinctive scientific and statistical methods of research to generate the knowledge and the means necessary to bridge shortfalls or gaps in the ability of that community's basic social structures (such as their systems of individual and public health) to effectively, efficiently, or equitably safeguard and advance the basic interests of that community's members.

A shortfall of this kind obtains when a threat to the basic interests of community members cannot be more effectively, efficiently, or equitably addressed through the application of existing knowledge and resources. Such threats may be novel in the sense that their cause is unknown or there are no established effective means of addressing them. Alternatively, such threats can be novel in the sense that established effective means of addressing them exist, but there is significant conflict or uncertainty about their relative merits under conditions that are attainable and sustainable in the host community.

The human development approach to international research retains the responsiveness requirement, recast to reflect a broader scope for research ethics and its role in shaping the strategic environment in which various parties to the research enterprise interact. Within this framework, the responsiveness requirement operates on two levels. At the system level it is understood as a duty that applies to a wide range of stakeholders to create and sustain a system of knowledge production in which the strategic environment aligns the interests of stakeholders with research that addresses those shortfalls in the basic institutions in LMICs that represent development priorities for host communities. This includes strengthening the capacity of LMICs to conduct research that addresses their distinctive development priorities. At the level of research review, the human development approach endorses a strong but defeasible requirement limiting research initiatives in LMIC contexts to those that are organized, designed, and conducted to produce the information necessary to expand the capacity of the host community's basic social structures to address threats to the basic interests of community members that constitute development priorities for those communities.[1]

The human development approach also retains the requirement of reasonable availability. At the system level, this is understood as a broad-based duty that applies to a wide range of stakeholders to ensure that resources of various kinds are in place so that the knowledge and the means that are developed in research can be incorporated into the basic social structures of host communities. At the level of research review, this translates into a duty to verify that such prior agreements are in place.

Finally, the human development approach holds that research must be conducted on terms that respect the status of study participants and host community members as free and equal persons. To do this, research must be consistent with the principle of equal concern (§6.2.2). The local de jure

---

[1] For a slightly different defense of a similar claim, see Flory and Kitcher (2004, 38–39).

interpretation of the standard of care holds that study participants should not receive a level of care for their basic interests that falls below what experts judge to be the most effective strategy for addressing the need in question under conditions that are attainable and sustainable in basic social systems—such as the local health systems—where the intervention in question will be deployed. Research in which the standard of care provided to participants satisfies this requirement is consistent with the principle of equal concern and is thus consistent with equal respect for the status of study participants and community members as free and equal persons.

Studies that meet the conditions of responsiveness, with credible assurance of reasonable availability, and that provide at least the local de jure standard of care satisfy conditions of justice. They represent an avenue for advancing the common good of LMIC community members on terms that respect the status of those who make these advances possible as free and equal persons.

9.3 Basic Interests and Moral Claims on Basic Social Institutions

9.3.1 Justice and Basic Social Structures

In contrast to the myopia of orthodox research ethics, in which the research activity is severed from its relationship to larger social structures and purposes, the human development approach understands research as an activity that calls into operation basic social institutions in a community and that has as its proper moral function generating the information those institutions need to better fulfill their proper social function. Research is thus a cooperative social activity that is constrained by and beholden to prior moral claims of justice on the part of the community members whose basic interests it shapes and impacts.

The human development approach treats justice as fundamentally concerned with the basic social structures of a society and whether they work to secure for all community members the fair value of their basic human capacities (Rawls 1971; Korsgaard 1993; Anderson 1999; Nussbaum 1999; Sen 1999b). It also recognizes, however, that in the nonideal world in which we live, the basic social institutions of most communities fall short of the requirements of justice. This shortfall is the motivation for a larger project of human development that takes these basic social structures as its focus.

In particular, the goal of this long-term, multisectoral project is to establish and foster, for every community, basic social structures that are organized around, and function in the service of, the common good of that community's members (Nussbaum 1999; Sen 1999b).

There are two reasons why the human development approach requires that international research initiatives must be evaluated in terms of the way they draw on and impact the basic social institutions of a community.[2] I state these reasons briefly here and then elaborate on each in §9.3.2 and §9.3.3.

First, the basic social structures of a community consist in the political, legal, social, economic, and health-related institutions that determine the distribution of fundamental rights and liberties and that set the terms on which individuals can access all-purpose goods and resources such as food, shelter, education, and productive employment, as well as health services necessary to protect, preserve, or restore the ability to function. These institutions are basic because they represent the background institutions, rules, entitlements, and restrictions within which other social interactions take place (Rawls 2001, 10).

These institutions have a deep and pervasive impact on the life prospects of those they govern because they regulate how rights and liberties are distributed and the terms on which community members can access individual and social opportunity. They determine the terms on which community members have access to education, productive employment, to the political process, control over their person and their personal environment, and protection of their basic human rights. As a result, how these structures operate is an important social determinant of health (Sen 1981, 1999b; Drèze and Sen 1989). More important than the sheer economic wealth of a community is whether the community directs its resources to creating and sustaining social conditions that promote the ability of community members to develop and exercise their basic intellectual, affective, and social capacities in the service of formulating, pursuing, and revising a life plan of their own (Daniels et al. 1999; Sen 1999b). Because the health

---

[2] It is worth emphasizing again that the human development approach is not a quixotic effort to lump the moral responsibility for addressing all injustice onto the shoulders of researchers or the research enterprise (see chapter 4 note 23). Rather, the goal is to specify the unique role that research can play in within a just division of social labor and to articulate criteria that can be used to promote research that advances those ends and to avoid research that detracts from them.

status of individuals is affected by a matrix of political, social, and economic factors, the project of creating and sustaining the conditions that foster health requires a coordinated, multisectoral approach that is sensitive to these interrelationships.

Second, this network of social institutions itself represents a division of social labor in which responsibility for safeguarding the basic interests of people in different spheres of life (e.g., education, health care, criminal justice) is delegated to identifiable parties. If all persons are morally equal to the extent that they share the same higher-order interest in having real freedom to formulate, pursue, and revise a reasonable life plan of their own (§4.5.3), then every community bears a responsibility of justice to ensure that its educational, economic, legal, political, criminal justice, and health-related social institutions work to realize this goal for all community members. In every community, in other words, there is a duty to ensure that this division of social labor works to produce what Henry Shue refers to as "full coverage" to the legitimate claims of community members (1988).

International research is to be evaluated against this background conception of justice and human development. It advances the goals of human development when it works to expand the capacity of a community's basic social systems to more effectively, efficiently and equitably secure or advance the basic interests of its members.

9.3.2 Social Determinants of Health and Prior Moral Claims

Members of a community have prior moral claims on the basic social structures of their community because those structures have such a profound impact on their rights, liberties, and health. Social structures that are not organized around or that do not function in the service of the common good create conditions in which some are denied effective opportunities to develop and exercise their basic capacities while others enjoy a rich array of opportunities and resources that support individual achievement (Daniels et al. 1999; Marmot and Bell 2012). Very often, these are also the conditions under which avoidable sickness, disease, and premature mortality flourish (Marmot and Wilkinson 2005; Commission on Social Determinants of Health 2008). When individuals in such conditions lack access to the basic building blocks of social and economic opportunity and healthy living, the harms that result cannot be dismissed as accidents of nature or justified by reference to the common good. They represent a failure to use the state's control over basic social structures to advance the interests of community members. Those who suffer in these cases can legitimately claim, as a strict obligation of justice, an entitlement to relief from such hardships.

To illustrate this point, consider some parallels between the health needs of LMIC populations and Amartya Sen's groundbreaking work on famine (Sen 1981; Drèze and Sen 1989). Famines are commonly viewed as natural disasters caused principally by a combination of poverty and poor food production. Sen showed, however, that these factors alone do not account for the occurrence of famines. For example, in 1979–1981 and 1983–1984, Sudan and Ethiopia experienced declines in food production of 11% or 12% and, like a number of other countries in sub-Saharan Africa, suffered massive famines. During the same period, however, food production declined by 17% in Botswana and by a precipitous 38% in Zimbabwe, yet these countries did not suffer the ravages of famine (Sen 1999b, 178–180).

According to Sen, the reason for this difference in outcomes can be traced to differences in the social and political structures of these countries. Botswana and Zimbabwe had rudimentary democratic social institutions that enabled them to stave off famine. They implemented a series of social support programs targeted at enhancing the economic purchasing power of affected groups while also supplementing food supplies. Mass starvation occurred in Sudan and Ethiopia because the dictatorial regimes in those nations failed to take such relatively simple social and economic steps to safeguard their citizens' interests.

These lessons should inform our view of sickness and disease more generally (Benatar 1998, 2001, 2002, Van Niekerk, A. A. (2002).). For example, HIV/AIDS has had a devastating impact on many populations in sub-Saharan Africa. In some nations, during the 1990s, as much as 30% of the population was HIV positive. In sharp contrast, during that same period, Senegal was able to limit both the prevalence of HIV/AIDS and the rate of new infections to about 1% of the population. The principal cause of Senegal's success lies not in advanced technology or great wealth, but in the government's long-standing, grassroots investment in its human resources. In Senegal, information about HIV/AIDS and many other sexually transmitted diseases has been disseminated through an assortment of educational programs. Empowering individuals with information and opportunities for activism enhances the public's capacities for communal interaction, free expression, and political participation and so creates a social context in which people can more effectively safeguard and secure their welfare.

This focus on education and activism has been further enhanced by the judicious use of scarce resources. Senegal closely monitors its blood supply and distributes millions of condoms free of charge. It invests in monitoring and treating many sexually transmitted diseases, especially in target populations such as commercial sex workers, young people, truck drivers, and the spouses of migrant workers. Additionally, as part of a program of perinatal care, it was one of the first countries to offer antiretroviral drugs to pregnant women, although on a very limited basis. This multisectoral approach to HIV/AIDS, and to public health in general, has halved HIV prevalence and illustrates the positive health effects of policies that strive to protect citizens' basic capacities for agency and welfare (Kharsany and Karim 2016).

The terms on which the basic social structures of a community are organized have a profound and far-reaching effect on the ability of community members to secure and advance their basic interests. Because every community member is equal insofar as they share the higher-order interest in having real freedom to formulate, pursue, and revise a life plan of their own, every community member has a moral claim to a set of basic social structures that are organized around the goal of securing this interest. As a result, resources that domestic authorities are willing to make available to various actors—including the parties who would use those resources for research purposes—may not be "available" in a more fundamental moral sense: those who control them have a prior moral obligation to deploy them in the service of ends that better advance the goals of human development (§4.8.2).

The same is true for other ways in which authorities might use the power of their offices. Regimes can fail to serve the common good by neglecting basic social institutions altogether, by misappropriating or misdirecting the time and energies of their personnel, or by inappropriately restricting or occupying important institutional spaces. These failures can violate prior moral claims that constrain the ways in which important social institutions can exercise authority and allocate various human and material resources (Gostin 2010). These prior claims—of all citizens to a set of basic social structures that secure and advance their basic interests, and of citizens whose interests are set back by failures or deficiencies in these basic social structures—shape and limit the terms on which research in a community can be conducted.

9.3.3 Full Coverage to Moral Claims

Because the basic interests of community members define the space of equality and because those with equal claims are equally deserving of assistance, efforts to secure and advance these interests must strive to satisfy the requirement of full coverage. A social arrangement, a policy, or an initiative satisfies the condition of full coverage to the extent that it addresses the interest of every party with a legitimate claim. As Shue (1988) notes, the duty of full coverage is often best achieved through a division of social labor in which specific parties are assigned particular duties and prerogatives that are jointly necessary to meet the conditions of full coverage.

For Rawls (1971, 7; 2001, 10), the basic social institutions of society represent exactly this sort of social division of labor. Their purpose is to assigns specific responsibilities, duties, permissions, and prerogatives to identified parties who are delegated specific tasks for meeting particular needs under specific terms and constraints. This division of labor thus seeks to increase the coverage of rights, resources, services, and opportunities provided to community members to secure their higher-order interest in having real freedom to formulate, pursue, and revise a life plan on terms that are consistent with the real freedom of their compatriots to do the same.

The health-related institutions of a community, including its public health and healthcare institutions, contribute to the process of human development in two fundamental ways. First, sickness, injury, and disease can undermine the ability of persons to exercise those basic cognitive and affective abilities they need to take full advantage of opportunities in various spheres of life, such as personal, social, economic, and political spheres (Daniels 1985). Sickness and disease can hinder education, frustrate full participation in the social and political life of a community, and reduce access to employment and economic opportunity. These deprivations, in turn, can produce compounding effects that hamper a person's ability to advance their own interests, including their health, educational, social, and economic interests (Bloom and Canning 2000; Jamison et al. 2013). Health systems promote human development through prevention efforts to reduce the probability that health-related threats materialize, through ameliorative efforts to mitigate the harmful effects of sickness and disease when they do occur, and by making available the knowledge and the means that individuals, clinicians, policy makers, and others require to make decisions about how to effectively safeguard and advance the basic interests of persons.

Second, although other elements of the basic social structures of the community provide individuals with important social determinants of health—education, nutrition, employment, access to social and political opportunity, and respect for basic human rights—health-related institutions address the health needs of individuals that persist in the face of these social determinants. Even if a just social order produces widespread health benefits for community members (Daniels et al. 1999; Sreenivasan 2007), residual sickness, injury, and disease can nevertheless impair the ability of afflicted individuals to realize the fair value of their basic abilities. The systems of individual and public health provide an infrastructure for addressing these residual needs.

To meet the duty of full coverage, health systems must be configured to make effective, efficient, and equitable use of existing knowledge and resources. Efforts to advance the goals of human development in health should first seek to close gaps in the ability of health systems to safeguard and secure the basic interests of community members by expanding their capacity to make use of existing knowledge and resources. Even a relatively modest increase in international aid targeted this way would transform the health needs of LMIC communities (Pogge 2002, 79). Roughly 90% of the avoidable mortality in LMICs stems from a handful of causes for which effective interventions already exist (Jhah et al. 2002). Making those interventions available through local health systems would have a transformative effect on individual health and opportunity (Jamison et al. 2013).

Even if these efforts are undertaken with new urgency and commitment, two broad categories of research with humans have an important role to play in advancing the goals of human development.[3] The first deals with the development of diagnostic, prophylactic (especially vaccine research), therapeutic, and vector control interventions. These interventions target health needs that persist in the face of such development efforts or represent strategies for addressing health needs that would significantly advance the ability of health systems to contribute to development goals. This type of research focuses on conditions of special importance to LMICs including HIV, malaria, tuberculosis, typhoid, kinetoplastids, parasitic worms, staphylococcal

---

[3] Discussing the increase in average life expectancy in LMICs and the decrease in cross-country inequalities in the last half century, Jamison et al. note, "Of much greater quantitative significance, however, have been the generation and diffusion of new knowledge and of low-cost, appropriate technologies. Increased access to knowledge and technology has accounted for perhaps as much as two-thirds of the impressive 2 percent per year rate of decline in under-five mortality rates" (2006, 4).

infections, diarrheal disease, and strategies for improving the ability of women and girls to avoid unplanned pregnancy and to reduce maternal and infant mortality (PATH 2014). It is also important to produce interventions that can be implemented at scale under conditions that are attainable and sustainable in LMIC contexts. An example of research of this kind in the context of vaccines includes research to produce formulations that require fewer doses; that are stable under hotter temperatures; that are effective against multiple strains of a pathogen, such as influenza; or that offer combined protection against multiple pathogens, such as a combined diarrheal vaccine against rotavirus, enterotoxigenic Escherichia coli, typhoid, and shigella (Jamison et al. 2013, 1940–1944). As the health needs of LMICs shift and non-communicable diseases account for an increasingly large share of the burden of disease, it will be important to develop interventions with similar utility for LMIC health systems.

The second category is health policy, health systems and implementation research. Establishing that interventions are effective against a particular condition is only a small part of the knowledge needed to use a set of interventions to improve the health of people on a large scale. Research in this category is necessary to determine whether and under what conditions interventions, whether newly developed or already established effective in a different context, can be deployed at scale in LMIC contexts in ways that increase the effectiveness, efficiency, or equity with which health systems are able to address the health needs of their populations. The same applies to research on individual and public health policies, programs, and health systems (Haines et al. 2004; Paina and Peters 2012; Alonge et al. 2019; Sheikh et al. 2020). This includes identifying and closing gaps in service provision; identifying and addressing impediments to intervention uptake, utilization, and adherence; and identifying and addressing shortfalls in the ability of current systems to secure and advance the health needs of populations that are marginalized, subject to exclusion or prejudice, or in some other respect historically underserved (Pratt and Hyder 2015).

9.3.4 Research and Basic Social Structures

The prior moral claims that citizens have to basic social structures that secure and advance the common good motivate the egalitarian research imperative and constrain the terms on which research with humans is morally permissible. In part, this is because research is a scheme of social cooperation that stands in a special relationship to the basic social structures of a community. Because of this relationship, research is entangled in a network of moral claims that shape both the permissible goals of research and the conditions on which research can be permissibly carried out.

First, as we saw in § 4.7.2–3, research stands in a special relationship to the basic structures of a community because it produces a unique public good. This public good is the information and means necessary to understand threats to the basic interests of community members, the causal processes involved in the lifecycle of such threats, to understand and develop alternative means of addressing those threats, and to clarify the relative merits of possible preventative or restorative strategies. The ability of a community's basic social structures, such as its institutions of individual and public health, to effectively, efficiently, and equitably secure and advance the basic interests of community members thus depends on how the research enterprise is structured and functions (Easterlin 1999). In part, this is because myriad stakeholders rely on the information produced in research to make decisions that impact health and welfare, the use of scarce social resources, and the entitlements of community members.[4] It is also because research is often the only way to produce the information and the means necessary to bridge gaps in the ability of a community's basic social structures to safeguard and advance the basic interests of that community's members.

Second, the research enterprise calls into action the basic social institutions of a society.[5] This can involve legislative action or rule making to support research through public financing or to shape intellectual property rights or conditions for market access in order to align the incentives of private actors with the common good. Similar legislation or rule making might create

---

[4] A key insight of Wenner (2018) is that failure to enforce requirements that research must produce social value for host communities has led to the concentration of power in the hands of private actors to shape the system of evidence production in ways that advance their own interests, and the interests of a narrow band of identifiable parties, to the detriment of a wider swath of the population whose health needs are deemed less lucrative or otherwise less worthy of investigation.

[5] For arguments to the effect that considerations of justice arise from the fact that research frequently relies on social resources and that this is true even for research conducted by private entities, see London (2005), London et al. (2010), and Wendler and Rid (2017). Wenner (2018) associates these arguments with a transactional view of research which she rightly rejects. The point I want to emphasize here is that these resources are made available, not just to support individual research transactions, but to create the kind of infrastructure that supports research and that shapes the terms on which it is conducted. It raises issues of justice, then, because it represents the use of social authority and the creation of rules, institutions, and social systems that shape an activity that has the kind of profound impacts that Wenner describes.

social institutions with the mandate to conduct research, to support the conduct of research by others, to regulate the products of research, or to oversee different elements in the lifecycle of knowledge generation and product development, licensing, marketing, and sales. This can include enacting rules and regulations that set standards for regulatory approval or for ensuring the ethical conduct of scientifically sound research. It can involve shaping educational institutions and curricula to train and educate actors capable of engaging in research or engaging in one of the allied disciplines that support the research enterprise or take it as its subject matter.

All of these activities require the exercise of social authority for the purpose of creating a system of rules and institutions that allocate rights and privileges, divide responsibility, and allocate scarce material resources, human time, and attention to support research activities. The exercise of this authority and the institutions, laws, rules, and investments that it produces must be justifiable to community members as serving and advancing the common good.

Finally, in addition to being a form of social cooperation that serves important public purposes and requires the exercise of social authority and various forms of public support, research is also an activity that directly affects the basic interests of participants. For all of these reasons, it must be organized and carried out on terms that respect the status of its various participants as free and equal persons. In part, this reiterates the logic of appeals to the common good, namely, that social activities undertaken to advance the common good must be carried out on terms that respect the common good (§4.5.5). So, research activities undertaken with the goal of enhancing the ability of health systems to protect, restore, or promote the basic interests of community members must be carried out on terms that reflect equal concern for the basic interests of research stakeholders, including study participants.

In light of these moral claims, the human development approach holds that the research enterprise must function as part of a division of social labor in which it is the purpose of the basic social institutions of a community to discharge the duty of providing full coverage to the basic interests of community members. The distinctive role that research can play in this division of social labor is to use scientific and statistical methods to target and investigate the means of filling gaps in the ability of those social structures to meet those needs.[6] The research enterprise represents a permissible use

---

[6] Wenner makes a similar point when she says that "Clinical research is one aspect of an institutional structure that governs the health systems that are available to individuals, that individuals

of a community's social authority and scarce public resources and is a permissible target of social support when it functions to expand the capacity of the basic social structures of that community to more effectively, efficiently, or equitably safeguard and advance the basic interests of that community's members.

When it is not possible to address every such knowledge gap then the stakeholders who shape the direction and focus of research have a duty to ensure that mechanisms are in place to focus research activities on knowledge gaps that represent priorities for human development. Because this is a claim about the way that research must relate to the basic social institutions of a community, it holds for all research, including domestic research carried out in HIC contexts. In the context of international medical research, the human development approach holds that stakeholders who shape the direction and focus of scientific research have a duty to promote research that targets the priority health needs of LMIC populations and to ensure that all research is carried out in a way that is responsive to and aligned with those needs.

Recognizing the importance of research to development underscores that the egalitarian research imperative requires that HICs support the ability of LMICs to carry out research of this kind for themselves. In other words, it is not sufficient that research resources and expertise be controlled by HIC sponsors and deployed in LMIC settings (Sitthi-Amorn and Somrongthong 2000; Nuyens 2005). Rather, the goal is to create and sustain the infrastructure in LMICs to support research that addresses their development priorities (Pratt and Loff 2014; Pratt and Hyder 2015).

9.4 The Duty to Promote Human Development

9.4.1 Avoiding Three Moral Pitfalls

In chapter 3 I argued that Wertheimer's radical proposal to permit relationships of exploitation, unfairness and injustice was motivated, in part, by a frustration over the way that orthodox research ethics navigates three

cannot opt out of, and that will have deep and lasting impacts on their life prospects, their final ends and purposes, and the way that they think of themselves" (2018, 31).

moral pitfalls. In particular, when the requirements of responsiveness and reasonable availability are applied by IRBs at the time of protocol review, they can prevent LMIC populations from engaging in research that might offer those populations a net benefit without ensuring that a better alternative is waiting in the wings. The concern, then, is that strong prohibitions against exploitation and unfairness might avert unfair or disrespectful relationships while leaving host communities vulnerable to the ravages of lethal neglect.

Alternatively, efforts to avoid neglect by requiring researchers to discharge a duty to aid or a duty to rectify past histories of injustice appear to arbitrarily saddle a narrow group of actors with a demanding duty to rectify unjust conditions that are not of their making, or that are not solely of their making. Because the decision-making of parties such as lawmakers, ministers of health, regulatory agencies, or private philanthropies who shape the research agenda is treated as falling outside the purview of orthodox research ethics, there is a kind of conceptual pressure to revise research ethics standards in international research in a way that allows host communities to advance their interests to the greatest extent possible, given the offers they are likely to receive.

The human development approach rejects the presumption that IRBs represent the most appropriate institutional focus for issues of justice in research ethics and that the stakeholders who are party to the IRB process exhaust the set of stakeholders who bear important duties in this realm. Instead, it expands the purview of research ethics to consider the role of research as an element in a just social order and the requirements on its design and conduct necessary to fill this role. The goal is then to advocate for institutional frameworks, laws, policies, incentive structures, partnerships, treaties, and any other viable means necessary to bring the conduct of research in practice into better alignment with these conditions (Benatar and Singer 2000). The stakeholders who bear responsibility for these goals include political leaders, policy makers, corporate leadership, trade organizations, professional societies, international organizations, philanthropies, and others.

In that regard, the primary goal of this framework is not to limit research in LMICs but to expand it. It seeks not to articulate conditions for the ethical conduct of international research and then to hope that stakeholders are motivated to propose research that satisfies those criteria. Rather, the goal is to establish that there is a moral imperative to promote research that satisfies these criteria grounded in the ability of research to produce a unique public good that is intimately tied to the ability of a community's basic social structures to discharge their responsibilities to that community's members.

9.4.2 Human Development and the Egalitarian Research Imperative

The imperative to support research that advances the goals of development is grounded in the relationship between research and the basic social institutions of a community and the moral imperative to undertake a process of human development that takes those social institutions as its target. Every community has a strong moral obligation to support and promote the larger process of human development. This obligation has two foci. The first is inward looking and encompasses the obligation to ensure that the basic social structures of their own community are designed and function on terms that preserve and advance the fair value of every community member's basic interest in having real freedom to formulate, pursue, and revise a life plan of their own (Gostin 2010).

Even technologically advanced HICs have a duty to engage in a domestic process of human development because the rights of women, racial and ethnic minorities, people with disabilities, or other marginalized groups are often unrecognized, or may be recognized on paper but disregarded in practice in ways that detract from the ability of individuals in these classes to realize the fair value of their basic interests. In such cases, unequal treatment for basic interests and the profound consequences this can have for the life prospects of individuals translate into a duty of justice to reform laws, social policies, and institutional arrangements around the goal of securing the fair value of the basic interests of all community members. The same considerations apply to domestic authorities within LMICs who must often discharge this responsibility against a background of severe resource constraints.

The second focus is outward looking and encompasses the obligations that communities have to one another. This obligation has three components. I state each component briefly and then elaborate on them in turn. First, all communities have an obligation to respect and not to undermine just social arrangements, wherever they exist (Rawls 1971, 334; Simmons 1979, 147–156). This obligation is grounded, at least in part, in the important role that the basic social institutions of other communities play in securing the basic interests of the individuals in those communities. Since the basic interests of individuals define the space of moral equality, there is no reason that membership in one community should empower its members to be indifferent to, or malevolent toward, the social arrangements that influence the ability of others to enjoy the fair value of their basic interests.

Second, when a set of communities interact on terms that undermine the capacity of the basic social structures of a subset of communities to advance the common good of their constituent members, the communities that are advantaged by such interactions incur a duty to rectify the consequences of these interactions. Such duties of rectification can stem from ongoing relationships of explicit domination and extraction. They can also arise from social arrangements that may not have been intended to advance such goals but that nevertheless have created a niche that powerful parties have been able to exploit to these ends.

Third, independently of prior relationships, countries with sufficient wealth, political power, and influence have an obligation to assist other communities in creating and sustaining basic social arrangements that satisfy conditions of justice and advance the project of human development. This obligation stems from the importance of the basic interests that are frustrated by less-than-decent social institutions and the ability of affluent and influential communities to encourage and promote systems that better provide full coverage to the claims of those who suffer and toil under adverse social, economic, political, and health conditions.

The human development approach regards each of these outward looking considerations as sufficient to establish a duty to support the larger project of human development in LMICs. We can start with the third consideration and work backwards. Moral frameworks that take human welfare and agency as sources of moral claims recognize that claims of assistance can be grounded in the importance of the basic interests of persons that are frustrated by less-than-decent social institutions (Ruger 2018; Cullity 1994; Sen 1999b; Nussbaum 1996, Ashford 2003). Such frameworks can be consequentialist in nature, but they need not be since they can also ground rights-based frameworks, including accounts of the source and nature of human rights.[7] Likewise, although the importance of these interests is emphasized

---

[7] Sen (1999b) offers an account that has both consequentialist and rights-based components. Proponents of the interest theory of rights, such as Joseph Raz, argue that " 'X has a right' if and only if x can have rights, and other things being equal, an aspect of x's well-being (his interest) is a sufficient reason for holding some other person(s) to be under a duty" (1984, 195). Nussbaum argues that capabilities needed to live a distinctively human life ground human rights claims (1999).

in global egalitarian conceptions of justice (Beitz 1979; Nussbaum 1996; Shue 1996; Brock 2009; Jones 1999; Pogge 2002, 1994; Caney 2005) the moral importance of these interests are often recognized even within state-based or nationalist conceptions of the global order. From the claim that individuals and states might owe special duties to their fellow citizens (e.g., Tamir 1993, 2019; Miller 1995, 2007; Gans 2003), it does not follow that such individuals or states do not also have a duty to aid others. For example, although Rawls rejects a global egalitarian framework that would extend justice as fairness to all people, regardless of national borders, he still holds that well-ordered societies have a duty to assist burdened peoples (Rawls 1999, 105–113).

Moreover, the importance of different aspects of what I am calling the basic interests of persons are reflected in the mission statements of international organizations and help to motivate global development initiatives, such as the millennium development goals, where research has also been recognized as an important element for advancing those goals (Jamison et al. 2013; PATH 2014). In that respect, the moral imperative to respond to threats to the basic interests of persons—whether formulated in consequentialist terms or in human rights language—is already recognized in some international policy and programs. In this respect, the human development approach seeks to bring research ethics into better alignment with ethical considerations whose relevance to policy and practice is already recognized though imperfectly supported and realized in practice.

The duty to aid is bolstered by prior relationships that generate special duties of rectification.[8] Many LMICs continue to struggle from the legacy of extractive relationships including colonial rule and post-colonial turmoil. Part of the enduring legacy of colonialism is the extent to which the interests of colonial powers shaped local policies and institutions in colonized territories, often to the detriment of those populations (Turshen 1977; Manderson 2002; Pearson 2018). To amass wealth and secure access to natural resources and raw materials, colonial powers co-opted the social structures of colonized peoples and fostered social divisions that could be exploited to prevent unified insurrection. Although foreign governments were most directly

---

[8] This argument is briefly explored in the context of international research in Crouch and Arras (1998) and Benatar (1998, 2001). For a clear exposition of duties of rectification, see Nozick (1977).

involved in colonial rule, the focus of that rule was often geared at enabling firms to exploit the material and human resources of colonized peoples. The extractive economic systems that colonial powers created were thus exploited by a range of stakeholders, from foreign trading partners to private firms across a variety of industries.

For example, recognizing and supporting what Pogge calls the "international resource privilege" creates a strategic environment in which any group that succeeds in wresting control of the national government in a developing country is recognized as having the legitimate authority "to borrow in the name of its people and to confer legal ownership rights for the country's resources" (Pogge 2002, 73). The existence of this privilege provides not only a powerful incentive for the unscrupulous to seize power, but also a convenient mechanism for consolidating power and then wielding it for the enrichment of a privileged few.[9] Employing power in this way saddles LMICs with disastrous long-term debt and prevents most of the population from sharing in the benefits generated by their country's natural resources. Instead, the benefits are enjoyed primarily by ruling elites and by governments and corporations in HICs who prop up such regimes in exchange for strategic alliances, the sale of military equipment or other large-industry commodities (e.g., airplanes, oil and gas services), and cheap access to raw materials and human resources. Although the global resource privilege is a policy of governments to recognize the authority of other governments, it enables trade among private firms who sell their products and services.

Similarly, one reason drugs are so scarce in LMIC populations is their cost. Many individual pharmaceutical companies played an active role in the negotiation of the Agreement on Trade-Related Aspects of Intellectual Property Rights (TRIPS agreement) at the World Trade Organization. The pharmaceutical lobby has used its considerable influence on US and EU trade representatives to enforce patent protections and intellectual property rights even though the TRIPS agreement allows countries to produce or import generic versions of beneficial medications in cases of national emergency. The pharmaceutical industry has aggressively pressed for trade sanctions or taken legal action against countries that have tried to implement this emergency clause (Barry and Raworth 2002; Schüklenk and Ashcroft 2002). In doing so, it has blocked legitimate efforts to provide

---

[9] Pogge (2002b, chapters 4, 6).

medicines to some of the populations that need them most (Pierson and Millum 2018).

Although specific governments and corporations may owe particularly strong duties of rectification to specific groups whom they directly wrong, the policies and practices of colonial rule and post-colonial exploitation have provided, and in some cases continue to provide, benefits to a wide range of governments and private entities. This includes the citizens of the countries in whose name colonial rule was undertaken and the shareholders in the firms in whose interests profits were maximized.[10]

Because duties of rectification are also owed equally to all parties who are affected, and because the effects of these systems have been widespread, priority should be given to strategies for redress that provide full coverage to those who have been affected. At a minimum, the targets for such a duty include eliminating the global and domestic structures in LMICs that perpetuate extractive relationships and establishing in their place structures that promote human development.

This view of development also provides a needed corrective to what amounts to an inappropriately narrow focus on inequalities in income or wealth in the literature on global justice. For example, a common theme in this literature is that international development requires a significant transfer of wealth from developed to developing nations. Transferring a greater share of wealth to LMIC populations would supposedly alleviate the conditions of poverty that provide the ecological niche in which sickness and disease flourish. Similarly, greater economic prosperity would provide the extremely poor with a broader range of opportunities and the resources necessary to meet more of their most basic needs.[11] To be sure, the development and maintenance of basic social structures are not cost free, and failure to provide monetary and socio-political support for the reform or expansion of such structures will impede a community's ability to achieve full coverage. But whether a transfer of resources will improve the social and economic

---

[10] Statist or nationalist theories of global justice hold that inequalities between states are not morally impermissible, as such, since these inequalities can reflect morally important differences, such as the willingness of certain people to invest time and effort in practices or innovations that turn out to be particularly advantageous. But Miller argues persuasively that such a view of national responsibility is a double-edged sword: it protects advantages won through fair means, but it renders citizens of such states liable for remedial duties tied to past state action (Miller 2007, 265–266).

[11] Sreenivasan claims that "Any plausible and complete ideal of international distributive justice . . . will at least require better-off states to transfer *one percent of their gross domestic product* (GDP) to worse off states" (2002). See also Pogge (2001).

conditions of community members depends crucially on the ends to which such resources are employed.

Without reforms to global institutions and the basic structures of LMIC communities, filling the pockets of regimes that do not employ existing resources to safeguard and secure the basic interests of all citizens does not guarantee that additional resources will trickle down to community members. For these reasons, even if those in the developing world are owed a greater share of global resources, international aid and development must target more than financial transfers. It must focus on improving those elements of the host community's basic social structure that affect individual agency and social opportunity, while taking interim steps to mitigate the adverse effects of existing social structures on the health and welfare of those who are subject to them. This dual focus on resources as well as individual agency and social opportunity is central to the kind of multisectoral approach that defines the human development view.

Finally, even if one does not recognize a duty to aid, or if one recognizes such a duty but believes it will not soon be honored on a large scale, the human development approach provides a more equitable foundation for collaborative partnership between communities. It permits research that targets knowledge gaps in HIC health systems to be carried out in partnership with LMICs under the conditions that the host community suffers from the same knowledge gap, regards its closure as an important policy goal, that the strategies or interventions being evaluated can be implemented on terms that are attainable and sustainable in LMIC communities, and there are reasonable commitments in place to ensure that the knowledge, policies, practices, or interventions vindicated in such research will be incorporated into the health systems of LMIC partners.

Together, concern for the basic interests of burdened peoples and recognition of the complex of extractive relationships that are part of the legacy of colonialism and post-colonial exploitation provide a network of reasons for policy makers in HICs to take affirmative steps to support and advance the basic social structures of LMICs. Although the bulk of these efforts should focus on the provision of existing knowledge, practices, and interventions, research with human participants still has a valuable role to play in this process. But it cannot play that role without concerted effort on the part of a range of stakeholders whose duties, obligations, and influence on research are not traditionally represented within research ethics (Pratt et al. 2012).

9.4.3 Responsiveness and Reasonable Availability as System-Level Concerns

Within the human development approach, the responsiveness and reasonable availability requirements help to ensure that research satisfies the social value requirement and so discharges the first part of the egalitarian research imperative. In this view, a necessary condition of responsiveness is that research must be designed to produce the information and the means that are necessary to expand the capacity of host community health systems to more effectively, efficiently, or equitably safeguard or advance the basic interests of that community's members. In this regard, the 2016 CIOMS guidelines are correct when they assert that, "Where communities or policy-makers have determined that research on particular health needs constitutes a public health priority, studies that address such needs seek to provide social value to the community or population and are therefore responsive to their health needs" (CIOMS 2016, Guideline 2). The cognate requirement of reasonable availability is necessary to ensure that research of this kind translates into concrete improvements in the capacity of local health systems to advance the basic interests of that community's members.

Even when research is designed to expand the capacity of local health systems to address local health needs, those needs can vary in terms of their importance. Earlier versions of the CIOMS guidelines required research to be "responsive to the health needs and the priorities of the population or community in which it is to be carried out" (CIOMS 2002, Guideline 10). But the 2016 revision of those guidelines holds that research must be "responsive to the health needs or priorities of the communities or populations where the research will be conducted" (CIOMS 2016, Guideline 2). The open question is whether research satisfies the condition of responsiveness if it is designed to generate "new knowledge about the best means of addressing a health condition present in that community or region" even if that health condition does not constitute a public health priority for the relevant communities (CIOMS 2016, Guideline 2). From the language of the commentary in the CIOMS guidelines, it appears that it can.

Within the human development approach, the responsiveness and reasonable availability requirements operate on two levels. At the system level, they reflect the imperative to strengthen research capacity in LMICs, to increase the amount of research that addresses shortfalls in the ability of local health systems to address needs that represent priorities for development, and to ensure that processes are in place to translate new knowledge and interventions into improved practices and procedures. This focus on capacity building and priority health needs reflects the strong claim on the part of community members to basic social systems that provide full coverage to the basic interests of all community members. When all such needs cannot be met, then these moral claims translate into a requirement to ensure that development efforts address needs that represent priorities for development.

This moral claim operates at the system level in the sense that it indicates the goals that should be advanced by incentives that structure the strategic environment in which various stakeholders in research act. I have argued here that research ethics plays a critical role in shaping the strategic environment in which various parties act. It does this, in part, by influencing the rules and the terms on which various practices or conduct is permitted. In chapters 2 and 8, for example, we saw that the conditions for permitting various kinds of studies can alter the portfolio of research proposed in a community because those conditions play a direct and an indirect role in determining whose interests drive the research agenda. In chapter 7 we saw that prospective review before committees of diverse representation alters the incentives that researchers face in ways that can improve the quality of research and its ethical acceptability. But we also saw that IRB review is not a viable forum for addressing all of the incentives that shape the research enterprise (e.g., §4.9).

Promoting responsiveness at the systems level requires engaging a wider range of stakeholders about questions that must be addressed long before individual protocols are composed and submitted for IRB review. A significant portion of these efforts should focus on promoting a legitimate process of priority setting for research and developing mechanisms for global health governance within which stakeholders can be accountable for funding research that addresses these priorities (Ruger 2018). For at least three decades, some organizations and communities have advanced a process of priority setting under various headings (Dye et al. 2013) including "essential national health research."[12] In this process, stakeholders seek to identify and prioritize research according to a range of relevant factors including prevalence, severity, economic impact, cost effectiveness, effects on equity, social justice, and so on. This process has met with varying degrees of success (McGregor,

Henderson, and Kaldor 2014) and faces numerous challenges, including ensuring that such processes are representative and fair (Pratt, Zion, and Loff 2012; Pratt and de Vries 2018).

Nevertheless, promoting this process is important to enable communities to exercise important rights to self-determination in forging a strategy to advance the goals of development. Such rights are not unlimited, since they are constrained by the prior claims of community members and the recognition that those who suffer the greatest shortfalls in their basic capabilities can have a strong claim to approaches that give priority to their basic interests. Nevertheless, even within these constraints there is likely to be a range of strategies for promoting development that are not clearly dominated by some viable alternative. Within this range, communities have an interest in determining their own development priorities. This latitude stems from several sources of legitimate diversity.

The first involves diversity in metrics that assign value to various aspects of health problems and procedures for decision-making that take these valuations as inputs. Quality-adjusted life years (QALYs) and disability-adjusted life years (DALYS) are two examples of metrics that are sometimes used to assign value to health states. These particular metrics assign value in a way that allows the relative value of all health states to be compared. However, their valuations do not always agree. These measures also have ethical shortcomings that are widely discussed (Arnesen and Nord 1999; Gold et al. 2002; Anand and Hanson 2004), and many alternatives have been proposed. Similarly, cost-effectiveness analysis (CEA) is an example of a procedure for combining this information in order to make decisions. Despite its popularity, CEA is a largely consequentialist framework that has been subject to criticism for its propensity to produce results that conflict with considerations of equity (Brock 2004). After reflective consideration of these issues, different communities might reasonably adopt different metrics for valuing health states and different procedures for decision-making (McGregor et al. 2014).

A second kind of diversity relates to diversity in the strategies available for advancing health-related goals. Some health conditions may be more amenable to control through prevention and improvements in the social determinants of health than others. In such cases, communities may have to determine how to divide social resources between broad-based improvements in living conditions, prevention measures that involve investments in social determinants of health, prevention measures that are more directly medical in nature, treatments for those who contract or de-velop the health problem in question, and steps that can be taken outside the realm of health care to support the ability of persons to function in the face of disability. Because the adverse effects of health conditions on the ability of persons to function can depend on the availability of various kinds of sup-port or alternative means of restoring functioning, health conditions can differ in terms of the variety of options available for mitigating their effects or restoring lost functions associated with the condition, and these conditions can vary across different communities both within LMICs and across them.

These various considerations can overlap with social and political back-ground conditions to create a matrix of combinations in which some health needs can raise special issues of equity and social justice. For example, health conditions that are prevalent in children from predominantly poor neighborhoods populated by groups who have traditionally been subject to social exclusion or oppression may affect only a subset of the population, but if they produce long-term harms that reinforce particularly pernicious histories of neglect or persecution then addressing those health conditions might be of particular urgency from the standpoint of equity in human development.

A third kind of diversity relates to the reasonable diversity of values re-garding strategies for development. For example, Drèze and Senn (1989) distinguish two broad strategies for reducing mortality and fostering human development in LMIC settings. A "growth-mediated" process aims to encourage economic growth in order to generate the means to reinvest into basic social services. On this approach, social resources are invested in expanding the social and economic opportunities available to those who can seize them, and the benefits of increased economic activity are used to build out social services to expand the share of the population who is capable of taking advantage of these opportunities. In contrast, a "support-led" process focuses on expanding educational opportunity and access to individual and public health services with the goal of enhancing the ability of individuals to create and take advantage of social opportunities.

Between the extremes of growth-mediated and support-led approaches to development lie a range of alternatives that assign differential relative im-portance to investments in particular social sectors. It may be the case that some health conditions are so important to a particular community that they will remain priorities for research no matter which approach a community adopts for reducing avoidable morbidity and mortality. It may also be the case that different health conditions will emerge as more or less important under different approaches to human development.

Even if a set of countries shares the same health needs, differences in infrastructure, technological development, and other aspects in this matrix of features, along with the reasonable pluralism of values in decent societies, might entail that if those communities engage in a fair process of priority setting for research, they would generate different lists of research priorities. In such cases, different knowledge gaps might emerge as more or less important depending on the strategies such societies pursue for advancing human development.

At the system level, the responsiveness requirement represents a goal to be advanced through institutional design, incentive systems, capacity building, and global health governance. This reflects the role of reasonable pluralism in determining permissible strategies of development and the autonomy interest of communities in selecting development strategies from this range of permissible options.

Ensuring that research can satisfy this requirement, and that research that satisfies this requirement actually advances the health needs of host communities requires strengthening the capacity of LMICs to complete the arc of translation. This is the process in which new knowledge, practices, or procedures are propagated through health systems to improve their ability to secure and advance the basic interests of community members. Such capacity building requires establishing or strengthening the institutions, norms, material, and human resources necessary to complete the arc of translation. It also requires a system of global health governance with established pathways to support this process.

It is the nature of some branches of research, such as new product development, given the current state of scientific knowledge, that the majority of studies do not establish that a novel intervention is sufficiently safe and effective that it merits use in clinical practice. As a result, the proponents of the fair benefits approach are correct when they assert that many studies, especially early phase research, will not produce a product that can be made reasonably available to host community members. But this does not mean that such studies only have social value if they serve as a conduit to some other, more tangible range of benefits. Rather, it shows only that the application of science in these areas often takes time to bear fruit and that new medical interventions are more like a pearl that results from the gradual accretion of knowledge over time, than they are like products manufactured in a factory.

The important point is that medical and public health knowledge is a public good and that communities with the capacity to produce this knowledge over time, especially when it is relevant to the health priorities of that community, benefit from this gradual and continual improvement in knowledge. These benefits include an increased knowledge base that supports further intervention development activities and that supports the decision-making of policy makers, practitioners, and patients. In this respect, well-designed studies that produce negative results are nevertheless a crucial part of the intervention development process, generating information that can be relevant to future development efforts and also to clinical practice (London and Kimmelman 2015; Kimmelman and London 2015).

When research is organized as an ongoing portfolio of inquiries in which individual studies are part of larger trajectories of inquiry, it is easier to ensure that early phase studies, and individual studies that produce negative results nevertheless contribute to an important public good for host communities. That is because the knowledge these studies produce contributes to a larger ongoing inquiry that takes place against a credible background assurance that the knowledge they produce and any practices, procedures, or products they vindicate will be incorporated into local health systems. When these conditions are met, such studies satisfy requirements of justice because they represent important elements within the kind of extended and careful study that is necessary to close shortfalls in the ability of that community's basic social systems to secure the basic interests of community members.

9.4.4 Misaligned Research and Injustice

At the level of protocol review, the human development approach recognizes a strong but defeasible requirement to limit research in LMIC settings to studies that address shortfalls in basic social systems that represent priorities for development. This requirement reflects the prior claims of community members, as outlined earlier, but it also reflects the role of protocol review in influencing stakeholder behavior. In particular, as we saw in chapter 7, the knowledge that protocols will be evaluated using particular criteria shapes the strategic environment in which researchers and sponsors act. The terms on which studies of various kinds are approved and permitted thus influences the nature of the protocols that are likely to be submitted for review.

Prohibiting research that does not align with the development priorities of host communities is not sufficient to promote research that does align with those priorities—that is a goal that must be addressed at a system level. But such a prohibition is likely necessary to reduce the use of LMICs as locations for research that perpetuates the fundamentally extractive practice of co-opting the basic social institutions of host communities to generate evidence and information that, if it is of genuine social value at all, is of value for communities that already enjoy extensive benefits from the fruits of scientific inquiry.

When research is untethered from the common good of host communities or the explicit project of generating the information necessary to aid less-advantaged communities in the process of human development, it can perpetuate injustice. In part, this is because clinical trials play a critical role in generating medical consensus, influencing practice behavior, and shaping patient demand (London, Kimmelman, and Carlisle 2012).

This is powerfully illustrated by Adriana Petryna's portrait of the ways in which communities that host international research are not simply temporary homes for transient research projects; they are also emerging markets for new interventions. In such contexts, clinical trials are not merely exercises in scientific inquiry; they are powerful tools for shaping the opinions, preferences, and behavior of physicians, patients, and a nexus of other actors—such as lawyers, judges, and politicians—who administer or oversee entitlement programs or other mechanisms by which citizens make claims on shared health resources. Nor are research environments separate ecosystems from the local medical and public health systems of the communities in which such trials take place. Rather, they are the means by which information is generated that is supported by and that feeds back into those social systems. As a result, Petryna argues that clinical trials are "operative environments that redistribute public health resources and occasion new and often tense medical and social fields" (2009, 30).

One particularly powerful illustration of the dangers of research that is misaligned with local priorities occurs when communities are used to "salvage" interventions whose therapeutic potential has been cast into doubt. Petryna reports the case of the pseudonymous Brazilian researcher "Dr. Santos" who was tasked with the job of securing approval for a new antidepressant that had failed to show superiority to a placebo in a phase III trial. At first, Dr. Santos planned to double the dose of the drug and combine it with a powerful hypnotic. However, this possibility was foreclosed by the passage of a Brazilian law prohibiting such combined drug formulations. Instead, Dr. Santos worked to place the drug on the Brazilian market for the treatment of "a mild form of depression—a 'made-up' illness as she called it" (Petryna 2009, 124).

Even if study participants, researchers, and host communities were to benefit from hosting and participating in such research in ways that do not derive from the social value of the information it produces, such research is morally objectionable. Private parties syphon scarce social resources to their own purposes while producing evidence that hampers the efficacy of care that health systems provide. Diversifying treatment practice without the benefit of increased efficacy hampers the efficiency with which health systems can address the many health needs of community members. Directing resources away from more effective avenues of care can also exacerbate inequities within health systems, especially if such decisions reduce the resources available to meet the needs of underserved populations.

Enforcing the requirement of reasonable availability without a credible assurance that research is responsive to the priority shortfalls of host community social systems would produce a similar effect. It would require expending resources and allocating time and effort to procuring and delivering an intervention that may not produce sufficient social value to justify these efforts. Doing so allows individual actors to profit from activities that subvert the prior claims of community members to basic social systems that are effective, efficient, and equitable.

It might appear possible to avoid these pitfalls by permitting research to be carried out in LMICs without the goal of influencing local health systems and without a requirement of reasonable availability. But this proposal faces several problems.

First, even if such studies are not intended to influence local health systems, they are conducted with the goal of influencing the decisions of providers, policy makers, and other stakeholders, even if those stakeholders do not reside in the host community (Wenner 2018). The globalization of clinical research allows contract research organizations to shop for populations of research participants with very specific disease characteristics. This makes it possible to quickly execute in practice trials that generate information from populations that can have very different characteristics from the patients likely to be the ultimate recipients of the intervention in the target population—the population where the intervention is likely to be sold and utilized. This can leave significant uncertainty about the external validity of this information for target populations—uncertainty about whether therapeutic or protective effects seen in such trials will materialize in populations with different comorbidities, whether adverse events in such populations will alter the net clinical value of the intervention, whether additional interventions are necessary to promote the clinical value of the intervention in the target population, and whether the intervention has sufficient clinical value relative to established alternatives that it ought to be incorporated into practice. Firms may have an interest in quickly generating a signal of efficacy so they can reap the benefits of earlier market access. But if this process offloads the costs and risks of reducing significant residual uncertainty onto the health systems of the target community, then such research can be objectionable on the grounds of justice (§4.9).

Second, such activities are often not separate from local medical and public health ecosystems. They frequently draw scarce social, material, and human resources away from prevention, primary care, and public health (Sitthi-Amorn and Somrongthong 2000). Lucrative ecosystems that support research activities unmoored from the goal of expanding the capacity of local health systems to address local health needs can subvert the common good of both host and target communities. In the worst cases, such trials enable sponsors to assemble what amount to made-up populations to produce interventions for what amount to made-up diseases, drawing real resources from the health systems of both host and target populations in order to generate unbelievable profits for pharmaceutical companies.

Finally, even in the best case, this proposal perpetuates a strategic environment in which parties who already play an outsized role in shaping the global research agenda are permitted to use LMIC populations to produce information that primarily benefits already advantaged populations. As long as this remains an option, powerful parties who stand to profit from its exploitation will allocate time, energy, and resources to doing so. As I indicated previously, forbidding such practices alone does not ensure that these resources are redirected in ways that promote human development for LMICs. But independent efforts to promote human development in LMICs, including efforts to focus research on LMIC priorities, may be hampered if such practices are sanctioned and permitted.

Requiring studies to generate information that addresses a shortfall in LMIC health systems is sufficient to rule out studies like the Surfaxin trial (§2.6.8). Although that study focused on a need that is represented in host communities, it was not designed to generate information that was necessary to close a knowledge gap necessary to enable health systems in those communities to better address acute respiratory distress in premature infants. Those communities lacked effective treatments for that condition that could be effectively and efficiently implemented under conditions that were attainable and sustainable. Several surfactant replacement treatments had been established as effective for treating acute respiratory distress in premature infants in HIC settings. But a variety of factors, including poverty and lack of infrastructure, prevented those countries from implementing those treatments on a widespread basis. There was nothing about Surfaxin or the question the trial was designed to answer that would generate information that would enable LMIC health systems to better address this medical need on a widespread basis.

Nevertheless, the requirement that research be responsive to health needs that represent development priorities for host communities is defeasible in that the presumption in favor of this restriction might be relaxed under certain conditions. One such condition obtains when communities have not articulated actionable research priorities. This may be because they have not articulated priorities for research or because those priorities are so vague that it is not clear how they provide actionable guidance to stakeholders. In such cases, review committees should, nevertheless, require assurance that the study or studies under review are part of a larger trajectory of research that is likely to advance the capacity of local institutions to safeguard or advance the basic interests of community members and that communities regard such research as sufficiently important that they are likely to support its uptake into local health systems if it is successful.

Another condition might include research that represents a low-cost, fortuitous opportunity. For instance, in the course of a research partnership that is responsive to a shared research priority of a set of communities, an opportunity to study a new question might be identified. Given existing research infrastructure it would be relatively easy to study this new question. It is possible that the new question is a research priority for some but not all of the communities with centers participating in the initial collaboration. It is also possible that this isn't a research priority for any of these communities but that it nevertheless addresses a knowledge gap that they share. Such research might also arise because the science in a particular area has matured to the point where it might be possible to close a knowledge gap that doesn't fall under any existing research priority.

Within the human development approach, such research might be permissible, but only under the conditions that permitting it does not undermine or impede the ability of host communities to mount and to secure support for research that addresses their research priorities, and that conducting such research in the presence of a requirement of reasonable availability does not detract from the ability of local health systems to function effectively, efficiently, or equitably. Having said that, the close connections between research and the institutions of individual and public health in a community provide important reasons to be wary of attempting to increase the benefits that are available to communities or study participants by permitting the conduct of research that does not address a question that represents a health priority for the host community.

9.5 The Standard of Care

9.5.1 The Local De Jure Standard of Care, Social Value, and Equal Concern

It is an advantage of the human development approach that it uses a single coherent framework to evaluate domestic research in HICs, domestic research in LMICs, and cross-national research between entities from HICs and populations in LMICs. In all of these cases, research should represent an avenue through which community members can advance the common good under terms that provide credible social assurance that their status as free and equal persons will not be compromised in the process. In chapter 6 I argued that the integrative approach to risk assessment and management provides a framework for ensuring that research designed to satisfy the social value requirement is consistent with the principle of equal concern (§6.2). Research is consistent with the principle of equal concern if it satisfies the requirements of no unnecessary risk (§6.3.1), special concern for basic interests (§6.3.2), and social consistency (§6.3.3). The human development approach makes clear that, in all cases, these criteria are to be understood against the background of the local de jure standard of care.

The local de jure standard of care states that participants in research are entitled to a level of care for their basic interests that does not fall below what experts judge to be the most effective strategy for preserving or advancing those interests under conditions that are attainable and sustainable in their community (§2.6.2). This phrasing reflects the fact that there may be reasonable diversity among experts about which practices, policies, or interventions represent the best way of preventing, treating, or ameliorating a threat to a person's basic interests. In such cases, respect for the status of individuals as free and equal persons requires that their treatment not be substandard or inferior to the options that are regarded as best by at least a reasonable minority of experts.

This interpretation of the standard of care reflects the deep moral claim that all community members have to conditions that provide real freedom to formulate, pursue, and revise a life plan and the special role that the basic social structures of a community play in meeting this claim. Individuals have a just claim on the basic structures of their community to use established knowledge, practices, policies, and interventions to safeguard and advance their basic interests on terms that reflect the duty of full coverage. This just claim correlates with a duty on the part of the basic social institutions of their community to provide the best means of safeguarding and advancing their basic interests, consistent with the equal regard for this same interest on the part of their compatriots.[13]

The requirements of the integrative approach are to be understood against this baseline set of claims. In particular, special concern for basic interests holds that if the basic interests of research participants are threatened or impaired (for example, by sickness, injury, or disease), participants must be provided a level of care and protection for their basic interests that does not fall below what at least a reasonable minority of experts in the relevant field(s) (e.g., experts from the medical or public health community) would regard as the most beneficial method of response. When there is uncertainty or conflict in the expert community about how best to secure and advance the basic interests of persons, research that is designed to resolve this uncertainty has a strong, prima facia claim to social value. When the uncertainty in question relates to a shortfall that represents a development priority for host communities, and research takes place in a context of credible assurance of reasonable availability, then research satisfies conditions of justice.

Within the cognitive ecosystem of orthodox research ethics, the idea that domestic research in HICs is governed by the local de jure standard of care may seem odd. But this does not reflect a shortcoming in that standard of

---

[13] For a comprehensive and insightful discussion of the relationship between this formulation of the standard of care and the rights of community members see MacKay (2018). See also Kukla (2007).

care; it reflects the difficulties of understanding the role of research in a just social order within the parochialism of orthodox research ethics.

It is worth emphasizing, therefore, that only the local de jure standard of care ensures that research tracks both the social value requirement and the principle of equal concern. One fundamental reason for this is that knowledge about how to safeguard and advance the basic interests of persons cannot achieve that goal under the requirement of full coverage if it does not augment the capacity of basic social institutions. This is because these institutions are responsible for dividing social labor and using social authority and resources to safeguard and advance the basic interests of community members. Both the local de facto and the global de jure standards of care permit research that violates these principles and that is therefore objectionable on the grounds of injustice.

9.5.2 The Local De Facto Standard of Care and Prior Moral Claims

The local de facto standard artificially separates current practice from the knowledge regarding the way the various resources in a community—including existing medical knowledge—could be used to effectively, efficiently, or more equitably safeguard the health interests of individuals in that community. As a result, studies designed to test interventions against this baseline can deviate from both the social value requirement and the principle of equal concern.

Studies that use the local de facto standard of care can lack social value, in part, because conditions reflected in current practice may not reveal knowledge gaps at all. To see this, consider that marginalized or oppressed groups are often denied access to practices, policies, or interventions that are safe and effective and that could be deployed within the economic and infrastructure requirements that prevail in the larger community.[14] In such cases, the local de facto standard of care falls below what could be achieved by extending existing services and the various benefits of social inclusion to members of these groups.

To the extent that health problems in a group or population are the product of prejudice, antipathy, neglect, or exclusion, they represent the

---

[14] See Annas and Grodin (1998) for some examples.

ravages produced from denying individuals various forms of social support (including equitable access to health services) and not uncertainty about how best to secure the interests of those people. Designing a study to assess whether some intervention A is superior to the local de facto standard of care B will not be relevant to the host community if there is an alternative C (extending existing social and health services to members of this disadvantaged group) that is preferable to both and that could be safely and effectively implemented under conditions that are attainable and sustainable in the host community.[15]

Moreover, this is the case even if C is not currently provided to individuals with the particular condition in question. If it is clear that C is the best alternative for addressing a problem and that the conditions necessary for its safe and effective delivery are attainable and sustainable in that community, then there is no knowledge gap to fill. The local de facto standard of care cannot capture this insight since it presupposes that the relevant normative baseline against which proposals are to be evaluated is the state of affairs that would obtain if no research were to be conducted.

Similarly, randomizing individuals to the local de facto standard of care can violate the principle of equal concern. When the status quo reflects antipathy, indifference, or deprivation, replicating that level of care within a study perpetuates the larger deprivations those groups experience in society. Doing so shows less concern for the basic interests of participants (and for members of marginalized groups outside of the trial) than for members of more advantaged groups who live under the same social institutions. In such cases, study participants have claim to more or better than the local de facto standard of care precisely because better alternatives are attainable and sustainable under social arrangements in which their basic social institutions better approximate the demands of full coverage.

9.5.3 The Global De Jure Standard of Care Is Fundamentally Confused

In §2.6 we saw that arguments against the local de facto standard of care are often seen as favoring the global de jure standard of care, which uses the judgments of experts to determine the baseline level of care that must be provided to participants in research using global centers of excellence as the

---

[15] Such studies violate concern for welfare (§6.2.1) and the principle of equal concern (§6.2.1).

relevant reference point for such assessments. One rationale for this choice of reference point is that it allows us to distinguish situations in which we do not know how to solve a problem (and therefore require new knowledge) from those cases in which we possess the know-how but lack the resources to put this know-how into practice. So understood, a focus on what can be achieved in global centers of excellence is intended to help stakeholders avoid conducting research that exploits conditions of poverty and deprivation.

However, although the motivation for this interpretation is important, the concept of a global de jure standard of care is fundamentally confused. It artificially separates research from its relationship to the basic social structures of a community that are required to translate knowledge, interventions, and practices into actions that secure or advance the basic interests of individuals. As a result, either it ignores the extent to which every community, including those that are home to global centers of excellence, must meet the basic interests of community members under resource constraints, or it incorrectly assumes that what can be achieved under one set of such constraints should be normative for all communities, regardless of the constraints under which they must meet the basic interests of their members. We can elaborate each horn of this dilemma in turn.

On the first horn of the dilemma, if the global de jure standard is interpreted as identifying the best level of care that can be attained in global centers of excellence regardless of resource constraints, then it is not normative for any community. Framed in these terms, this formulation of the standard of care would include practices that require all resources to be dedicated to solving a single problem. Clearly, tremendous strides could be made in reducing HIV transmission, for example, if all resources were dedicated to this end. But the practices that would bring about these achievements are not normative as a baseline standard of care even in HIC centers of excellence. The reason is that every community must use its scarce social, human, and economic resources to address the full range of threats to the ability of individuals to develop and exercise the capacities they need to formulate, pursue, and revise a reasonable life plan. Moreover, health-related social structures are only one element in a larger network of social structures that must work together to safeguard the basic interests of community members. Not only would it be unjust for communities to dedicate all of their resources to addressing a single problem, but also they must not focus solely on problems in one particular domain, such as health.

Turning to the second horn of the dilemma, if the practices and interventions labeled as the global de jure standard of care are normative for the communities that are served by global centers of excellence, then this status is explained by the fact that they constitute the local de jure standard of care for those communities. Individuals in those communities would be wronged if they were denied such interventions or practices because those practices can be effectively implemented on a sustainable basis within the health systems of those communities.

To use an example from chapter 2, the 076 protocol became the standard of care in HICs because it represented the most effective intervention for preventing perinatal HIV transmission that could be deployed under conditions that are attainable and sustainable in those countries. Moreover, it had this status, in part, because the protocol was formulated against a background set of assumptions that hold, or can be established, in the HICs that hosted that research. These assumptions include the economic conditions and the type of infrastructure that would be available in the contexts in which this intervention would be delivered. Against this background, for example, early identification of pregnancy is consistent with routine medical practice. Intravenous medication can be delivered safely and effectively on a routine basis. The widespread availability of clean, potable water allows women who refrain from breast feeding to provide safe alternatives to their infants.

The status of the 076 protocol as the local de jure standard of care for HIC communities explains the conditions under which using this intervention as the normative baseline for research supports the social value requirement in those communities. The 076 protocol could be safely and effectively implemented in health systems in HICs to reduce perinatal HIV transmission. To expand the capacity of those health systems to better address this health need, a comparator would have to offer a more effective, efficient, or equitable way of addressing this same health need. If there is credible uncertainty or conflicting expert judgment about the relative merits of the 076 protocol in comparison to an alternative or a set of alternatives, then research that reduces or resolves this uncertainty can play a valuable role in enhancing the capacity of those health systems to better meet the needs of the people who rely on them.

Treating this intervention as the normative baseline for research in HICs also satisfies the principle of equal concern. But it does so because it satisfies the conditions of the local de jure standard of care, namely, it reflects the judgment of the relevant experts about the best diagnostic, prophylactic, or therapeutic intervention for this condition that can be delivered effectively under conditions that are attainable and sustainable in the target population. It does not violate the principle of equal concern to allow participants to be random-ized to a set of interventions as long as there is conflict or uncertainty among the relevant set of experts about the relative merits of the interventions in that set and the local de jure standard of care. In other words, nobody in such a trial is made worse off relative to the other participants in the trial or to the members of the larger community who rely on this set of health systems to safeguard and advance their basic interests.

It would violate the principle of equal concern, however, if some study participants are randomized to interventions or practices that fall below the local de jure standard of care. The reason is that all community members have a just claim on the basic social structures of their community to practices that safeguard and advance their basic interests, consistent with the requirement of full coverage.

Now consider some community that is not served by one of these global centers of excellence. Does it make sense to hold that the same interventions that are required in those centers of excellence must also be provided to indi-viduals in different communities? The answer is clearly "yes it does" if it is the case that the same intervention can be safely and effectively deployed in this new community under conditions that are attainable and sustainable in that community. But this is simply to say that when another community can attain and sustain the conditions necessary to safely and effectively deliver that same practice, procedure, or intervention then using it as a comparator against which new interventions are tested ensures that those studies satisfy the social value requirement and the principle of equal concern. The same intervention must be provided to study participants in these two different communities for the same reasons, and these reasons are captured by the local de jure standard of care.

In contrast, the global de jure standard of care says that an intervention that experts judge to be the best way of safeguarding the basic interests of individuals in one place, under one set of background social, economic, and political conditions, must be provided to study participants in any commu-nity, regardless of differences in the background social, economic, or political conditions in the target community. So, even if it is not the case that the inter-vention in question can be safely and effectively deployed under conditions that are attainable and sustainable in a different community, the global de jure standard of care says that it must still serve as the comparator against which any alternative intervention will be tested. But, in doing so, this re-quirement is now divorced from both the social value requirement and the principle of equal concern.

It is divorced from the social value requirement because the global de jure standard of care effectively requires every social community to test new interventions, policies, or practices against a baseline that can be wildly different from what can be attained and sustained in that community. If the information that is generated from such studies is relevant to any community, it is most likely to be relevant to the already more advantaged communities that are served by those global centers of excellence. This not only permits research in LMIC settings that is designed to produce information to expand the capabilities of social structures that advance the basic interests of already more advantaged communities, it prohibits research that does otherwise (§2.6.4). This standard of care effectively prohibits communities from conducting research that is most directly relevant to the capacity of their own health systems to safeguard and advance the basic interests of their own community members.

This argument also assumes that it would be possible to implement the intervention that serves as the global de jure standard of care in all studies, regardless of background social, economic, or epidemiological conditions, in a way that would preserve its safety and efficacy. In other words, if an intervention was shown to be safe and effective in resource-intensive HIC contexts, then this position assumes that it is possible to create a comparable clinical context in LMIC settings that preserves the intervention's safety and efficacy. But this may not be possible. For example, if the background health status of HIC and LMIC populations is sufficiently different—if LMIC residents have higher rates of medical conditions that were absent in trials of the intervention in question in HICs—then the rate of adverse events may differ significantly between these two populations. Such a difference can affect both the safety and efficacy profile of the interventions provided. If this is the case, then a study that compares a novel intervention against the global de jure standard of care might generate information that is not relevant to any community. In particular, if we cannot ensure that the conditions necessary to preserve the safety and efficacy of the control intervention are in place, then it is difficult, if not impossible, to interpret the findings of such a study. In the worst case, for example, if the control intervention is positively harmful, then the investigational intervention might appear to be superior even though it is merely ineffective.

Studies that use the global de jure standard of care are disconnected from the principle of equal concern to the extent that the interventions provided to at least some participants far exceed what is attainable and sustainable in the larger community. This might not appear to be a significant problem since providing higher-quality care to study participants advances the interests of those individuals, and prohibiting this merely out of a concern for equality might represent a morally objectionable instance of "leveling down." As long as nobody in a study is denied a level of care and concern to which they are entitled, then we should be very careful about forbidding the provision of extra benefits to some study participants (MacKay 2020).

Although concerns about leveling down are legitimate, it is important to bear in mind three points. First, it is worth emphasizing that this argument is most compelling when the relevant baseline is set by the local de jure standard of care. If inequalities in the standard of care provided to study participants or between study participants and community members are permissible as long as nobody is deprived of a level of care to which they are entitled, then we need an independent account of the baseline of care to which study participants are entitled. The local de jure standard provides a compelling account of that entitlement.

Second, the local de jure standard reflects the claims that community members can make against their shared social institutions given the duty of full coverage. If some study participants occasionally receive a higher level of care for their basic interests than what is attainable and sustainable in the broader community, such isolated cases may not result in others being denied a level of care or concern to which they are entitled.

However, the systematic provision of a standard of care that is higher than the local de jure standard raises questions about the extent to which the research enterprise is functioning on terms that are consistent with the duty of full coverage. The local de jure standard of care and the principle of equal concern help to ensure that the research enterprise functions efficiently and equitably within a larger social division of labor in which scarce social resources are enmeshed in a network of prior claims. If such a system prevents more research from being conducted, or siphons resources from the provision of goods or services to which community members are entitled, then the higher standard of care may benefit participants but at the price of leaving other legitimate claims of community members unmet or addressed with less efficacy or efficiency than is feasible.

Finally, it is also worth emphasizing that the principle of equal concern is closely connected to the epistemic goals of research and the social value requirement. Evidence generated against a baseline that more closely reflects what is attainable and sustainable outside the trial is likely to have greater direct relevance for the stakeholders who rely on this information to discharge important social responsibilities. These responsibilities include making decisions about how to use scarce time, effort, and human and material resources to effectively, efficiently, and equitably address the many different needs of community members. If the standard of care within a trial is not normative for the host community, then establishing the merits of alternative interventions relative to this baseline does not directly address the uncertainties that are most relevant to the decisions facing key stakeholders in that community (§6.6).

In many ways, these points reiterate key themes that run throughout this book. First, the provision of benefits to study participants raises issues of fairness, but those issues are not simply a matter of the amount of benefit provided. The social function of research is to produce information that is a public good and the social value of that information for host communities depends on its alignment with and relevance to a normative baseline that reflects the prior moral claims of community members. These prior moral claims implicate issues of justice because they relate to basic social institutions that have a responsibility to make effective, efficient, and equitable use of existing knowledge and resources. The local de jure standard of care tracks this baseline.

Second, research ethics needs to be sensitive to the way that the parochial interests of different parties to the research enterprise can align or conflict with the common good. Enriching the standard of care available in individual trials can be a way of inducing people to participate in studies they might not otherwise consider. But if the baseline created in such trials is most directly relevant to more advantaged communities, then such research can represent an extractive relationship in which social arrangements in less advantaged communities are co-opted to generate social value for already more advantaged groups.

9.6 Justice and the Process of Human Development

9.6.1 The Standard of Care and Just Moral Baselines

We said in chapter 2 that debates about the standard of care sometimes feel like proxy wars for larger philosophical positions that exert their influence from offstage. The arguments from the previous section allow us to explain one way in which this might be the case. This, in turn, can help to avoid an important confusion and to bring into better focus distinct ways in which research activities can contribute to the process of moving toward a more just social order.

The confusion in question involves the following distinct claims. The first claim is about the relationship between the standard of care and the basic social structures of the communities that are affected by that research. In particular, I argued in the previous section that only the local de jure standard of care ensures that research advances the common good of host communities while respecting the status of study participants and community members as free and equal persons.

The second claim is about whether the conditions that are attainable and sustainable in a community are themselves morally defensible. In particular, we saw that the local de facto standard of care was problematic because the level of care that individuals actually receive in a community might not reflect the level of care that is attainable and sustainable under a social order in which the community's basic social institutions make more efficient and equitable use of existing knowledge and resources. But, in a world of widespread injustice, there may be an analogous gap between the conditions that can be attained and sustained in a particular community if its basic social structures made a more effective use of existing knowledge and resources and the conditions that could be attained and sustained if that same community also enjoyed a larger and fairer share of resources.

This last point might be seen as calling into question the normative status of the local de jure standard of care. For example, if one held a strict, global egalitarian view according to which national boundaries are morally arbitrary and there is a strong duty to redistribute global resources, then one might think that this would entail support for the global de jure standard of care. The reason is that equalizing resources would equalize the baseline of care that individuals receive, regardless of where they are located, and that the global de jure standard of care might be expected to capture this baseline.

It is a mistake to think that the second claim stands in this relationship to the first. To begin with, the global de jure standard of care is still vulnerable to the original dilemma that I posed earlier. Either that position can identify practices as the standard of care that would not be normative for any community or it identifies standards that are normative but only to the extent that it effectively uses the local de jure standard of care for some paradigm community as the normative standard for all other communities. Global egalitarian theories of justice seek to reduce the gap in infrastructure between HICs and LMICs. Even so, the specific interventions, policies, or practices that constitute the local de jure standard of care for one community would only be normative for those other communities if they also share priority health needs.

It is true, however, that vindicating the local de jure interpretation as the best way of understanding the standard of care does not settle the issue raised in the second claim. In particular, what is attainable and sustainable in a community depends on the resources that can be allocated to solving a problem and this, in turn, can depend on at least two factors. One is the share of resources a community can legitimately claim and legitimately expect to receive within the relevant window of time. The other is how those resources can be legitimately used to address the problem in question, given that communities can adopt different strategies for development in light of the factors discussed in §9.4.3. Different theories of global justice can have important consequences for this first factor since they might entail that communities have a just claim to greater or lesser shares of resources.

The point I want to emphasize here is that the close connection between what is attainable and sustainable in LMIC communities and larger theories of global justice does not undermine the status of the local de jure interpretation of the standard of care. That is because the local de jure standard captures the important relationship between the principle of equal concern and the background conditions against which communities are constrained to safeguard and advance the basic interests of their constituent members. The fact that changes in the resources available to LMICs might alter this baseline underscores the importance of situating international research initiatives within the larger context of human development and the efforts to improve the baseline circumstances in LMICs that it entails.

9.6.2 Research on the Way to a More Just Social Order

In previous chapters we said that the minimalist approach to justice is latent in the conceptual ecosystem of orthodox research ethics and that this is due, in part, to the desire to preserve the practical utility of research ethics. If perennial questions of global, social, and distributive justice have to be settled before questions of research ethics can be addressed, then the worry is that the urgent business of regulating research with humans will be undermined. Because the approach to research ethics outlined in this book explicitly situates research within a larger conception of political and distributive jus- tice, the concerns of the last section might seem to pose a particularly urgent and thorny problem.

It is fitting to close this discussion, therefore, by addressing these worries. I will begin by addressing the narrow issue raised in the previous section and then turn to more general concerns.

The first point I want to make is that the human development approach and the egalitarian research imperative understand research as one social activity within a much larger, multisectoral division of labor aimed at moving communities toward a more just social order. In particular, research plays this role when it addresses uncertainty or conflicting expert assessments about the best ways to secure and advance the basic interests of persons. These questions must be formulated relative to what is attainable and sustainable within the basic social institutions of the host community for the very pragmatic reason that those institutions structure the environment within which individuals are constrained to live and to act and against which public officials, healthcare providers, public health agents, and others must discharge their concrete social and moral obligations to community members.

In that respect, the focus of the human development approach and the egalitarian research imperative on eliminating shortfalls in the capacity of a community's basic social institutions to secure and advance the basic interests of that community's members does not necessarily presuppose the truth or falsity of any particular conception of global or distributive justice. Even if global egalitarians are correct and there is nothing morally sacrosanct about national boundaries or national identities, it does not follow that education, security for basic rights and interests, environmental and public health, and the panoply of health services on which individuals depend can be delivered independently of the basic social structures of society on terms that satisfy the requirement of full coverage. Rather, it follows only that the vast majority of the world has a strong moral claim to basic social structures that do a much better job of advancing their basic interests than they do now.

The second point I want to make is that because the human development approach recognizes a moral responsibility, both domestically and internationally, to engage in a larger process of human development, arguments about the extent of such duties—about when such duties have been fulfilled and about the extent of the transfers that this requires—do not pose a radical challenge for the application of this framework. In part, this is because the process of meeting development goals and discharging duties of justice is likely to be extended over time. Additionally, the entitlements that are in force for decisions within research ethics must reflect the extent to which what *ought* to be done is constrained by what *can* be achieved within relevant time horizons.

Host communities face uncertainty about how best to meet the distinctive needs of their members as the development process unfolds, including how best to allocate new resources for advancing development goals across different sectors. Because there is likely to be room for reasonable pluralism about alternative strategies for achieving development goals, as we argued in §9.4.3, this point illustrates the importance of foregrounding discussions about development priorities and identifying knowledge gaps that are likely to persist across sufficient periods of time for research to represent an attractive strategy for closing those gaps.

During this process, communities must still strive to provide full coverage to the basic interests of their members. In that respect, there may be cases in which the rate of social and economic development calls into question the social value of research that is too closely tied to a baseline of care that is likely to be superseded before such research could meaningfully advance the goals of human development. In other cases, however, differences in endemic diseases, infrastructure, and development priorities might entail that particular research initiatives represent a valuable investment in an effort to address threats to the basic interests of persons that might frustrate development and that are unlikely to be met more quickly, more easily, or more equitably through the application of existing resources.

To use a concrete example, imagine a case similar to the short-course zidovudine studies discussed in chapter 2. In that context, Crouch and Arras (1998) argued persuasively that in order to determine the standard of care for a short-course zidovudine study, it is not sufficient to establish that there are circumstances under which an intervention like the 076 Protocol could be effectively deployed in LMIC settings. This is not sufficient, they argued, because such conditions might be attainable, but not be sustainable in the sense of being consistent with a just allocation of resources in that community. Moreover, they argued that this might be the case even if we grant that such communities are entitled to a larger share of resources than they already enjoy.

To simplify matters, we can say that if a community would not implement the 076 Protocol in the near future, even if the process of development were accelerated, because of concerns about that community's ability to meet the relevant need on terms that satisfy the requirements of full coverage, then it would be permissible to compare the short-course against whatever intervention is regarded as the best alternative under those conditions. If no such alternative exists, then the claim is that if it is morally permissible for that community not to implement the 076 Protocol in practice, even under a more just resource allocation, then it is morally permissible to evaluate the merits of a short course against a placebo control, as long as it is the case that the host community is prepared to implement this alternative intervention if its merits are confirmed in testing.

The point for our present purposes is that this reasoning may play out differently for different communities. For LMICs with a more robust health infrastructure, the 076 Protocol might be both attainable and sustainable under social and economic circumstances that are likely to prevail in the near term. In that case, it might be permissible to test a short course against the 076 Protocol in a trial designed to establish whether a cheaper, more portable, easier to implement alternative might represent a more effective and efficient way to address perinatal HIV transmission on terms that are consistent with full coverage. Here, the difference is that if the short course fails to meet the relevant benchmarks, the host community is committed to implementing the 076 Protocol on a widespread basis.

This last point illustrates that the application of the same normative requirements (using a single moral standard to make different decisions) can produce different outcomes in different cases. It is not an embarrassment that a placebo control may be morally permissible in research that is carried out in one place but not in another if this result follows from the sound application of just moral principles. The example provided a moment ago is intended to illustrate merely how such variation in what is morally permissible might be possible. In contrast, it is an embarrassment to require that clinical trials adopt the same design if this comes at the cost of frustrating the morally legitimate goals of human development.

The idea that judgments about what is attainable and sustainable in a community must be made against a larger background understanding of the development priorities of a community may be particularly jarring to Americans. In part, this is because Americans are particularly resistant to recognizing the extent to which healthcare budgets are limited. Nevertheless, public entitlement programs, such as Medicare or Medicaid, and private insurance plans may not cover certain forms of treatment because such decisions conflict with the efficient and equitable allocation of shared resources. Citizens of nations with national health services are more familiar, and often more comfortable, with the idea that not all established effective interventions must be provided in such systems.

If it is consistent with principles of justice to limit access to established effective care out of concerns for the just allocation of scarce resources, then it must also be consistent with principles of justice to ensure that research is carried out against a moral baseline that reflects the legitimate entitlements of community members (London 2019).

Finally, one of the main contentions of the present work is that research with humans has an important role to play in improving the ability of social systems, such as public and individual health systems, to effectively, efficiently, and equitably advance the basic interests of community members. Failing to appreciate the relationship between the research activity and these larger social structures can undermine and frustrate these goals. It allows powerful parties to co-opt social resources and social systems to advance the parochial ends of profit, promotion, or individual benefit without a guarantee that these rewards attach to activities that also promote the common good. Although this is dramatized by research that crosses national boundaries, the same concerns apply to domestic research as well.

Situating research within a larger social context, where it is evaluated in light of and beholden to larger social purposes, is more demanding. It will require a reconceptualization of the audience that research ethics addresses and the social institutions and stakeholders who fall within the legitimate boundaries of the field, and a widening of the menu of mechanisms that might be used to shape stakeholder behavior. Nevertheless, this complexity is not an avoidable nuisance. It reflects the complexity of the social systems within which research is embedded, into which it feeds, and that influence the incentives for stakeholders who advance the many different objectives out of which the larger tapestry of cooperation is woven.

References

Advisory Committee on Human Radiation Experiments. (1996). *Final report of the Advisory Committee on Human Radiation Experiments* [R. Faden, Chair]. Oxford University Press.

Akerlof, G. A. (1970). The market for "lemons": Quality uncertainty and the market mechanism. *Quarterly Journal of Economics, 84*(3), 488–500.

Alonge, O., Rodriguez, D. C., Brandes, N., Geng, E., Reveiz, L., & Peters, D. H. (2019). How is implementation research applied to advance health in low-income and middle-income countries? *BMJ Global Health, 4*(2), e001257.

Altman, L. K. (1972). Auto-experimentation: An unappreciated tradition in medical science. *New England Journal of Medicine, 286*(7), 346–352.

Anand, S., & Hanson K. (2004). Disability-adjusted life years: A critical review. In S. Anand, F. Peter, & A. Sen (Eds.), *Public health, ethics, and equity* (pp. 183–199). Oxford University Press.

Anderson, E. S. (1999). What is the point of equality? *Ethics, 109,* 287–337.

Anderson, J. A., & Weijer, C. (2002). The research subject as wage earner. *Theoretical Medicine and Bioethics, 23*(4), 359–376.

Angell, M. (1997). The ethics of clinical research in the Third World. *New England Journal of Medicine, 337*(12), 847–849.

Angus, D. C., Alexander, B. M., Berry, S., Buxton, M., Lewis, R., Paoloni, M., Webb, S. A. R., Arnold, S., Barker, A., Berry, D. A., Bonten, M. J. M., Brophy, M., Butler, C., Cloughesy, T. F., Derde, L. P. G., Esserman, L. J., Ferguson, R., Fiore, L., Gaffey, S. C., . . . & Woodcock, J. (2019). Adaptive platform trials: Definition, design, conduct and reporting considerations. *Nature Reviews: Drug Discovery, 18*(10), 797–808.

Annas, G. J., & Grodin, M. A. (1991). Treating the troops [Commentary]. *The Hastings Center Report, 21*(2), 24–27.

Annas, G. J., & Grodin M. A. (Eds.). (1992). *The Nazi doctors and the Nuremberg Code: Human rights in human experimentation.* Oxford University Press.

Annas, G. J., & Grodin, M. A. (1998). Human rights and maternal-fetal HIV transmission prevention trials in Africa. *American Journal of Public Health, 88*(4), 560–563.

Applbaum, A. I. (1999). *Ethics for adversaries: The morality of roles in public and professional life.* Princeton University Press.

Aquinas, T. (2005). *Aquinas: Disputed questions on the virtues* (E. M. Atkins & T. Williams, Eds.). Cambridge University Press.

Arendt, H. (1973). *The origins of totalitarianism.* Harcourt Brace Jovanovich.

Aristotle. Nicomachean ethics. (1984). In J. Barnes (Ed.), *Complete works of Aristotle, Vol. 1: The revised Oxford translation.* Princeton University Press.

Arnesen, T., & Nord, E. (1999). The value of DALY life: Problems with ethics and validity of disability adjusted life years. *British Medical Journal, 319,* 1423–1425.

Arras, J. D. (2008). The Jewish chronic disease hospital case. In E. J. Emanuel, C. C. Grady, R. A. Crouch, R. K. Lie, F. G. Miller, & D. D. Wendler (Eds.), *The Oxford textbook of clinical research ethics* (pp. 73–79). Oxford University Press.

Arrow, K. J. (1951). *Social choice and individual values.* (Cowles Commission Monograph No. 12.). Wiley & Sons.

Ashcroft, R. (1999). Equipoise, knowledge and ethics in clinical research and practice. *Bioethics, 13*(3–4), 314–326.

Ashford, E. (2003). The demandingness of Scanlon's contractualism. *Ethics, 113*(2), 273–302.

Athanasiou, E., London, A. J., & Zollman, K. J. (2015). Dignity and the value of rejecting profitable but insulting offers. *Mind, 124*(494), 409–448.

Attaran, A. (1999). Human rights and biomedical research funding for the developing world: Discovering state obligations under the right for health. *Health and Human Rights, 4*(1), 26–58.

Ballantyne, A. (2010). How to do research fairly in an unjust world. *American Journal of Bioethics, 10*(6), 26–35.

Barry, B. (1982). Humanity and justice in global perspective. In J. W. Chapman & J. R. Pennock (Eds.), *Ethics, economics, and the law; Nomos 24* (pp. 219–252). New York University Press.

Barry, B. (1989). *Theories of justice: A treatise on social justice* (Vol. 16). University of California Press.

Barry, C., & Raworth, K. (2002). Access to medicines and the rhetoric of responsibility. *Ethics & International Affairs, 16*(2), 57–70.

Basu, A., & Gujral, K. (2020). Evidence generation, decision making, and consequent growth in health disparities. *Proceedings of the National Academy of Sciences, 117*(25), 14042–14051.

Beauchamp, T. L., & Childress, J. F. (2001). *Principles of biomedical ethics.* Oxford University Press.

Beecher, H. K. (1966). Ethics and clinical research. *The New England Journal of Medicine, 274,* 1354–1360.

Beitz, C. R. (1979). *Political theory and international relations.* Princeton University Press.

Benatar, S. R. (1998). Global disparities in health and human rights: A critical commentary. *American Journal of Public Health, 88*(2), 295–300.

Benatar, S. R. (2001). Justice and medical research: A global perspective. *Bioethics, 15*(4), 333–340.

Benatar, S. R. (2002). The HIV/AIDS pandemic: A sign of instability in a complex global system. *The Journal of Medicine and Philosophy, 27*(2), 163–177.

Benatar, S. R., & Singer, P. A. (2000). A new look at international research ethics. *British Medical Journal, 321*(7264), 824–826.

Benatar, S. R., Daar, A. S., & Singer, P. A. (2003). Global health ethics: The rationale. *International Affairs, 79*(1), 107–138.

Berry, D. A. (2011). Adaptive clinical trials: The promise and the caution. *Journal of Clinical Oncology, 29*(6), 606–609.

Bledsoe, C. H., Sherin, B., Galinsky, A. G., & Headley, N. M. (2007). Regulating creativity: Research and survival in the IRB iron cage. *Northwestern University Law Review, 101,* 593–641.

Bloom, D. E., & Canning, D. (2000). The health and wealth of nations. *Science, 287*(5456), 1207–1209.

Brandt, A. M. (1978). Racism and research: The case of the Tuskegee Syphilis Study. *Hastings Center Report*, 8(6), 21–29.

Brassington, I. (2007). John Harris' argument for a duty to research. *Bioethics*, 21(3), 160–168.

Brassington, I. (2011). Defending the duty to research? *Bioethics*, 25(1), 21–26.

Brazier, M. (2008). Exploitation and enrichment: The paradox of medical experimentation. *Journal of Medical Ethics*, 34(3), 180–183.

Brennan, G., & Lomasky, L. (2006). Against reviving republicanism. *Politics, Philosophy & Economics*, 5(2), 221–252.

Brennan, T. A. (1999). Proposed revisions to the Declaration of Helsinki—Will they weaken the ethical principles underlying human research? *The New England Journal of Medicine*, 341(7), 527–531.

Brink, D. O. (1989). *Moral realism and the foundations of ethics.* Cambridge University Press.

Brink, D. O. (1992). Mill's deliberative utilitarianism. *Philosophy & Public Affairs*, 21(1), 67–103.

Brock, D. (2004). Ethical issues in the use of cost effectiveness analysis for the prioritization of health care resources. In S. Anand, F. Peter, & A. Sen (Eds.), *Public health, ethics, and equity* (pp. 201–224). Oxford University Press.

Brock, G. (2009). *Global justice: A cosmopolitan account.* Oxford University Press.

Brody, H., & Miller, F. G. (1998). The internal morality of medicine: Explication and application to managed care. *The Journal of Medicine and Philosophy*, 23(4), 384–410.

Brody, H., & Miller, F. G. (2003). The clinician-investigator: Unavoidable but manageable tension. *Kennedy Institute of Ethics Journal*, 13(4), 329–346.

Calabresi, G. (1969). Reflections on medical experimentation in humans. *Daedalus*, 98(2), 387–405.

Callahan, D. (1990). *What kind of life: The limits of medical progress.* Simon and Schuster.

Callahan, D. (2000). Death and the research imperative. *The New England Journal of Medicine*, 342(9), 654–656.

Callahan, D. (2003). *What price better health: Hazards of the research imperative.* University of California Press.

Caney, S. (2005). *Justice beyond borders: A global political theory.* Oxford University Press.

Caplan, A. L. (1984). Is there a duty to serve as a subject in biomedical research? *IRB: Ethics & Human Research*, 6(5), 1–5.

Carpenter, D. (2009). Confidence games: How does regulation constitute markets? In E. J. Balleisen & D. A. Moss (Eds.), *Government and markets: Toward a new theory of regulation* (pp. 164–190). Cambridge University Press.

Centers for Disease Control and Prevention. (2003). Update: Adverse events following smallpox vaccination—United States 2003. *JAMA*, 289(20), 2642.

Chan, S., & Harris, J. (2009). Free riders and pious sons—Why science research remains obligatory. *Bioethics*, 23(3), 161–171.

Chard, J. A., & Lilford, R. J. (1998). The use of equipoise in clinical trials. *Social Science & Medicine*, 47(7), 891–898.

Cogburn, C. D. (2019). Culture, race and health: Implications for racial inequalities and population health. *Milbank Quarterly*, 97(3), 736–761.

Columbia Law School. (2009, November 24). The Threat to Academic Freedom on Campus [Press release]. Retrieved from https://www.law.columbia.edu/news/archive/threat-academic-freedom-campus

Commission on Health Research for Development. (1990). *Health research: Essential link to equity in development*. Oxford University Press.

Commission on Social Determinants of Health. (2008). *Closing the gap in a generation: Health equity through action on the social determinants of health: Final report of the Commission on Social Determinants of Health*. World Health Organization.

Cooley, D. R. (2001). Distributive justice and clinical trials in the third world. *Theoretical Medicine, 22*, 151–167.

Council for International Organizations of Medical Sciences. (2002). *International Ethical Guidelines for Biomedical Research Involving Human Subjects*. Retrieved from: https://cioms.ch/publications/product/international-ethical-guidelines-for-biomedical-research-involving-human-subjects-2/

Council for International Organizations of Medical Sciences. (2016). *International Ethical Guidelines for Health-Related Research Involving Humans*. Retrieved from: https://cioms.ch/wp-content/uploads/2017/01/WEB-CIOMS-EthicalGuidelines.pdf.

Council on Health Research for Development (COHRED). (2007). Are international health research programmes doing enough to develop research systems and skills in low and middle incomes countries? Available: http://www.cohred.org/wp-content/uploads/2013/08/4.ResponsibleVerticalProgrammingLOWRES.pdf.   Accessed December 2020.

Crouch, R. A., & Arras, J. D. (1998). AZT trials and tribulations. *The Hastings Center Report, 28*(6), 26–34.

Cullity, G. (1994). International aid and the scope of kindness. *Ethics, 105*(1), 99–127.

Cullity, G. (2004). *The moral demands of affluence*. Oxford University Press.

Daniels, N. (1985). *Just health care*. Cambridge University Press.

Daniels, N. (1990). Equality of What: Welfare, resources, or capabilities? *Philosophy and Phenomenological Research, 50*, 273–296.

Daniels, N., Kennedy, B. P., & Kawachi, I. (1999). Why justice is good for our health: The social determinants of health inequalities. *Daedalus, 128*(4), 215–251.

Dickert, N., & C. Grady. (1999). What's the price of a research subject? Approaches to payment for research participation. *New England Journal of Medicine, 341*(3), 198–203.

Dingwall, R. (2008). The ethical case against ethical regulation in humanities and social science research. *Twenty-First Century Society, 3*(1), 1–12.

Donagan, A. (1977). Informed consent in therapy and experimentation. *The Journal of Medicine and Philosophy, 2*(4), 307–329.

Dresser, R. (1992). Wanted single, white male for medical research. *The Hastings Center Report, 22*(1), 24–29.

Drèze, J., & Sen, A. (1989). *Hunger and public action*. Clarendon Press.

Dworkin, G. (1972). Paternalism. *The Monist, 56*(1), 64–84.

Dwyer-Lindgren, L., Bertozzi-Villa A., Stubbs R. W., Morozoff, C., Mackenbach, J. P., van Lenthe, F. J., Mokdad, A. H., & Murray, C. (2017). Inequalities in life expectancy among US counties, 1980 to 2014: Temporal trends and key drivers. *JAMA Internal Medicine, 177*(7), 1003–1011.

Dye, C., Boerman T., Evans D., Harries A. D., Lienhardt C., McManus J, Pang T, Terry R, Zachariah R. (2013). *The world health report 2013: Research for universal health coverage*. World Health Organization.

Easterlin, R. A. (1999). How beneficent is the market? A look at the modern history of mortality. *European Review of Economic History, 3*(3), 257–294.

Edwards, S. K. L., & Wilson J. (2012). Hard paternalism, fairness and clinical research: Why not? *Bioethics, 26*(2), 68–75.

Eisenberg, L. (1977). The social imperatives of medical research. *Science, 198*(4322), 1105–1110.

Emanuel, E. J. (2008). Benefits to host countries. In E. J. Emanuel, C. C. Grady, R. A. Crouch, R. K. Lie, F. G. Miller, & D. D. Wendler (Eds.), *The Oxford textbook of clinical research ethics* (pp. 719–728). Oxford University Press.

Emanuel, E. J., Wendler, D., & Grady, C. (2000). What makes clinical research ethical? *JAMA, 283*(20), 2701–2711.

Enkin, M. W. (2000). Clinical equipoise and not the uncertainty principle is the moral underpinning of the randomised controlled trial: Against. *British Medical Journal, 321*(7263), 756–758.

Eyal, N., & Lipsitch, M. (2017). Vaccine testing for emerging infections: The case for individual randomisation. *Journal of Medical Ethics, 43*(9), 625–631.

Fauber, J. (2012, January 3). BMJ: Discipline researchers who withhold research results. *MedPage Today*. Retrieved from https://www.medpagetoday.com/publichealthpolicy/clinicaltrials/30482.

Finnis, J. (2011). *Natural law and natural rights*. Oxford University Press.

Fishkin, J. S. (1982). *The limits of obligation*. Yale University Press.

Flory, J. H., & Kitcher, P. (2004). Global health and the scientific research agenda. *Philosophy & Public Affairs, 32*(1), 36–65.

Forde, A. T., Sims M., Muntner P., Lewis T, Onwuka A, Moore K, Ruox A. V. (2020). Discrimination and hypertension risk among African Americans in the Jackson heart study. *Hypertension, 76*(3), 715–723.

Francis, D.P. (1998). To the editor, *New England Journal of Medicine 338*, 837.

Freedman, B. (1987). Equipoise and the ethics of clinical research. *New England Journal of Medicine, 317*, 141–145.

Freedman, B. (1990). Placebo-controlled trials and the logic of clinical purpose. *IRB: Ethics & Human Research, 12*(6), 1–6.

Freedman, B., Weijer, C., & Glass, K. C. (1996). Placebo orthodoxy in clinical research I: Empirical and methodological myths. *The Journal of Law, Medicine & Ethics, 24*(3), 243–251.

Freeman, S. (1990). Reason and agreement in social contract views. *Philosophy & Public Affairs, (19)*2, 122–157.

Freeman, S. (2000). Deliberative democracy: A sympathetic comment. *Philosophy & Public Affairs, 29*(4), 371–418.

Freeman, S. (2006). Distributive Justice and *The Law of Peoples*. In R. Martin & D. A. Reidy (Eds.), *Rawls's law of peoples: A realistic utopia?* (pp. 243–260). Blackwell Publishing.

Freidenfelds, L., & Brandt, A. M. (1996). Commentary: Research ethics after World War II: The insular culture of biomedicine. *Kennedy Institute of Ethics Journal, 6*(3), 239–243.

Fried, C. (1974). *Medical experimentation: Personal integrity and public policy*. North-Holland Publishing.

Galston, W. A. (2004). Liberal Pluralism: The implications of value pluralism for political theory and practice. Cambridge University Press.

Gans, C. (2003). *The limits of nationalism*. Cambridge University Press.

Genest, C., McConway, K. J., & Schervish, M. J. (1986). Characterization of externally Bayesian pooling operators. *The Annals of Statistics, 14*(2), 487–501.

Gifford, F. (1986). The conflict between randomized clinical trials and the therapeutic obligation. *The Journal of Medicine and Philosophy, 11*(4), 347–366.

Glantz, L. H., Annas, G. J., Grodin, M. A., & Mariner, W. K. (1998). Research in developing countries: Taking "benefit" seriously. *The Hastings Center Report, 28*(6), 38–42.

Glickman, S. W., McHutchison, J. G., Peterson, E. D., Cairns, C. B., Harrington, R. A., Califf, R. M., & Schulman, K. A. (2009). Ethical and scientific implications of the globalization of clinical research. *New England Journal of Medicine, 360,* 816–823. doi:10.1056/NEJMsb0803929

Gold, M. R., Stevenson D., & Fryback, D. G. (2002). HALYS and QALYS and DALYS, oh my: Similarities and differences in summary measures of population health. *Annual Review of Public Health, 23,* 115–134.

Goldman, A. H. (1980). *The moral foundations of professional ethics.* Rowman and Littlefield.

Goodman, S. N. (2007). Stopping at nothing? Some dilemmas of data monitoring in clinical trials. *Annals of Internal Medicine, 146*(12), 882–887.

Gostin, L. O. (2010). What duties do poor countries have for the health of their own people? *Hastings Center Report, 40*(2), 9–10.

Grady, C. (1998). Science in the service of healing. *The Hastings Center Report, 28*(6), 34–38.

Green, A. (2014). Remembering health workers who died from Ebola in 2014. *The Lancet, 384*(9961), 2201–2206.

Haines, A., Kuruvilla, S., & Borchert M. (2004). Bridging the implementation gap between knowledge and action for health. *Bulletin of the World Health Organization, 82,* 724–732.

Hardin, G. (1968). The tragedy of the commons. *Science, 162*(3859), 1243–1248.

Hardin, R. (1988). *Morality within the limits of reason.* University of Chicago Press.

Harris, J. (2005). Scientific research is a moral duty. *Journal of Medical Ethics, 31*(4), 242–248. doi:10.1136/jme.2005.011973

Hellman, D. (2002). Evidence, belief, and action: The failure of equipoise to resolve the ethical tension in the randomized clinical trial. *The Journal of Law, Medicine & Ethics, 30*(3), 375–380.

Herper, M., & Riglin, E. (2020). "Data show panic and disorganization dominate the study of Covid-19 drugs" STAT News. July 6, 2020. https://www.statnews.com/ 2020/07/06/data-show-panic-and-disorganization-domin- ate-the-study-of-covid-19-drugs/.

Herrera, C. D. (2003). Universal compulsory service in medical research. *Theoretical Medicine and Bioethics, 24*(3), 215–231.

Heyd, D. (1996). Experimentation on trial: Why should one take part in medical research? Jahrbuch fur Recht und Ethik/ Annual Review of Law and Ethics 4: 189–204.

Heymann, D. L. (2000). *The urgency of a massive effort against infectious diseases, statement before the Committee on International Relations, US House of Representatives,* 1–141. 106ᵗʰ Congress.

Hill, A. B. (1963). Medical ethics and controlled trials. *British Medical Journal, 1*(5337), 1043–1049.

Hobbes, T. (1985). *Leviathan.* Penguin Group.

Holm, S. (2020). Belmont in Europe: A mostly indirect influence. *Perspectives in Biology and Medicine, 63*(2), 262–276.

Hull, D. L. (1988). *Science as a process: An evolutionary account of the social and conceptual development of science.* University of Chicago Press.

Hyman, D. A. (2007). Institutional review boards: Is this the least worst we can do. *Northwestern University Law Review, 101,* 749–774.

IJsselmuiden, C. B. (1998). New England Journal of Medicine 338(12), 838.

Institute of Medicine. (2007). *Rewarding provider performance: Aligning incentives in Medicare, pathways to quality health care.* The National Academies Press.

Jamison, D. T., Breman, J. G., Measham, A. R., Alleyne, G., Claeson, M., Evans, D. B., Jha, P., Mills, A., and Musgrove, P. (Eds.). (2006). *Disease control proprieties in developing countries* (2nd ed.). The World Bank.

Jamison, D. T., Summers, L. H., Alleyne, G., Arrow, K. J., Berkley, S., Binagwaho, A., Bustreo, F., Evans, D., Feachem, R. G., Frenk, J., Ghosh, G., Goldie, S. J., Guo, Y., Gupta, S., Horton, R., Kruk, M. E., Mahmoud, A., Mohohlo, L. K., Ncube, M., . . . Yamey, G. (2013). Global health 2035: A world converging within a generation. *Lancet, 382,* 1898–1955.

Jansen, L. A., & Wall, S. (2009). Paternalism and fairness in clinical research. *Bioethics, 23*(3), 172–182.

Jha, P., Mills, A., Hanson, K., Kumaranayake, L., Conteh, L., Kurowski, C., Nguyen, S. N., Cruz, V. O., Ranson, K., Vaz, L. M., Yu, S., Morton, O., & Sachs, J. D. (2002). Improving the health of the global poor. *Science, 295*(5562), 2036–2039.

Jonas, H. (1969). Philosophical reflections on experimenting with human subjects. *Daedalus 98*(2), 219–247.

Jones, C. (1999). *Global justice: Defending cosmopolitanism.* Oxford University Press.

Jones, J. H. (1993). *Bad blood.* Free Press.

Jones, J. H. (2008). The Tuskegee syphilis experiment. In E. J. Emanuel, C. C. Grady, R. A. Crouch, R. K. Lie, F. G. Miller, & D. D. Wendler (Eds.), *The Oxford textbook of clinical research ethics* (pp. 86–96). Oxford University Press.

Kadane, J. B. (Ed.). (1996). *Bayesian methods and ethics in a clinical trial design.* John Wiley & Sons.

Kagan, S. (1997). *Normative ethics.* Westview Press.

Kahn, J. P., Mastroianni, A. C., & Sugarman, J. (Eds.). (1998). *Beyond consent: Seeking justice in research.* Oxford University Press.

Katz, J., Capron, A. M., & Glass, E. S. (1972). *Experimentation with human beings: The authority of the investigator, subject, professions, and state in the human experimentation process.* Russell Sage Foundation.

Kharsany, A. B., & Karim, Q. A. (2016). HIV infection and AIDS in sub-Saharan Africa: Current status, challenges and opportunities. *The open AIDS journal, 10*, 34.

Kimmelman, J. (2012), A theoretical framework for early human studies: Uncertainty, intervention ensembles, and boundaries. *Trials, 13*(1), 173.

Kimmelman, J., Carlisle, B., & Gönen, M. (2017). Drug development at the portfolio level is important for policy, care decisions and human protections. *JAMA, 318*(11), 1003–1004.

Kimmelman, J., & London, A. J. (2011). Predicting harms and benefits in translational trials: Ethics, evidence, and uncertainty. *PLoS Medicine, 8*(3), e1001010.

Kimmelman, J., & London, A. J. (2015). The structure of clinical translation: efficiency, information, and ethics. *Hastings Center Report, 45*(2), 27–39.

Kimmelman, J., Weijer, C., & Meslin, E. M. (2009). Helsinki Discords: FDA, Ethics, and International Drug Trials. *The Lancet, 373*(9657), 13–14.

Kitcher, P. (1995). *The advancement of science: Science without legend, objectivity without illusions.* Oxford University Press.

Klemperer, P. (2004). *Auctions: Theory and practice.* Princeton University Press.

Korsgaard, C. (1993). G. A. Cohen: Equality of what? On welfare, goods and capabilities. Amartya Sen: Capability and well-Being. In M. C. Nussbaum & A. Sen (Eds.), *The quality of life* (pp. 54–61). Oxford University Press.

Kukla, R. (2007). Resituating the principle of equipoise: Justice and access to care in nonideal conditions. *Kennedy Institute of Ethics Journal, 17*(3), 171–202.

Laage, T., Loewy, J. W., Menon, S., Miller, E. R., Pulkstenis, E., Kan-Dobrosky, N., & Coffey, C. (2017). Ethical considerations in adaptive design clinical trials. *Therapeutic Innovation & Regulatory Science, 51*(2), 190–199.

Lasagna, L. (1971). Some ethical problems in clinical investigation. In E. Mendelsohn, J. P. Swazey, & I. Taviss (Eds.), *Human aspects of biomedical innovation* (pp. 98–110). Harvard University Press.

Lederer, S. (1995). *Subjected to science: Human experimentation in America before the Second World War.* Johns Hopkins University Press.

Lederer, S. (2008). Walter Reed and the yellow fever experiments. In E. J. Emanuel, C. C. Grady, R. A. Crouch, R. K. Lie, F. G. Miller, & D. D. Wendler (Eds.), *The Oxford textbook of clinical research ethics* (pp. 9–17). Oxford University Press.

Lemmens, T., & Elliott, C. (1999). Guinea pigs on the payroll: The ethics of paying research subjects. *Accountability in Research, 7*(1): 3–20.

Leon, A. C. (2001). Can placebo controls reduce the number of non-responders in clinical trials? A power-analytic perspective. *Clinical Therapeutics, 23*(4), 596–603.

Levi, I. (1986). *Hard choices: Decision making under unresolved conflict.* Cambridge University Press.

Levine, C. (1998). Placebos and HIV: Lessons learned. *The Hastings Center Report, 28*(6), 43–48.

Levine, R. J. (1998). The "best proven therapeutic method" standard in clinical trials in technologically developing countries. *IRB: Ethics & Human Research, 20*(1), 5–9.

Levine, R. J. (1999). The need to revise the Declaration of Helsinki. *New England Journal of Medicine, 341*, 531–534.

Lewis, R. J. (2016). The pragmatic clinical trial in a learning health care system. *Clinical Trials, 13*(5), 484–492.

Lin, J., Lin, L. A., & Sandkoh, S. (2016). A general overview of adaptive randomization design for clinical trials. *Journal of Biometrics and Biostatistics, 7*(2), 294.

London, A. J. (2000a). Thrasymachus and managed care: How not to think about the craft of medicine. In Mark G Kuczewski (Ed.) *Bioethics: Ancient themes in contemporary issues,* 131–154. MIT Press.

London, A. J. (2000b). The ambiguity and the exigency: Clarifying "standard of care" arguments in international research. *The Journal of Medicine and Philosophy, 25*(4), 379–397.

London, A. J. (2001). Equipoise and international human-subjects research. *Bioethics, 15*(4), 312–332.

London, A. J. (2003). Threats to the common good: Biochemical weapons and human subjects research. *Hastings Center Report, 33*(5), 17–25.

London, A. J. (2005). Justice and the human development approach to international research. *Hastings Center Report, 35*(1), 24–37.

London, A. J. (2006a). Reasonable risks in clinical research: A critique and a proposal for the integrative approach. *Statistics in Medicine, 25*(17), 2869–2885.

London, A. J. (2006b). Sham surgery and reasonable risks. In D. Benatar (Ed.), *Cutting to the core: Exploring the ethics of contested surgeries* (pp. 211–228). Rowman & Littlefield Publishers.

London, A. J. (2007a). Clinical equipoise: Foundational requirement or fundamental error? In B. Steinbock (Ed.), *The Oxford handbook of bioethics* (pp. 571–596). Oxford University Press.

London, A. J. (2007b). Two dogmas of research ethics and the integrative approach to human-subjects research. *The Journal of Medicine and Philosophy, 32*(2), 99–116.

London, A. J. (2008). Responsiveness to host community health needs. In E. J. Emanuel, C. C. Grady, R. A. Crouch, R. K. Lie, F. G. Miller, & D. D. Wendler (Eds.), *The Oxford textbook of clinical research ethics* (pp. 737–744). Oxford University Press.

London, A. J. (2009). Clinical research in a public health crisis: The integrative approach to managing uncertainty and mitigating conflict. *Seton Hall Law Review, 39*(4), 1173–1202.

London, A. J. (2012). A non-paternalistic model of research ethics and oversight: Assessing the benefits of prospective review. *The Journal of Law, Medicine & Ethics, 40*(4), 930–944.

London, A. J. (2019). Social value, clinical equipoise, and research in a public health emergency. *Bioethics, 33*(3), 326–334.

London, A. J. (2020). Self-defeating codes of medical ethics and how to fix them: Failures in COVID-19 response and beyond. *The American Journal of Bioethics, 21*(1), 4–13.

London, A. J., & Kadane, J. B. (2002). Placebos that harm: Sham surgery controls in clinical trials. *Statistical Methods in Medical Research, 11*(5), 413–427.

London, A. J., & Kadane, J. B. (2003). Sham surgery and genuine standards of care: Can the two be reconciled? *American Journal of Bioethics, 3*(4), 61–64.

London, A. J., & Kimmelman, J. (2008). Justice in translation: From bench to bedside in the developing world. *The Lancet, 372*(9632), 82–85.

London, A. J., & Kimmelman, J. (2015). Why clinical translation cannot succeed without failure. *eLife* (4), e12844.

London, A. J., & Kimmelman, J. (2016). Accelerated drug approval and health inequality. *JAMA Internal Medicine, 176*(7), 883–884.

London, A. J., & Kimmelman J. (2019). Clinical trial portfolios: A critical oversight in human research ethics, drug regulation, and policy. *Hastings Center Report, 49*(4), 31–41.

London, A. J., Kimmelman, J., & Carlisle, B. (2012). Rethinking research ethics: The case of postmarketing trials. *Science, 336*(6081), 544–545.

London, A. J., Kimmelman, J., & Emborg, M. E. (2010). Beyond access vs. protection in trials of innovative therapies. *Science, 328*(5980), 829–830.

London, A. J., & Zollman, K. J. (2010). Research at the auction block: Problems for the fair benefits approach to international research. *Hastings Center Report, 40*(4), 34–45.

Lurie, P., & Wolfe, S. M. (1997). Unethical trials of interventions to reduce perinatal transmission of the human immunodeficiency virus in developing countries. *New England Journal of Medicine, 337*(12), 853–856.

Lynch, H. F. (2014). Human research subjects as human research workers. *Yale Journal of Health Policy, Law, and Ethics, 14*(1), 122–193.

MacKay, D. (2018). The ethics of public policy RCTs: The principle of policy equipoise. *Bioethics, 32*(1), 59–67.

MacKay, D. (2020). Government policy experiments and the ethics of randomization. *Philosophy and Public Affairs 48*(4), 319–352.

Macklin, R. (2001). After Helsinki: Unresolved issues in international research. *Kennedy Institute of Ethics Journal, 11*(1), 17–36.

Macklin, R. (2004). *Double standards in medical research in developing countries*. Cambridge University Press.

Malmqvist, E. (2019). "Paid to endure": Paid research participation, passivity, and the goods of work. *The American Journal of Bioethics, 19*(9), 11–20.

Malone, R. E., Yerger, V. B., McGruder, C., & Froelicher, E. (2006). "It's like Tuskegee in reverse": A case study of ethical tensions in institutional review board review of community-based participatory research. *American Journal of Public Health, 96*(11), 1914–1919.

Manderson, L. (2002). *Sickness and the state: Health and illness in colonial Malaya, 1870–1940*. Cambridge University Press.

Marmot, M., & Bell, R. (2012). Fair society, healthy lives. *Public Health, 126*, S4–S10.

Marmot, M., & Wilkinson, R. (Eds.). (2005). *Social determinants of health*. Oxford University Press.

Marquis, D. (1983). Leaving therapy to chance. *Hastings Center Report, 13*(4), 40–47.

McDermott, W. (1967). Opening comments on the changing mores of biomedical research. *Annals of Internal Medicine, 67* (Suppl. 7), 39–42.

McGregor S., Henderson K. J., & Kaldor J. M. (2014). How are health research priorities set in low and middle income countries? A systematic review of published reports. *PLoS ONE, 9*(10), e108787.

McManus, J., & Saywell, T. (2001). The lure to cure. *Far Eastern Economic Review, 164*(5), 32–37.

Mello, M. M., & Brennan, T. A. (2001). The controversy over high-dose chemotherapy with autologous bone marrow transplant for breast cancer. *Health Affairs, 20*(5), 101–117.

Menikoff, J., & Richards, E. P. (2006). *What the doctor didn't say: The hidden truth about medical research*. Oxford University Press.

Meurer, W. J., Lewis, R. J., & Berry, D. A. (2012). Adaptive clinical trials: A partial remedy for the therapeutic misconception? *JAMA, 307*(22), 2377–2378.

Mill, J. S. (1880). *On liberty*. Longmans, Green, Reader and Dyer.

Miller, D. (1995). *On nationality*. Oxford University Press.

Miller. D. (2007). *National responsibility and global justice*. Oxford University Press.

Miller, F. G. (2003). Sham surgery: An ethical analysis. *American Journal of Bioethics, 3*(4), 41–48.

Miller, F. G., & Brody, H. (2002). What makes placebo-controlled trials unethical? *The American Journal of Bioethics, 2*(2), 3–9.

Miller, F. G., & Brody, H. (2003). A critique of clinical equipoise: Therapeutic misconception in the ethics of clinical trials. *Hastings Center Report, 33*(3), 19–28.

Miller, F. G., & Brody, H. (2007). Clinical equipoise and the incoherence of research ethics. *The Journal of Medicine and Philosophy, 32*(2), 151–165.

Miller, F. G. & Grady, C. (2001). The ethical challenge of infection-inducing challenge experiments. *Clinical Infectious Diseases, 33*(7), 1028–1033.

Miller, F. G., & Wertheimer, A. (2007). Facing up to paternalism in research ethics. *Hastings Center Report, 37*(3), 24–34.

Miller, P. B., & Weijer, C. (2003). Rehabilitating equipoise. *Kennedy Institute of Ethics Journal, 13*(2), 93–118.

Miller, P. B., & Weijer, C. (2006a). Fiduciary obligation in clinical research. *The Journal of Law, Medicine & Ethics, 34*(2), 424–440.

Miller, P. B., & Weijer, C. (2006b). Trust based obligations of the state and physician-researchers to patient-subjects. *Journal of Medical Ethics, 32*(9), 542–547.

Moreno, J. D. (1999). *Undue risk: Secret state experiments on humans.* W. H. Freeman.

Moss, J. (2007). If institutional review boards were declared unconstitutional, they would have to be reinvented. *Northwestern University Law Review, 101,* 801–807.

Mueller, J. H. (2007). Ignorance is neither bliss nor ethical. *Northwestern University Law Review, 101,* 809–836.

Muldoon, R. (2013). Diversity and the division of cognitive labor. *Philosophy Compass, 8*(2), 117–125.

Myerson, R. B. (1981). Optimal auction design. *Mathematics of Operations Research, 6*(1): 58–73.

Nagel T. (1991). Equality and Partiality. Oxford University Press.

Narens, L., & Luce, R. D. (1983). How we may have been misled into believing in the interpersonal comparability of utility. *Theory and Decision, 15*(3), 247–260.

National Commission for the Protection of Human Subjects of Biomedical and Behavioral Research. (1979). *The Belmont report: Ethical principles and guidelines for the protection of human subjects of research.* Retrieved from https://www.hhs.gov/ohrp/regulations-and-policy/belmont-report/read-the-belmont-report/index.html.

Neuringer, A. (1981). Self-experimentation: A call for change. *Behaviorism, 9*(1), 79–94.

Nozick, R. (1974). *Anarchy, state, and utopia.* Basic Books.

Nussbaum, M. (1996). Patriotism and cosmopolitanism. In J. Cohen (Ed.), *For love of country: Debating the limits of patriotism* (pp. 3–17). Beacon Press.

Nussbaum, M. C. (1999). Women and equality: The capabilities approach. *International Labour Review, 138*(3), 227–245.

Nussbaum, M. C. (2000). *Women and human development: The capabilities approach.* Cambridge University Press.

Nuyens, Y. (2005). *No development without research: A challenge for capacity strengthening.* Global Forum for Health Research.

Paina, L., & Peters D. H. (2012). Understanding pathways for scaling up health services through the lens of complex adaptive systems. *Health Policy and Planning, 27,* 365–373.

Parfit, D. (1984). *Reasons and persons.* Oxford University Press.

Participants in the 2001 Conference on Ethical Aspects of Research in Developing Countries. (2002). Fair benefits for research in developing countries. *Science 298*(5601), 2133–2134.

Participants in the 2001 Conference on Ethical Aspects of Research in Developing Countries. (2004). Moral standards for research in developing countries: From "reasonable availability" to "fair benefits." *Hastings Center Report, 34*(3), 17–27.

PATH. (2014). *The role of research and innovation for health in the post-2015 development agenda: Bridging the divide between the richest and poorest within a generation.* COHRED, Global Health Technologies Coalition, International AIDS Vaccine Initiative, PATH.

Pearson, J. L. (2018). *The colonial politics of global health: France and the United Nations in postwar Africa.* Harvard University Press.

Peto, R., & Baigent, C. (1998). Trials: The next 50 years: large scale randomised evidence of moderate benefits. *British Medical Journal, 317,* 1170–1171.

Peto, R., Pike, M., Armitage, P., Breslow, N. E., Cox, D. R., Howard, S. V., Mantel, N., McPherson, K., Peto, J., & Smith, P. G. (1976). Design and analysis of randomized clinical trials requiring prolonged observation of each patient. I. Introduction and design. *British Journal of Cancer, 34*(6), 585–612.

Petryna, A. (2007). Clinical trials offshored: On private sector science and public health. *BioSocieties 2*(1): 21–40.

Petryna, A. (2009). *When experiments travel: Clinical trials and the global search for human subjects*. Princeton University Press.

Pettit, P. (1997). *Republicanism: A theory of freedom and government*. Oxford University Press.

Pettit, P. (2004). The common good. In K. M. Dowding, R. E. Goodin, C. Pateman, & B. Barry (Eds.), *Justice and democracy: Essays for Brian Barry* (pp. 150–169). Cambridge University Press.

Pierson, L., & Millum, J. (2018). Health research priority setting: The duties of individual funders. *American Journal of Bioethics, 18*(11), 6–17.

Pogge, T. W. (1994). An egalitarian law of peoples. *Philosophy & Public Affairs, 23*(3), 195–224.

Pogge, T. W. (2001). Eradicating systemic poverty: Brief for a global resources dividend. *Journal of Human Development, 2*(1), 59–77.

Pogge, T. W. (2002a). Responsibilities for poverty-related ill health. *Ethics & International Affairs, 16*(2), 71–79.

Pogge, T. W. (2002b). *World poverty and human rights*. Polity Press.

Potts, M. (2000). Thinking about vaginal microbicide testing. *American Journal of Public Health, 90*(2), 188–190.

Pratt, B., & de Vries, J. (2018). Community engagement in global health research that advances health equity. *Bioethics, 32*, 454–463.

Pratt, B., & Hyder, A. A. (2015). Global justice and health systems research in low- and middle-income countries. *Journal of Law, Medicine & Ethics, 43*(1), 143–161.

Pratt, B., & Loff, B. (2014). A framework to link international clinical research to the promotion of justice in global health. *Bioethics, 28*(8), 387–396.

Pratt, B., Zion, D., & Loff, B. (2012). Evaluating the capacity of theories of justice to serve as a justice framework for international clinical research. *The American Journal of Bioethics, 12*(11), 30–41.

President's Council on Bioethics. (2009). *Session 2: National ethics committees: Mission, functions, philosophies, and modus operandi* [Presentation]. Retrieved from https://bioethicsarchive.georgetown.edu/pcbe/transcripts/march09/session2.html.

Protection of Human Subjects, 45 C.F.R. § 46 (2009). US Department of Health and Human Services.

Rajczi, A. (2004). Making risk-benefit assessments of medical research protocols. *Journal of Law, Medicine & Ethics, 32*(2), 338–348.

Ramsey, P. (1976). The enforcement of morals: Nontherapeutic research on children. *Hastings Center Report, 6*(4), 21–30.

Rawls, J. (1971). *A theory of justice*. Harvard University Press.

Rawls, J. (1982). Social unity and the primary goods. In A. Sen, B. Williams, & B. A. O. Williams (Eds.), *Utilitarianism and beyond* (pp. 159–185). Cambridge University Press.

Rawls, J. (1999). *The law of peoples*. Harvard University Press.

Rawls, J. (2001). *Justice as fairness: A restatement*. Harvard University Press.

Raz, J. (1984). On the nature of rights. *Mind, 93*(370), 194–214.

Rehnquist, J. (2001). *The globalization of clinical trials: a growing challenge in protecting human subjects*. (DHHS Publication No. OEI-01-00-00190). U.S. Department of Health and Human Services, Office of Inspector General Report.

Renfro, L. A., & Sargent, D. J. (2017). Statistical controversies in clinical research: Basket trials, umbrella trials, and other master protocols: A review and examples. *Annals of Oncology, 28*(1), 34–43.

Resnik, D. B. (2001). Developing drugs for the developing world: An economic, legal, moral, and political dilemma. *Developing World Bioethics*, *1*(1), 11–32.

Reverby, S. M. (2009). *Examining Tuskegee: The infamous syphilis study and its legacy.* University of North Carolina Press.

Reverby, S. M. (2011). "Normal exposure" and inoculation syphilis: A PHS "Tuskegee" doctor in Guatemala, 1946–1948. *Journal of Policy History*, *23*(1), 6–28.

Rhodes, R. (2008). In defense of the duty to participate in biomedical research. *American Journal of Bioethics*, *8*(10), 37–38.

Rid, A., & Wendler, D. (2010). Risk–benefit assessment in medical research—critical review and open questions. *Law, Probability & Risk*, *9*(3–4), 151–177.

Ridley, M., Rao, G., Schilbach, F., & Patel, V. (2020). Poverty, depression, and anxiety: Causal evidence and mechanisms. *Science*, *370*(1289), eaay0214.

Riley, J. G., & Samuelson, W. F. (1981). Optimal auctions. *The American Economic Review*, *71*(3), 381–392.

Rothman, D. J. (1991). *Strangers at the bedside: A history of how law and bioethics transformed medical decision making.* Basic Books.

Rothman, D. J., & Rothman, S. M. (1984). *The Willowbrook wars.* Harper and Row.

Rowberg, R. E. (1998). Federal R & D funding: A concise history. Congressional Research Service, the Library of Congress.

Różyńska, J. (2018). What makes clinical labour different? The case of human guinea pigging. *Journal of Medical Ethics*, *44*, 638–642.

Rubin, J. Z., Pruitt, D. G., & Kim, S. H. (1994). *Social conflict: Escalation, stalemate, and settlement.* Mcgraw-Hill Book Company.

Ruger, J. P. (2018). *Global health justice and governance.* Oxford University Press.

Sackett, D. L. (2000). Equipoise, a term whose time (if it ever came) has surely gone. *Canadian Medical Association Journal*, *163*(7), 835–836.

Salim, S. and K. Abdool (1998). Placebo controls in HIV perinatal transmission trials: A South African's viewpoint, *American Journal of Public Health* 88, 564–566.

Savage, L. J. (1972). *The foundations of statistics.* Courier Corporation.

Saville, B. R., & Berry, S. M. (2016). Efficiencies of platform clinical trials: A vision of the future. *Clinical Trials*, *13*(3), 358–366.

Saxman, S. B. (2015). Ethical considerations for outcome-adaptive trial designs: A clinical researcher's perspective. *Bioethics*, *29*(2), 59–65.

Schaefer, G. O., Emanuel, E. J., & Wertheimer, A. (2009). The obligation to participate in biomedical research. *JAMA*, *302*(1), 67–72. doi:10.1001/jama.2009.931

Scheffler, S. (1994). *The rejection of consequentialism: A philosophical investigation of the considerations underlying rival moral conceptions.* Oxford University Press.

Schneider, C. (2009). Session 2: National Ethics Committees: Mission, Functions, Philosophies, and Modus Operandi (Meeting of the President's Council on Bioethics, Washington, DC, March 12, 2009). http://bioethics.georgetown.edu/pcbe/transcripts/march09/session2.html.

Schüklenk, U., & Ashcroft, R. E. (2002). Affordable access to essential medications in developing countries: Conflicts between ethical and economic imperatives. *The Journal of Medicine and Philosophy*, *27*(2), 179–195.

Seidenfeld, T., Schervish, M. J., & Kadane, J. B. (2010). Coherent choice functions under uncertainty. *Synthese*, *172*(1), 157–176.

Sen, A. (1979). Utilitarianism and welfarism. *The Journal of Philosophy*, *76*(9), 463–489.

Sen, A. (1981). *Poverty and Famines.* Oxford: Clarendon Press.

Sen, A. (1982). Equality of what? In A. Sen (Ed.), *Choice, welfare, and measurement* (pp. 353–369). Harvard University Press.

Sen, A. (1999a). *Commodities and capabilities.* Oxford University Press.

Sen, A. (1999b). *Development as freedom.* Anchor Books.

Senn, S. (2001). The misunderstood placebo. *Applied Clinical Trials, 10*(5), 40–46.

Shah, S. (2002). Globalizing clinical research. *The Nation, 275*(1), 23–28.

Shah, S. (2003). Globalization of clinical research by the pharmaceutical industry. *International Journal of Health Services, 33*(1), 29–36.

Shamoo, A., & Resnik, D. B. (2009). *Responsible conduct of research.* Oxford University Press.

Sheikh, K., Hargreaves J., Khan M., & Mounier-Jack S. (2020). Implementation research in LMICs—evolution through innovation. *Health Policy and Planning, 35* (Issue Supplement 2), ii1–ii3.

Shue, H. (1988). Mediating duties. *Ethics, 98*(4), 687–704.

Shue, H. (1996). *Basic rights: Subsistence, affluence, and U.S. foreign policy* (2nd ed.). Princeton University Press.

Sidgwick, H. (1930). *The methods of ethics* (7th ed.). Macmillan and Co.

Simmons, A. J. (1979). *Moral principles and political obligations.* Princeton University Press.

Singer, P. (1972). Famine, affluence, and morality. *Philosophy & Public Affairs, (1)*3, 229–243.

Singer, P. A., & Benatar, S. R. (2001). Beyond Helsinki: A vision for global health ethics. *British Medical Journal, 322*, 747–748. doi:https://doi.org/10.1136/bmj.322.7289.747

Sitthi-Amorn, C., & Somrongthong, R. (2000). Strengthening health research capacity in developing countries: a critical element for achieving health equity. *British Medical Journal, 321*, 813–817.

Skyrms, B. (2004). *The stag hunt and the evolution of social structure.* Cambridge University Press.

Sobel, D. (2007). The importance of the demandingness objection. *Philosopher's Imprint 7*(8),1–17.

Sofaer, N., & Strech, D. (2011). Reasons why post-trial access to trial drugs should, or need not be ensured to research participants: a systematic review. *Public Health Ethics, 4*(2), 160–184.

Solomon, M. (1992). Scientific rationality and human reasoning. *Philosophy of Science, 59*(3), 439–455.

Sreenivasan, G. (2002). International justice and health: A proposal. *Ethics & International Affairs, 16*(2), 81–90.

Sreenivasan, G. (2007). Health care and equality of opportunity. *Hastings Center Report, 37*(2), 21–31.

Stadtmauer, E. A., O'Neill, A., Goldstein, L. J., Crilley, P. A., Mangan, K. F., Ingle, J. N., Brodsky, I., Martino, S., Lazarus, H. M., Erban, J. K., Sickles, C., & Glick, J. H. (2000). Conventional-dose chemotherapy compared with high-dose chemotherapy plus autologous hematopoietic stem-cell transplantation for metastatic breast cancer. *New England Journal of Medicine, 342*(15), 1069–1076.

Suntharalingam, G., Perry, M. R., Ward, S., Brett, S. J., Castello-Cortes, A., Brunner, M. D., & Panoskaltsis, N. (2006). Cytokine storm in a phase 1 trial of the anti-CD28 monoclonal antibody TGN1412. *New England Journal of Medicine, 355*(10), 1018–1028.

Tamir, Y. (1993). *Liberal nationalism, press.* Princeton University Press.

Tamir, Y. (2019). *Why nationalism.* Princeton University Press.

Taylor, C. (1979). Atomism. In A. Kontos (Ed.), *Powers, possessions and freedom: Essays in honour of C. B. Macpherson* (pp. 39–61). University of Toronto Press.

Temple, R., & Ellenberg, S. S. (2000). Placebo-controlled trials and active-control trials in the evaluation of new treatments. Part 1: Ethical and scientific issues. *Annals of Internal Medicine, 133*(6), 455–463.

Thiers, F. A., Sinskey, A. J., & Berndt, E. R. (2008). Trends in the globalization of clinical trials. *Nature Reviews Drug Discovery, 7*, 13–14.

Trials of war criminals before the Nuernberg Military Tribunals under control council law no. 10. Volume II: "The medical case" (1949). Washington: US Government Printing Office.

Trusheim, M. R., Shrier, A. A., Antonijevic, Z., Beckman, R. A., Campbell, R. K., Chen, C., Flaherty, K. T., Loewy, J., Lacombe, D., Madhavan, S., Selker, H. P., & Esserman, L. J. (2016). PIPELINEs: Creating comparable clinical knowledge efficiently by linking trial platforms. *Clinical Pharmacology & Therapeutics, 100*(6), 713–729.

Turshen, M. (1977). The impact of colonialism on health and health services in Tanzania. *International Journal of Health Services, 7*(1), 7–35.

U.S. Department of Health and Human Services. (2018). Code of Federal Regulations: Title 45, Public Welfare; Part 46, Protection of Human Subjects. Washington, DC: https://www.ecfr.gov/cgi-bin/retrieveECFR?gp=&SID=83cd09e1c0f5c6937cd9d7513160fc3f&pitd=20180719&n=pt45.1.46&r=PART&ty=HTML.

U.S. Public Health Service. (1973). *Final report of the Tuskegee Syphilis Study Ad Hoc Advisory Panel.* U.S. Department of Health, Education, and Welfare.

Van Niekerk, A. A. (2002). Moral and social complexities of AIDS in Africa. *The Journal of Medicine and Philosophy, 27*(2), 143–162.

Varmus, H., & Satcher, D. (1997). Ethiccal complexities of conducting research in developing countries. New England Journal of Medicine 337: 1003–1005.

Washington, H. A. (2006). Medical apartheid: The dark history of medical experimentation on black Americans from colonial times to the present. Harlem Moon.

Wayne, K., & Glass, K. C. (2010). The research imperative revisited: Considerations for advancing the debate surrounding medical research as moral imperative. *Perspectives in Biology and Medicine, 53*(3), 373–387.

Weijer, C. (1999). Thinking clearly about research risk: Implications of the work of Benjamin Freedman. *IRB: A Review of Human Subjects Research, 21*(6), 1–5.

Weijer, C. (2000). The ethical analysis of risk. *The Journal of Law, Medicine & Ethics, 28*(4), 344–361.

Weijer, C., & Crouch, R. A. (1999). Why should we include women and minorities in randomized controlled trials? *Journal of Clinical Ethics, 100*(2), 79–87.

Weijer, C., & LeBlanc, G. J. (2006). The balm of Gilead: Is the provision of treatment to those who seroconvert in HIV prevention trials a matter of moral obligation or moral negotiation? *The Journal of Law, Medicine & Ethics, 34*(4), 793–808.

Weijer, C., & Miller, P. B. (2004). When are research risks reasonable in relation to anticipated benefits? *Nature Medicine, 10*(6), 570–573.

Wendler, D., & Miller, F. G. (2007). Assessing research risks systematically: The net risks test. *Journal of Medical Ethics, 33*(8), 481–6.

Weijer, C., Miller, P. B., & Graham, M. (2014). The duty of care and equipoise in randomized controlled trials. In J. D. Arras, E. Fenton, R. Kukla (Eds.), *The Routledge Companion to Bioethics* (pp. 200–214). Taylor and Francis.

Wendler, D., & Rid, A. (2017). In defense of a social value requirement for clinical research. *Bioethics, 31*(2), 77–86.

Wenner, D. M. (2016). Against permitted exploitation in developing world research agreements. *Developing World Bioethics, 16*(1), 36–44.

Wenner, D. M. (2018). The social value requirement in research from the transactional to the basic structure model of stakeholder obligations. *The Hastings Center Report, 48*(6), 25–32.

Wertheimer, A. (2008). Exploitation in clinical research. In J. S. Hawkins & E. J. Emanuel (Eds.), *Exploitation and developing countries: The ethics of clinical research* (pp. 63–104). Princeton University Press.

Wertheimer, A. (2010). *Rethinking the ethics of clinical research: Widening the lens.* Oxford University Press.

Whitney, S. N., & Schneider, C. E. (2011). A method to estimate the cost in lives of ethics board review of biomedical research. *Journal of Internal Medicine, 269*(4), 396–402.

Wolitz, R., Emanuel, E., & Shah, S. (2009). Rethinking the responsiveness requirement for international research. *The Lancet, 374*(9692), 847–849.

Woodward, B. (1999). Challenges to human subject protections in US medical research. *JAMA, 282*(20), 1947–1952.

World Health Organization. (1996). *Investing in health research and development: Report of the Ad Hoc Committee on Health Research Relating to Future Intervention Options.* WHO Geneva.

World Medical Association. (2000). *Declaration of Helsinki: Ethical principles for medical research involving human subjects.* Adopted by the 18th WMA General Assembly, Helsinki, Finland, June 1964, and amended by the 52nd WMA General Assembly, Edinburgh, Scotland, October 2000. https://www.wma.net/policies-post/wma-declaration-of-helsinki-ethical-principles-for-medical-research-involving-human-subjects

Zollman, K. J. (2010). The epistemic benefit of transient diversity. *Erkenntnis, 72*(1), 17–35.

Zwolinski, M. (2007). Sweatshops, choice, and exploitation. *Business Ethics Quarterly, 17*(4), 689–727.

Index

For the benefit of digital users, indexed terms that span two pages (e.g., 52–53) may, on occasion, appear on only one of those pages.

Figures are indicated by *f* following the page number